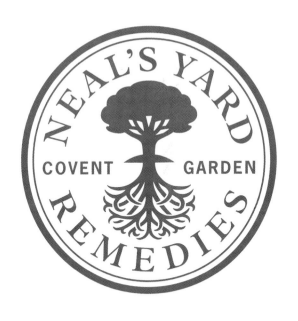

ESSENTIAL OILS

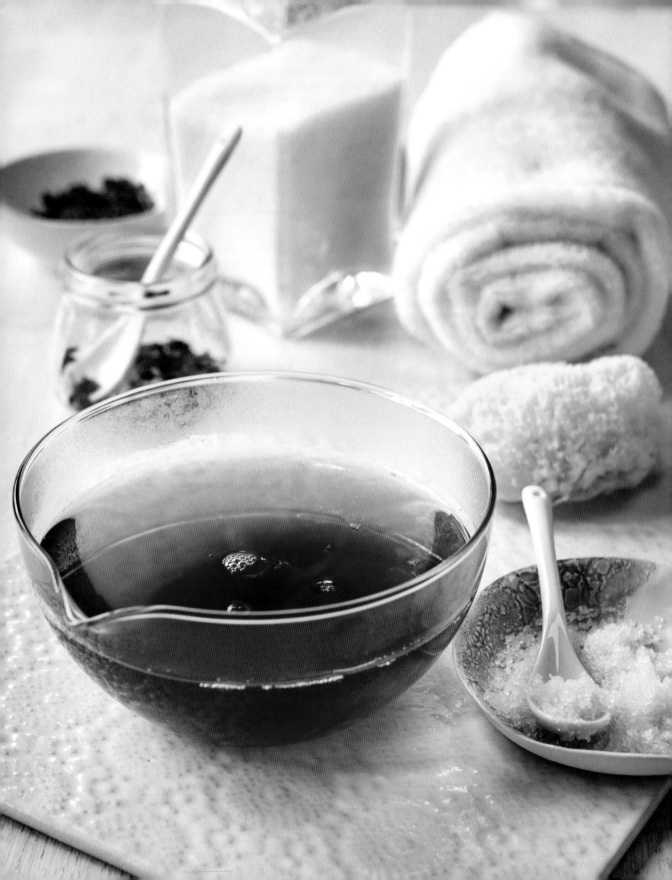

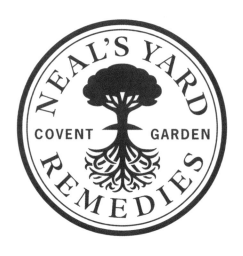

ESSENTIAL OILS

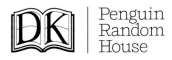

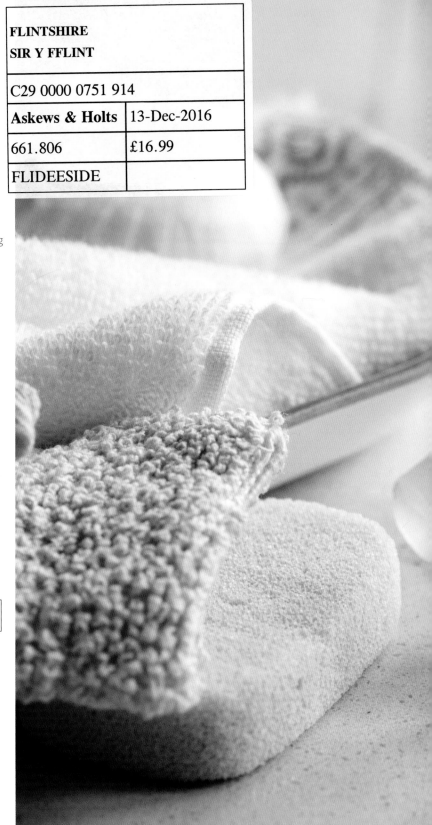

Editor Claire Cross
Senior Designer Collette Sadler
Design and Art Direction
Emma Forge and Tom Forge
Managing Editor Angela Wilkes
Managing Art Editor
Marianne Markham
Jacket Designer Harriet Yeomans
Senior Jacket Creative Nicola Powling
Senior Producer, Pre-Production
Tony Phipps
Art Director Maxine Pedliham
Publisher Mary-Clare Jerram

First published in Great Britain in 2016
by Dorling Kindersley Limited
80 Strand, London, WC2R 0RL

2 4 6 8 10 9 7 5 3 1

001 – 296393 – Oct/2016

A CIP catalogue record for this book is
available from the British Library.

DISCLAIMER See page 256.

ISBN 978-0-2412-7309-8

Printed and bound in China

All images © Dorling Kindersley Limited

A WORLD OF IDEAS:
SEE ALL THERE IS TO KNOW
For further information see:
www.dkimages.com

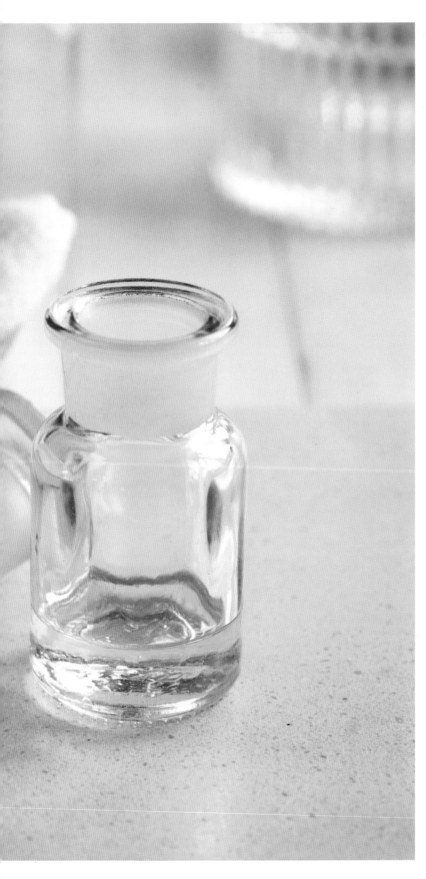

THE AUTHORS

Susan Curtis is a qualified homeopath and naturopath and is the Director of Natural Health for Neal's Yard Remedies. She is the author of numerous books including *Looking Good and Feeling Younger* and several books on essential oils, and co-author of *Natural Healing for Women*. Susan has two grown-up children and is passionate about helping people to live a more natural and healthy lifestyle.

Pat Thomas is a journalist, campaigner, and broadcaster. Her previous books include *Cleaning Yourself to Death, What's in this Stuff?*, and *Skin Deep*. Through her work she has led the way in exposing harmful chemicals in many everyday beauty products, as well as promoting natural alternatives that work. She is a former editor of *The Ecologist* magazine and is a trustee of the Organic Research Centre and editor of Neal's Yard Remedies' natural health website, *NYR Natural News*.

Fran Johnson is a passionate cosmetic scientist and aromatherapist, and has been part of the Product Development team at Neal's Yard Remedies since 2006, formulating therapeutic products for healing and wellbeing. She has written and teaches a number of Neal's Yard Remedies courses that cover aromatherapy, natural perfumery, and making cosmetic products.

Contents

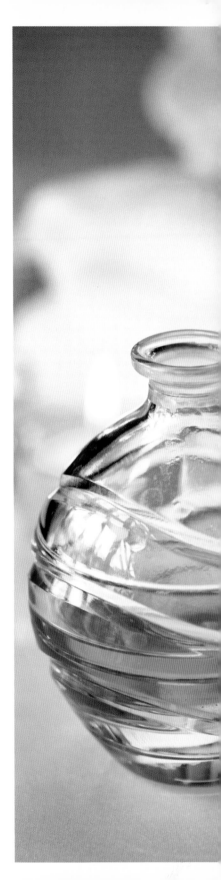

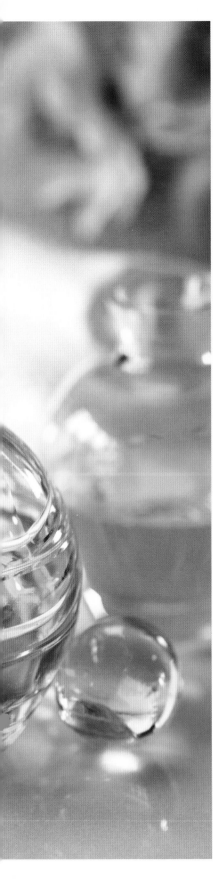

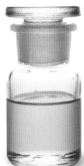

Introduction

Aromatic essential oils have been used for thousands of years as traditional remedies to enhance **health** and **wellbeing.** The ability of **fragrances** to affect mood and atmosphere has long been recognized, and different cultures have made use of the **aromatic** plants available to them for spiritual rituals and personal use. The appeal of essential oils has endured, and today, the practice of **aromatherapy** is well established in the lexicon of natural health.

Essential oils **today**

The essential oil trade emerged about 200 years ago for use in the perfumery and food industries. In recent years, an increased emphasis on holistic healing has led to a resurgence of interest in the traditional use of essential oils for health, wellbeing, and beauty.

Pleasurable and extremely versatile, essential oils can be used as remedies for ailments, incorporated into cosmetics and fragrances, and, increasingly, are used in the fast-growing trend for diffusing aromas to enhance living spaces and create a sense of wellbeing.

The growth of interest in essential oils also coincides with a rise in stress-related conditions associated with hectic modern-day living. With their ability to soothe body and mind, essential oils are especially helpful for combatting the effects of chronic stress.

At Neal's Yard Remedies, we have sold pure and natural essential oils since our first shop opened in 1981, and have witnessed, and been part of, the growth of interest in essential oils, as more and more people look to natural ingredients to improve their lifestyle and enhance wellbeing.

A greater understanding There is an art and a science to using essential oils. In the past few decades, the aromatherapy industry's understanding

Neroli essential oil, extracted from the delicate blossom, has an exquisite floral aroma.

of how to use oils and their properties has developed apace. Increasingly, the traditional use of oils in different cultures is being researched in laboratories, and clinical trials are being carried out to enhance our understanding of how and why oils act as they do.

In this book, we impart some of this knowledge to help you learn how to enjoy oils in your daily beauty regime and as part of an everyday healthy lifestyle. With a little knowledge and common sense, essential oils can be used by everyone. This book will help you become confident incorporating these wonderful plant essences into a more healthy and natural lifestyle.

Therapeutic oil blends, scented candles, and nourishing skin products are just some of the ways to enjoy aromatic essential oils.

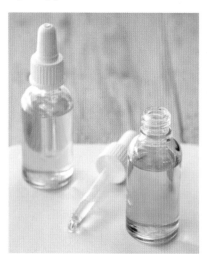

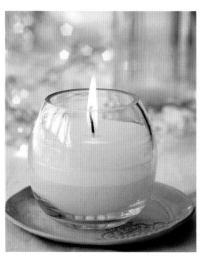

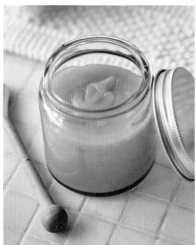

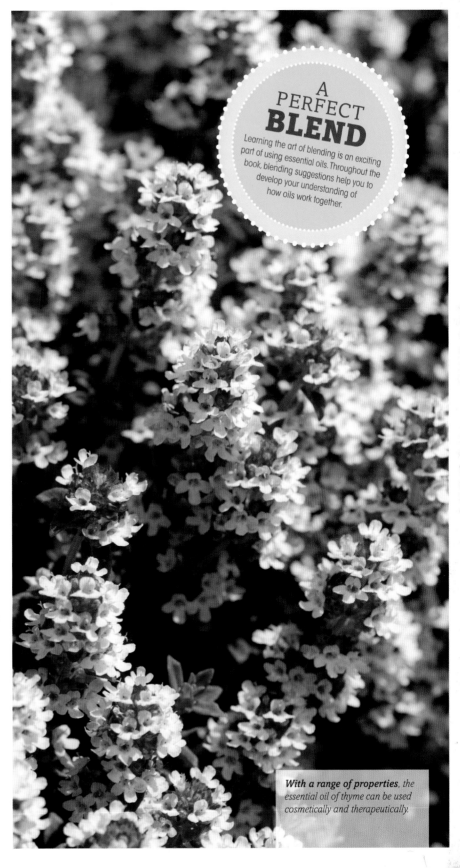

Versatile and a pleasure to use, essential oils are natural healers.

For serious or chronic health concerns, do seek medical advice and consult a professional aromatherapist.

Enjoying **essential oils**

At Neal's Yard Remedies, we believe an understanding of the plant that is the source of an oil is important to choose the best oil for your needs. The beautiful images in the A–Z section of this book, together with the plants' properties and suggestions for use, will help you develop an understanding and awareness of each plant and its oil.

Highly concentrated, essential oils are used in tiny amounts and need to be diluted before use in a base, or carrier, oil. A chapter on base oils guides you through some of the most popular oils and their properties.

We have developed a wide range of recipes and remedies for this book for health, beauty, and home. Simple instructions show you how to create aromatic blends and products, and tried-and-tested remedies will help you treat a range of common complaints.

So enjoy this introduction to essential oils and go on to create some wonderful products and experiences for you and your friends and family.

Susan Curtis, Director of Natural Health, Neal's Yard Remedies

With a range of properties, the essential oil of thyme can be used cosmetically and therapeutically.

Understanding
Essential Oils

Essential oils contain the **essence of nature.** Find out what exactly is in essential oils, how these complex substances work **holistically** to heal and balance body and mind, and how to ensure you are using the purest, **very best-quality** products.

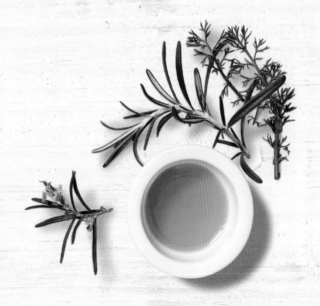

What are essential oils?

Aromatic essential oils are the **highly concentrated** essences derived from plants. Used today in **aromatherapy** and fragrances, they have a long history in **natural healing**. The oils harness a plant's **therapeutic** properties to restore **balance** to the mind, body, and spirit.

The plant's **essence**

The aromatic compounds in essential oils are thought to help plants survive, for example, by attracting pollinators and warding off fungus and bacteria. Once extracted, essential oils contain the essence of a plant in a very concentrated form, which means the essential oils often smell delightful and retain the plant's unique therapeutic benefits for our use.

Essential oils in aromatherapy

Today, there are around 150 essential oils used in aromatherapy. Each has a unique chemistry and properties that produce a distinct therapeutic, psychological, and physiological effect. As well as being anti-inflammatory, pain-relieving, decongesting, and antiseptic, oils can ease anxiety and lift the spirits. Their powerful constituents can have a profound physiological effect, restoring balance and vitality.

A single essential oil contains as many as 100 different chemical components.

Essential oil **sources**

Each plant contains essential oils. In some plants, oil is extracted from the dried seeds, peel or resin, while in others it is found in the leaves, roots, bark or flowers.

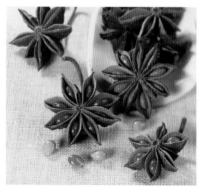

Both dried and fresh seeds can be pressed to extract the essential oils.

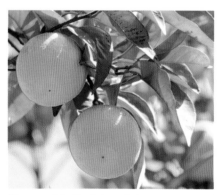

The essential oils of citrus fruits are concentrated mostly in the rinds.

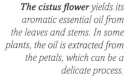

The cistus flower yields its aromatic essential oil from the leaves and stems. In some plants, the oil is extracted from the petals, which can be a delicate process.

What's in **an oil?**

A single essential oil can contain as many as 100 chemical components, which work together to give the oil its unique properties and aroma. Each component plays a role, but some are more dominant and determine how an oil will act on the body and mind.

The chemistry of oils Oils are made up of major, minor, and trace components. Menthol is an example of a major component, making up around 40 per cent of peppermint oil. These major components work with the more numerous minor and trace components and all contribute to an oil's aroma and therapeutic value.

Breaking oils down Each oil's component parts split into two further categories: oxygenated compounds and terpenes. Oxygenated compounds tend to be stronger smelling and longer lasting than terpenes. They include alcohols, which are antibacterial and found in oils such as ginger and juniper; esters, which can be antiseptic, found in oils such as basil and clove; and ketones, which regenerate cells, found in oils such as rose, camphor, and vetiver. Terpenes, found in oils such as myrrh, have a range of properties, but spoil quickly when exposed to air.

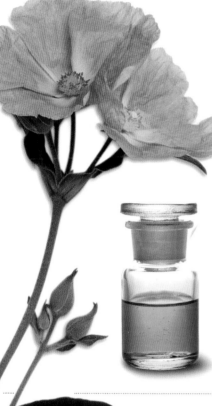

The amber-hued essential oil derived from the cistus plant is rich in oxygenated compounds.

The history of essential oils

Traditionally, highly concentrated oils from a variety of natural sources have been used to calm or stimulate the emotions and enhance wellbeing.

The use of scented oils in incense and candles has played a part in religious rituals throughout the ages, with many cultures believing the aromas could ward off evil or inspire us to new heights. The Egyptians used scented oils in burial rituals and as a symbol of status. The Greeks believed aromas connected them to the gods, while the Romans used scented oils for seduction.

The modern use of essential oils as a therapy began in the 1930s when the French chemist René-Maurice Gattefossé coined the term aromatherapy after finding that lavender oil helped heal his burned hand without scarring. In World War II, Dr Jean Valnet, a French army surgeon, used oils on wounded soldiers, while Austrian beauty therapist and biochemist Marguerite Maury prescribed oils and is credited with the idea of using essential oils in massage.

Whether lifting the spirits or healing wounds, aromatherapy is a safe and effective traditional practice with real relevance to our lives today.

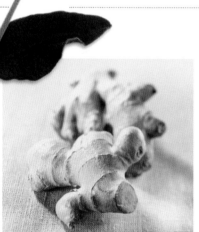

Plants such as ginger and plai produce a highly concentrated essential oil from the roots.

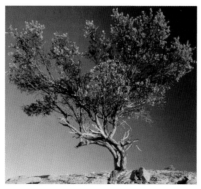

The resin from trees such as myrrh can be extracted and distilled into therapeutic oils.

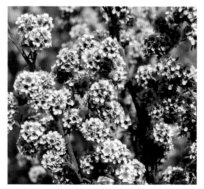

Some plants, such as fragonia, hold essential oil in the branches, as well as the leaves.

How essential oils work

Our sense of smell is more **sensitive** and immediate than any of our other senses, which is why aromas can be so evocative. Chemicals in a scent can trigger **physiological** responses and affect our mental state. These combined effects enable aromatic oils to work holistically on **mind**, **body**, and **spirit**, bringing **balance**, healing, and an often profound sense of wellbeing.

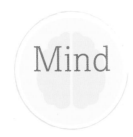

Mind

On the **mind**

Essential oils can be used to help promote a state of mind. For example, stimulating oils can be used to enhance focus, while oils that are calming enable us to relax and help to combat the effects of stress.

Enhance wellbeing and mood

Essential oils have many components that affect the nervous system, helping to lift mood and enhance wellbeing. For example, studies show that the compound linalool in lavender and clary sage reduces anxiety, while limonene, found in many citrus oils, can ease anxiety and lift depression. Chamomile and bergamot essential oils contain the compounds alpha- and beta-pinene, which also work as antidepressants, helping to lift the spirits and increase feelings of wellbeing.

When we feel anxious or depressed, it's not just our minds that are affected, our bodies can also suffer. For example, we tend to hold tension in our muscles when we are anxious. Many oils have both mood-enhancing properties and physiological effects so they treat

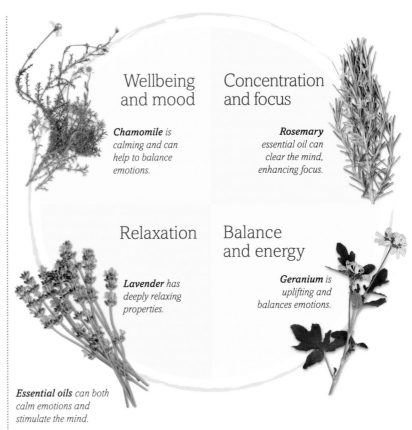

Wellbeing and mood

Chamomile is calming and can help to balance emotions.

Concentration and focus

Rosemary essential oil can clear the mind, enhancing focus.

Relaxation

Lavender has deeply relaxing properties.

Balance and energy

Geranium is uplifting and balances emotions.

Essential oils can both calm emotions and stimulate the mind.

both the mental and physical symptoms of stress and anxiety.

An aromatherapy massage adds the inherently relaxing benefits of touch to an oil's therapeutic effects, which can be profoundly calming and uplifting. Even without the benefit of touch, simply smelling a pleasant aroma, such as a mandarin or vanilla bean, can reduce stress-induced muscle tension.

Promote relaxation The relaxing effects of oils are well documented. How they help us relax is a complicated process thought to involve several parts of the brain. One theory is that linalool, found in oils such as lavender, regulates the neurohormone GABA (gamma-aminobutyric acid). This in turn regulates levels of adrenaline, noradrenaline, and dopamine.

Rose has an uplifting and calming aroma.

Improve concentration and focus

Some oils clear and refresh the mind. For example, inhaling rosemary essential oil has been shown to improve memory by up to 75 per cent. The oil contains the compound eucalyptol, which acts in a similar way to dementia drugs by increasing a neurotransmitter called acetylcholine that helps regulate brain activity.

Balance energy

Many essential oils can either relax or stimulate as needed and are called "adaptogens". These balance body systems in a process known as homeostasis, gently calming or stimulating. Adaptogens help the body to process stress by recharging the adrenal glands, which can be over-stimulated or exhausted from stress. Lavender, rose, and geranium are examples of adaptogens.

How oils work holistically

The concept of holistic healing involves treating the entire person so that the body, mind, and spirit are in harmony. This approach is very different to the conventional one that uses targeted drugs to tackle or suppress symptoms, but doesn't always address the root cause of a symptom.

Essential oils act on the mind and body to achieve deeper healing. For example, when relaxed, the body may be better at letting go of toxins and maintaining a healthy circulation. Inhaling black pepper oil gives physical and mental support to smokers trying to quit as the oil is decongesting and also helps to reduce cravings.

Black pepper essential oil

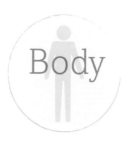

Body

On the **body**

Essential oils are natural healers, harnessing the medicinal properties that are traditionally associated with plants. For example, oils can be anti-inflammatory, antiseptic, and antifungal, and many essential oils are anti-microbial, helping to kill a whole variety of harmful micro-organisms to protect us against disease.

Work as antiseptics

Many essential oils have been shown to destroy the bacteria, viruses, and fungi that cause infection. One of the best known antiseptic essential oils, tea tree, is thought to be as effective as conventional treatments for athlete's foot, and recent research suggests that wounds infected with the *Staphylococcus aureus* bacterium heal faster when treated with tea tree oil than they do with conventional methods of treatment.

Chemical components, such as thymol found in thyme essential oil, menthol in peppermint, and eugenol in clove essential oil, to name but a few, have been shown to be powerfully antiseptic. Studies have demonstrated that inhaling these antiseptic essential oils can be as effective as applying them directly to the skin, and essential oil inhalation therapy has been used to treat the symptoms of bronchitis and acute sinusitis for many years.

In a world where many strains of bacteria are becoming resistant to conventional antibiotics, essential oils are beginning to be seen as a viable alternative.

Relieve pain and reduce inflammation

Essential oils are often used for their mild anaesthetic properties that can relieve localized pain. Oils such as thyme, rose, eucalyptus, clove, bergamot, and fennel have been shown to work on the body in a similar way to non-steroidal anti-inflammatory drugs (NSAIDs) such as ibuprofen, by inhibiting the enzymes in the body that cause inflammation, swelling, and pain. This analgesic effect makes these essential oils especially useful for soothing muscle and joint pains and for providing localized pain relief, for example from tension headaches and from sprains and strains.

Pain is often accompanied by inflammation. Many essential oils have anti-inflammatory properties. One notable example is frankincense. Several varieties of frankincense essential oil have been shown to inhibit the production of inflammatory proteins called cytokines and to prevent white blood cells, known as leukocytes, leaking into tissues, both of which cause inflammation.

Have a cleansing action

When functioning properly, our lungs, liver, digestive system, kidneys, and skin all help to remove waste products and toxins from the body. Negative factors such as stress, anxiety, poor diet, and lack of sleep can all interfere with this process. Essential oils often have detoxifying properties that help to cleanse the body and support a healthy excretory system.

For example, a chemical called D-limonene, found in citrus fruits such as oranges, lemons, mandarins, limes, and grapefruits, supports the healthy functioning the of the liver, as well as helping

Star anise has strong antiseptic properties.

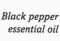

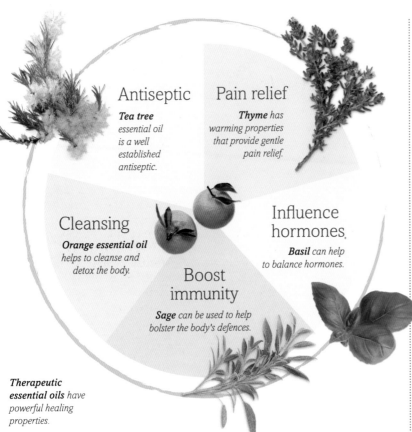

Antiseptic

Tea tree *essential oil is a well established antiseptic.*

Pain relief

Thyme *has warming properties that provide gentle pain relief.*

Cleansing

Orange essential oil *helps to cleanse and detox the body.*

Influence hormones

Basil *can help to balance hormones.*

Boost immunity

Sage *can be used to help bolster the body's defences.*

Therapeutic essential oils have powerful healing properties.

Influence hormones The endocrine system secretes hormones to regulate the body's processes. Essential oils can influence the action of hormones and smooth out imbalances. For example, relaxing rosemary has been shown to reduce levels of the stress hormone cortisol, and inhaling calming rose essential oil can help to decrease elevated levels of adrenaline. Several essential oils are thought to help regulate women's hormones during different stages of reproductive life. Lavandin essential oil is believed to help control hormone-induced mood fluctuations, and clary sage, fennel, basil, sage, cypress, and geranium have a similar balancing effect.

to regulate appetite and lower cholesterol. And juniper, grapefruit, rosemary, fennel, and cypress oils have a mild diuretic effect that helps to support the work of the kidneys by encouraging the elimination of excess water. Combining these oils with a gentle massage and body brush encourages the healthy circulation of blood and lymphatic fluid, and in turn the removal of waste.

Help boost immunity
Essential oils promote wellness by enhancing and strengthening our immune response to disease. Some essential oils actually stimulate the

production of disease-fighting white blood cells, such as phagocytes, T-cells, and B-cells, which are vital to the body's defences and immunity. In particular, eucalyptus and niaouli essential oils have been shown to encourage the process known as phagocytosis, where larger white blood cells called phagocytes engulf and then destroy, or deactivate, bacteria and viruses.

The compound linalool, which is found in high levels in essential oils such as lavender, sage, bay laurel, and eucalyptus has also been shown to increase the efficiency of the body's white blood cells.

The concept of synergy

Blending oils *can enhance their effects. For example, mixing an anti-viral oil with one that is anti-inflammatory provides more effective relief from coughs and colds. This is sometimes called synergy, but the concept of synergy goes deeper than blending.*

Often, the therapeutic benefit of an essential oil is attributed to one or two of its major components. But increasingly evidence shows that the benefits of oils come from the interaction of major and minor components. For example, thymol, a major component of thyme, is highly antibacterial. However, studies show that the whole essential oil has a greater antibacterial effect than the isolated component. There's still much to understand about how oils work synergistically, but it is clear that while science is geared towards using single compounds, whole oils have benefits that can't be replicated in the lab.

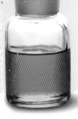

The components *in a single oil work together to greater effect.*

Essential oils work on the root cause as well as the symptom.

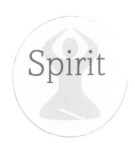

Spirit

On the **spirit**

Essential oils have been used for thousands of years to enhance spiritual practice. From their use in traditional ceremonies to supporting personal spiritual practices such as meditation, essential oils help to support spiritual attainment.

Promote spiritual pursuit

Essentials oils have been used for millennia to support prayer. Historically, oils such as frankincense, myrrh, cinnamon, cedarwood, and rose have been used in religious ceremonies. A well-chosen fragrance can calm breathing, settle and focus the mind, and create a sense of intent.

Enhance mindful practices

Aromas that calm the mind or help to lift the spirits, found in oils such as lavender, elemi, and bergamot, can be used to enhance focus during practices such as meditation, yoga, and breathing techniques.

Energy and chi
In some traditional practices, essential oils are used to clear blockages in the "chakras", believed to be the energy centres in the body that relate to specific glands and organs. Chakras are said to be connected by meridians, which are described as channels through which vital energy, or "chi", flows.

Blockages in these areas are thought to lead to poor health in the related part of the body. The illustration, right, shows the position of the seven chakras. Specific essential oils are associated with different chakras, or

centres, and are recommended to help bring balance and healing to these areas.

- **The crown chakra** at the top of the head governs the pineal gland and our "inner self". Oils such as frankincense, rose, jasmine, lavender, and elemi correspond with this area.
- **The brow chakra**, located just above and between the eyes, is connected to the pituitary gland and rules memory and mind. Oils such as myrrh, sandalwood, and jasmine can be used to treat blockages here.
- **The throat chakra** covers the area of the throat and the thyroid gland and relates to communication. Try lavender, chamomile, clary sage, cajuput, peppermint, geranium, and rosemary to treat this area.
- **The heart chakra**, located around the heart and upper body, affects wellbeing. Useful oils include rose, bergamot, lemon balm, chamomile,

neroli, sandalwood, and palmarosa.
- **The solar plexus chakra** includes organs in the upper abdomen and is connected to self-esteem. Try ginger, helichrysum, manuka, coriander, lavender, marjoram, and orange.
- **The sacral chakra**, located in the lower abdomen, is linked to the reproductive system and responds to essential oils such as sandalwood, jasmine, rose, ylang ylang, orange, and geranium.
- **The base chakra**, at the base of the spine, connects to our ability to feel grounded. Oils that help healing here include myrrh, cedarwood, patchouli, petitgrain, benzoin, carrot, and vetiver.

Cinnamon enhances meditation.

In some practices, oils are used to clear blockages in the "chakras", or energy centres, in the body

Chakras

- The crown chakra
- The brow chakra
- The throat chakra
- The heart chakra
- The solar plexus chakra
- The sacral chakra
- The base chakra

How essential oils are extracted

A plant's essential oils are contained in tiny sacs on the surface of a leaf or flower, and sometimes within bark, seeds, and roots. When you scratch a piece of lemon peel and get a spray with an **intense lemon fragrance**, you are breaking open the sacs on the peel's surface and **releasing** the lemon oil. And when you rub the leaves of a herb between your fingers to produce a smell, you are **breaking the vessels** to release the oil. Producing essential oils involves one of several methods to burst open the sacs and collect the oil.

18

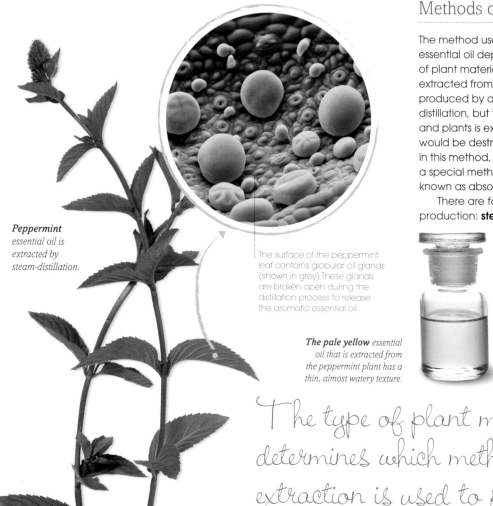

Peppermint essential oil is extracted by steam-distillation.

The surface of the peppermint leaf contains globular oil glands (shown in grey). These glands are broken open during the distillation process to release the aromatic essential oil.

The pale yellow essential oil that is extracted from the peppermint plant has a thin, almost watery texture.

Methods of **extraction**

The method used to produce an essential oil depends on the type of plant material that the oil is being extracted from. Most essential oils are produced by a process of steam-distillation, but the oil in some flowers and plants is extremely delicate and would be destroyed by the heat used in this method, so these plants require a special method of oil production known as absolute extraction.

There are four main methods of production: **steam-distillation**, the most widely used; **expression**, a simple method that is used to extract oil from rinds; **absolute extraction**, used for producing an oil from very delicate flowers; and **CO_2 extraction**, a new, evolving method.

The type of plant material determines which method of extraction is used to produce the essential oil.

Steam-distillation The most popular method for extracting essential oils is steam-distillation, a process used for herbs, roots, bark, and resins. This ancient method of extraction can be dated back around 5,000 years with the discovery of earthenware stills. Today, most stills are made of stainless steel or copper.

Firstly, the plant material is placed in a large container. Either steam is passed through the container, or water is added and heated to produce steam. As the plant material heats up, it gradually softens and pressure builds up on the surface of the plant, breaking open the tiny sacs that contain the plant's essential oil. The volatile oil rises up with the steam. The steam is then condensed, usually with cold water held in a coiling pipe, and collected in a vessel. Here, the oil and the water separate, with the oil rising and gathering on top of the water, ready to be tapped off and bottled.

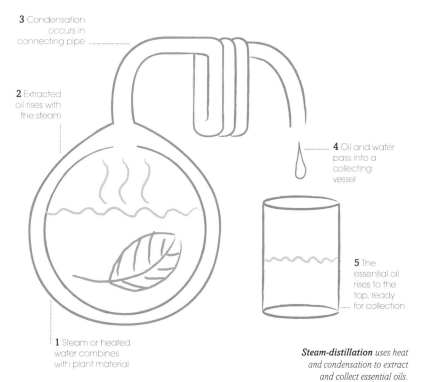

3 Condensation occurs in connecting pipe

2 Extracted oil rises with the steam

4 Oil and water pass into a collecting vessel

5 The essential oil rises to the top, ready for collection

1 Steam or heated water combines with plant material

Steam-distillation uses heat and condensation to extract and collect essential oils.

Expression The simplest way to extract an essential oil is to press the plant material and then collect the oil.

This method is used when the essential oils are found in the outer rind of a fruit and are easily released, as is the case with citrus peel. Citrus fruits, such as grapefruit, orange, lemon, and lime are mechanically pressed to extract their liquid, and then the watery juice is separated from the essential oil.

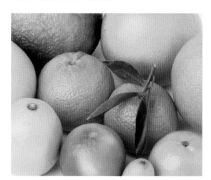

The outer rind of citrus fruits contains oil glands that can be pressed to extract the oil.

Absolute extraction The fragrance of extremely delicate flowers, such as jasmine or mimosa, is damaged by the heat involved in distillation, so these plants require a different method of extraction without steam or water. The result is a highly concentrated oil known as an absolute.

In Grasse, the perfumery capital of France, flower oils were traditionally hand-extracted using a time-consuming process known as

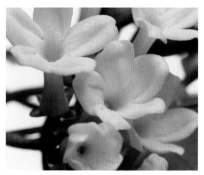

The oil from the delicate jasmine flower is obtained by solvent extraction.

enfleurage. Framed glass plates were covered with lard, and the flowers placed on top. After a few days, the lard absorbed the fragrant oil from the flower, which was then extracted by alcohol to produce the absolute.

Modern methods involve blending flowers with a solvent. The solvent is then removed to leave the absolute oil.

CO_2 extraction A new method of extraction called "supercritical carbon dioxide (CO_2) extraction" uses gas rather than heat. This involves putting CO_2 under pressure to convert it from a gas into a liquid that can be used as a solvent. The solvent diffuses through the plant material and extracts its aromatic constituents.

This method tends to produce additional constituents, and so more research is needed before it becomes widely used. However, it does produce an aroma closer to that of the actual plants than that acheived by other methods and so may grow in popularity.

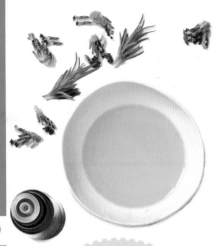

Choosing essential oils

It is not always easy, especially as a novice, to know whether or not you are buying a **pure**, **natural**, good-quality, **sustainable** essential oil. Being aware of what to look for can help you make a worthwhile purchase. The following guidelines set out key factors to consider when purchasing oils, helping you to assess **quality** and **provenance** and to choose the best oils for you.

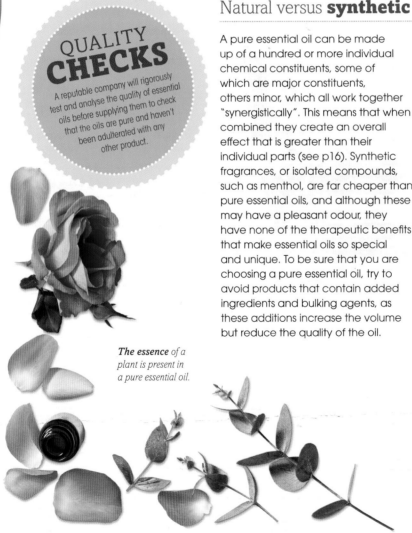

QUALITY CHECKS

A reputable company will rigorously test and analyse the quality of essential oils before supplying them to check that the oils are pure and haven't been adulterated with any other product.

The essence of a plant is present in a pure essential oil.

Natural versus **synthetic**

A pure essential oil can be made up of a hundred or more individual chemical constituents, some of which are major constituents, others minor, which all work together "synergistically". This means that when combined they create an overall effect that is greater than their individual parts (see p16). Synthetic fragrances, or isolated compounds, such as menthol, are far cheaper than pure essential oils, and although these may have a pleasant odour, they have none of the therapeutic benefits that make essential oils so special and unique. To be sure that you are choosing a pure essential oil, try to avoid products that contain added ingredients and bulking agents, as these additions increase the volume but reduce the quality of the oil.

Recognizing **quality**

Spend time researching companies and try to identify reputable ones that are likely to go to the most trouble to ensure their oils are of a high quality.

Company credentials Some companies have developed their own terminology to demonstrate that their oils are superior. For example, an oil may be described as being of "therapeutic" or "aromatherapy" grade, but ultimately these are marketing terms and not meaningful. It can be more helpful, though not a guarantee of quality, to check if a company is a member of a reputable association, such as the Aromatherapy Trade Council (ATC) in the United Kingdom or the National Association of Holistic Aromatherapy (NAHA) in the United States. Another way to check a company's credentials is to find out if it runs aromatherapy courses and/or has links with qualified aromatherapy practitioners, which indicates that the company has a deserved reputation.

All in the name If an essential oil is authentic, the botanical name should appear on the label, and compounds called chemotypes (substances that link oils to a specific plant variety), may

Ensure that you are buying a pure, natural, good-quality, sustainably produced essential oil.

also be listed. For example, thyme will list its botanical name *Thymus vulgaris*, and the label might also mention linalool or thymol, to indicate that the oil is from one botanical species. The label, or a company website, may also cite a country of origin, which indicates that it is a true plant oil.

Checking **sustainability**

Certain oils, such as sandalwood and rosewood, are now available only in limited amounts, or are unavailable, due to concerns about sustainability. Check the sustainability policy of a company before you buy an oil.

Endangered plants Some plants have been harvested almost to extinction. For example, spikenard (*Nardostachys jatamansi*) has a critically endangered status and so this oil should be avoided unless the supplier can guarantee that it is cultivated. You can check a plant's status at www.iucnredlist.org/search.

Supporting fair trade Fairtrade often ensures sustainability. Harvesting plants for oils can be an important source of income for some communities. With a conservation plan in place, plants are more likely to be protected as an important resource. Frankincense oil from Kenya, for example, is available as a FairWild source, a standard that protects the harvesting of wild species and ensures fair trading. When choosing oils, look

for Fairtrade or Fair for Life logos that suggest sustainability and help to ensure the benefits of producing an oil are felt by the people growing and harvesting the plants.

Choosing **organic**

Organic essential oils and base oils have a higher therapeutic value because they contain the highest levels of antioxidants and are less likely to have potentially toxic residues from pesticides and chemical fertilizers. Organic production also benefits farmers, their families, and communities, is kinder to the soil, and generally provides a more positive outlook for future crops, wildlife, and water sources. Check company literature to see if they support organic farming practices.

What's on the label?

Reading a label closely can help you to make an on-the-spot assessment of an essential oil. A label that has the following information suggests a high-quality oil:

The oils's botanical name and the part of the plant used.
The country of origin.
The distillation or packing date and/or expiration date.
The batch number and, if applicable, a chemotype (such as thymol).

Assessing **cost**

All essential oils require a large amount of plant matter to make just a small amount of oil. The price of an oil is connected to its yield from the plant matter, which can vary greatly, from less than 0.1 per cent to 25 per cent. For example, around 1,000kg (2,200lb) of hand-picked orange blossom produces just 1kg (2¼lb) of neroil oil – hence the high cost of exquisite neroli. In contrast, 1 tonne of cloves produces up to 200kg (440lb) clove oil, making this a less expensive oil.

Any company that sells all of their oils for the same price, or has prices that seem too good to be true, should be avoided. The good news is that because essential oils are so highly concentrated, just a small amount goes a long way, and only a few drops are used at a time. To ensure freshness, buy a small amount regularly, rather than large amounts that might go off before you use them.

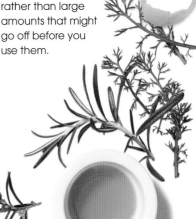

Europe

Europe is a major source *of essential oils. The range of climates means that a variety of plants can be grown, from citrus fruits in the hot and sunny climes of Spain and Italy to more frost-tolerant plants in northern European countries.*

Bosnia	Bay laurel
	Helichrysum
Bulgaria	Parsley
	Rose
	Valerian
France	Angelica
	Caraway
	Carrot
	Cedarwood
	Clary sage
	Cypress
	Fenugreek
	Juniper
	Lavender
	Lemon balm
	Mullein
	Oregano
	Pine
	Sage
	Tarragon
	Thyme
	Tuberose
	Violet
Germany	Chamomile (blue)
Hungary	Coriander
	Dill
	Fennel
	Roman Chamomile
	Savoury
	Yarrow
Italy	Bergamot
	Helichrysum
	Lemon
	Orange
Sweden	Birch
Spain	Cistus
	Eucal. globulus
	Lemon verbena
	Marjoram
	Rosemary
	Sage
United Kingdom	Lavender
	Peppermint
	Roman Chamomile
	Yarrow

Where do oils come from?

Essential oils are extracted from a wide range of plants worldwide. Where plants grow depends on factors such as their **tolerance to frost** and if there's sufficient **rainfall** or irrigation. Many oils **thrive** in Mediterranean areas and in subtropical and tropical climates.

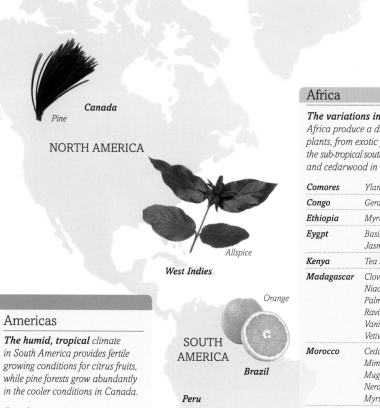

Canada
Pine

NORTH AMERICA

Allspice

West Indies

Americas

The humid, tropical *climate in South America provides fertile growing conditions for citrus fruits, while pine forests grow abundantly in the cooler conditions in Canada.*

Canada	Pine
Brazil	Eucal. citriodora
	Mandarin
	Orange
	Rosewood
Paraguay	Petitgrain
Peru	Lemon verbena
West Indies	Allspice
	Grapefruit
	Peppermint

Orange

SOUTH AMERICA

Brazil

Peru

Paraguay

Petitgrain

Africa

The variations in climate *across Africa produce a diverse range of plants, from exotic ylang ylang in the sub-tropical southeast, to myrtle and cedarwood in the north.*

Comores	Ylang ylang
Congo	Geranium
Ethiopia	Myrrh
Eygpt	Basil
	Jasmine
Kenya	Tea tree
Madagascar	Clove
	Niaouli
	Palmarosa
	Ravintsara
	Vanilla
	Vetiver
Morocco	Cedarwood
	Mimosa
	Mugwort
	Neroli
	Myrtle
Réunion	Geranium
Somalia	Frankincense
	Myrrh
South Africa	Buchu
	Euc. Radiata
	Lemongrass
Uganda	Palmarosa
Zimbabwe	Eucal. smithii
	Tagetes

How crops are **grown**

Traditionally, most essential oils were harvested from the wild, and this is still the case for some abundant species such as juniper. However, as aromatherapy grows in popularity, with markets expanding in countries such as the United States, there is increased pressure on plants grown in the wild, and it can be a struggle to keep up with demand. To ensure a continuous supply of oils, many plants are specially cultivated, with suppliers creating the soil conditions and irrigation needed to grow crops.

Asia

Essential oils from Asia are mainly from the south of the continent, where tropical conditions provide ideal growing conditions for spices such as cardamom and nutmeg.

China	Camphor
India	Cardamom
	Cumin
	Patchouli
	Sandalwood
Indonesia	Benzoin
	Citronella
	Galangal
	Nutmeg
Iran	Rose
Nepal	Wintergreen
Oman	Frankincense
Philippines	Elemi
Sri Lanka	Black pepper
	Cardamom
	Cinnamon
	Citronella
	Ginger
	Lime
Thailand	Plai
Turkey	Rose
Vietnam	Cajuput
	Litsea
	Star anise

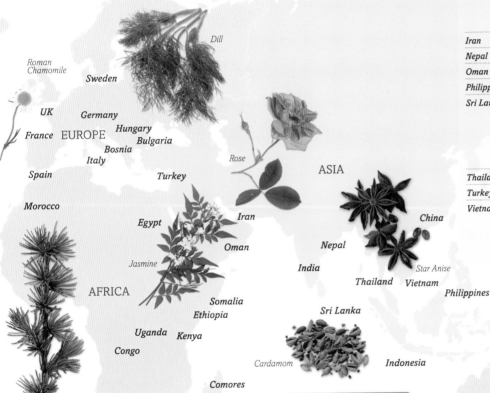

Roman Chamomile

Dill

Sweden

UK

Germany

France EUROPE **Hungary**

Bosnia **Bulgaria**

Italy

Spain

Turkey

Morocco

Rose

ASIA

Egypt

Iran

China

Jasmine

Oman

Nepal

AFRICA

India

Thailand **Vietnam**

Star Anise

Somalia

Ethiopia

Sri Lanka

Philippines

Uganda **Kenya**

Congo

Cardamom

Indonesia

Comores

Zimbabwe

Cedarwood

Réunion

Madagascar

South Africa

Australasia

*Much of **Australasia** is semi-arid, suitable for drought-resistant plants such as tea tree.*

Australia	Eucal. Globulus
	Fragonia
	Tea tree
New Zealand	Manuka

AUSTRALASIA

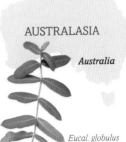

Australia

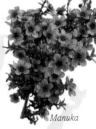

Manuka

New Zealand

Eucal. globulus

Using Essential Oils

Healing and enhancing, aromatic essential oils are a joy to use and easily incorporated into **health and beauty regimes**. Discover all the ways to enjoy essential oils, how to look after your oils, and how to treat these **concentrated substances** with care.

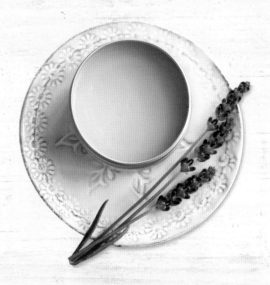

How essential oils enter the body

The quickest way to absorb essential oils is by **inhaling** their aroma, which has a direct effect on the brain. Oils can also be absorbed via the skin during a **massage**, in a **bath**, or in a cream. Both routes allow oils to enter the bloodstream, where their healing properties take effect.

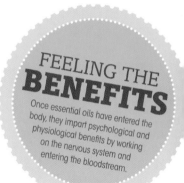

FEELING THE BENEFITS

Once essential oils have entered the body, they impart psychological and physiological benefits by working on the nervous system and entering the bloodstream.

Inhaling essential oils

Humans are believed to have the ability to distinguish between more than 10,000 different aromas. Of all the senses, smell has the most direct connection to the mind and effect on our emotions. In fact, our ability to perceive odour is so connected to our sense of wellbeing that those who have lost their sense of smell can be more prone to problems such as depression and anxiety. The entire concept of aromatherapy is rooted in how aromas directly interact with our brains and body chemistry.

Processing aromas This involves complex pathways in the brain. When we inhale a scent, we take in aromatic molecules that bind to "receptor" cells in the nasal passage. Here they send messages to the olfactory "bulb" in the forebrain and these are interpreted as a smell. Molecules are also inhaled into the lungs where they enter the blood.

The effects on the body Studies show that inhaling a scent has an immediate effect on the brain's activity. Scents breach the blood–brain barrier (the brain's protective membrane), accessing centres in the brain linked to conscious thought, and also reaching the limbic system – the brain's emotional switchboard, where memory and emotions reside, and impulses such as "fight or flight", nurturing, hunger, and arousal are controlled. The limbic system is also linked to hormones.

How the body **inhales an aroma**

When you inhale the aroma of an essential oil, it is processed rapidly by the brain so that you quickly receive the therapeutic benefits of the oil.

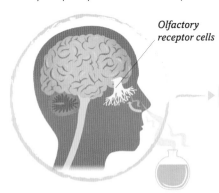

Olfactory receptor cells

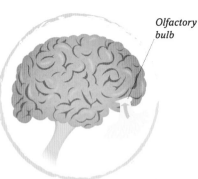

Olfactory bulb

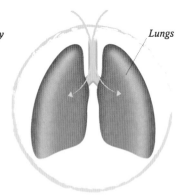

Lungs

1 Aromatic molecules travel up the nasal passage, where they bind to olfactory receptor cells in the nose. The cells send impulses to the olfactory bulb at the base of the forebrain.

2 The forebrain interprets the electrical impulses as a smell and rapidly processes and responds to the essential oil's unique aroma and properties.

Molecules are also inhaled directly from the nasal passages into the lungs, and from these enter the bloodstream, contributing to the healing effect of essential oils.

Essential oils impart their therapeutic effects on the body by being inhaled or absorbed into the skin.

Absorption into the skin

Diluted essential oils can be absorbed into the bloodstream via the skin. Many factors influence how much oil is absorbed, including skin type, the room's and the oil's temperature, and whether the base that the essential oil is mixed with is easily absorbed.

Therapeutic touch When essential oils are combined with massage, this enhances the healing effects of the oils as massage in itself can induce a state of deep relaxation. When you are stressed, physically or emotionally, your body is flooded with hormones that keep you awake and aware. In this "fight or flight" state, other processes, such as immunity, cellular repair, and the assimilation of nutrients from food, are shut down. The relaxing effect of a massage helps the body systems to start working effectively again.

During an aromatherapy massage you also inhale the aroma of the essential oil. Studies using either a plain base oil or an essential oil blend in a massage have shown that those receiving the essential oil blend usually experience greater therapeutic benefits. For example, a footbath with lavender essential oil is more relaxing and healing than a footbath with just warm water. Likewise, a massage with essential oils chosen for their specific healing properties has been shown to be more effective at healing and relieving pain from a range of causes, including post-surgical pain, cancer pain, and backache, than a massage with plain vegetable oil.

Diluting essential oils

Concentrated essences *Essential oils are highly concentrated plant essences, so as a general rule they should always be used diluted in a base oil, lotion, ointment or balm, or bath oil. In addition, while diluted oils can be used as mouthwashes and gargles, they should never be swallowed without the advice of a medically trained practitioner.*

Even when diluted, most leave-on essential oil skin preparations should avoid delicate areas of the body, such as the eyes and mucous membranes. If you have sensitive skin, or suffer from allergies, it is always good to perform a patch test of your chosen oil first. Never apply essential oils neat on babies or children. See pages 36–37 for safety guidelines.

Exceptions to the rule *Some essential oils, such as rose absolute, ylang ylang, jasmine, chamomile, tea tree, and lavender, are an exception to this rule and can be applied neat, as a scent. Likewise, tea tree can be used neat as emergency first aid for cuts, stings, and bites. Follow the guidelines in the A–Z section of this book.*

How the body **absorbs oils**

Oils can be absorbed into the bloodstream via application to the skin. During massage, you also gain therapeutic benefits from inhaling the aroma of oils.

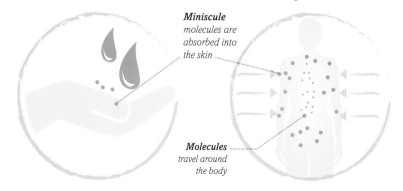

Miniscule molecules are absorbed into the skin

Molecules travel around the body

1 Tiny essential oil molecules are absorbed through the pores of the skin where they enter the bloodstream and start to take effect.

2 Once in the bloodstream, the oils travel around the body via the circulatory system. The therapeutic effects of the oils act on the body systems and promote healing.

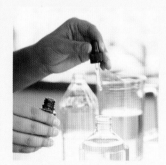

Always dilute *essential oils with a base oil before using, unless the oil's usage guidelines state otherwise.*

Applying essential oils

There are many ways to enjoy the benefits of essential oils. Languishing in a luxurious **aromatherapy** bath or enjoying an **oil-infused massage** are two popular methods. You can also disperse oils in the air, dab an oil balm on a **pulse point**, or sprinkle a few drops of oil on a tissue and **inhale** the scent deeply. Here are the main ways to enjoy your essential oils.

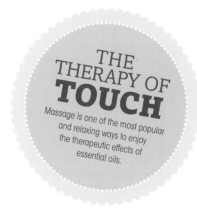

THE THERAPY OF TOUCH
Massage is one of the most popular and relaxing ways to enjoy the therapeutic effects of essential oils.

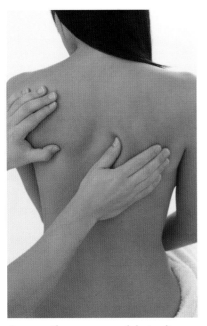

An aromatherapy massage helps to relieve tension in the body while delivering the benefits of your chosen blend of oils.

Massage

An essential oil massage has the added benefit of soothing touch. A massage from a trained aromatherapist is a wonderful treat, but you can just as easily enjoy a massage from a partner, or practise self-massage, which is a great way to nurture yourself and can become part of a daily skin- and health-care routine.

As essential oils are concentrated, they need diluting in a base, or carrier, oil (see pp148–61). For normal skin, try a light base, such as almond, grapeseed, apricot, coconut, sunflower, or canola. For dry skin, use heavier enriching oils, such as avocado, olive, wheatgerm, argan, and jojoba. Medicinal bases, such as neem, calendula, or St John's wort, provide therapeutic properties.

Mixing massage blends For a body massage, use a 2.5 per cent (for sensitive or damaged skin) to 5 per cent (for normal skin) dilution; for a facial massage use a 1 per cent dilution (see the dilutions chart on page 37). To make enough for a full-body massage, pour about 2 tablespoons base oil onto a saucer and add about 4–6 drops of your chosen essential oil, or oil blend.

Pulse point massage Pulse points are areas where blood vessels are close to the surface. Applying essential oils at these points speeds the oil's absorption.

When **to use**

Massage is ideal for addressing problems over a large surface area, for example, achy muscles and joints, digestive problems, and fluid retention. You can also home in on an area, for example, massaging the abdomen to relieve period pains or digestive upsets.

A therapeutic massage with essential oils is effective at creating a sense of calm and deep relaxation, and a feeling of being cared for.

To ease headaches, massage an essential oil balm onto the temples. You can also try massaging a balm into the pulse points on the wrist or neck to help you relax and unwind.

Mix essential oils with the base oil that best suits your needs.

Inhalation

Inhaling an essential oil, or a blend of oils, is a quick and easy way to enjoy the oils' benefits, and forms the basis of aromatherapy, as an essential oil's aroma is inhaled whichever method of application you use.

Tissue inhalation
The simplest way to inhale an essential oil is to sprinkle 2–3 drops of the oil onto a tissue and then inhale deeply. You can place the tissue in a plastic bag and carry it around with you to use as and when you wish. Similarly, you can sprinkle a few drops of a soothing essential oil onto your pillowcase (or a tissue to avoid staining) at night to help you relax and induce restful sleep.

Making a steam inhalation
Make a therapeutic steam inhalation by adding about 4–8 drops of your chosen oil, or oils, to a bowl of just-boiled water. Lean over the bowl and place a towel over your head to contain the vapours, then, with eyes closed, breathe deeply for 10 minutes, or until there is no more steam. Alternatively, you can buy a special inhaler cup.

For epilepsy or asthma sufferers, or with young children, use caution. Instead of leaning over a bowl and covering the head with a towel, simply place the bowl of hot water nearby and capture the wafts of steam.

When to use

Respiratory conditions, such as hay fever, colds, congested sinuses or a chesty cough, particularly benefit from inhalations. Steam inhalations also refresh and cleanse the skin.

Try an inhalation as a quick remedy to calm or invigorate the mind or lift the spirits.

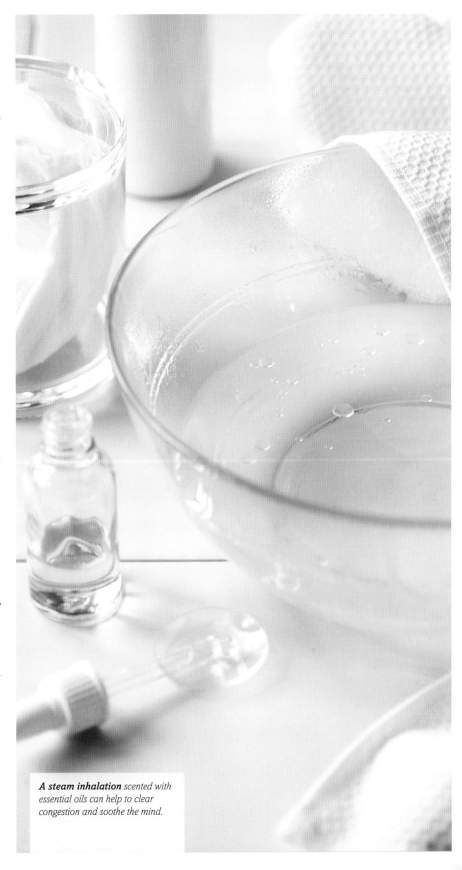

A steam inhalation scented with essential oils can help to clear congestion and soothe the mind.

Baths

Whether you are enjoying a leisurely warm bath or a quick shallow hand, foot or sitz bath (see below), adding essential oils to water is a hugely pleasurable and popular way to use them. The warmth of the water relaxes and soothes muscles, encouraging relaxation, and at the same time opens pores to help the essential oils penetrate the skin and enter the body more rapidly.

Adding oils to a bath Even though the essential oils will be diluted in the bath water, you still need to blend the oils in a base, or carrier, oil before adding them to the bath. This helps the oils to disperse in the water and also moisturizes the skin. For an average-sized bath, mix 4–6 drops of your chosen essential oil, or oils, with 1 tablespoon of a light base oil, such as sunflower, which contains waxes that act like an emulsifier, helping to disperse the oils evenly. You can also buy neutral, water-

dispersing base oils, or mix the essential oils with 1 tablespoon of full-fat milk – the fats in the milk work in a similar way to the base oil, helping to disperse the oils evenly. Aim to relax in the bath for at least 15 minutes. To get the full benefits of the oils, add them once the bath has been run as they can quickly evaporate in the heat.

Hand and foot baths Hand and foot baths are a great way to target smaller areas of the body quickly. A foot bath can treat a specific condition such as athletes' foot, or soothe tired, sore feet. If your ankles are swollen, try following a hot foot bath with a cool one to improve circulation. You can also use hot and cold baths for sore, swollen hands. Fill a bowl or basin (one large enough to take both your feet, or hands) with hot water, and add 4–6 of drops of your chosen oil to a base oil or milk, as for a normal bath. Soak the hands or feet for 10 minutes.

Sitz baths A sitz (shallow) bath is an excellent way to treat conditions such as thrush, haemorrhoids, and urinary infections, or to heal stitches after childbirth. Adding tea tree oil to a sitz bath is a classic treatment for thrush. To make the bath, half-fill the bath with warm water. Use the same method of dilution as for a large bath, and sit in the water for 10 minutes.

When **to use**

Aromatherapy baths are deeply relaxing and reviving. Make sure you give yourself plenty of time to lie back and enjoy the therapeutic soak.

A sitz bath can bring immediate relief to conditions such as thrush or haemorrhoids, while a hand or foot bath is best for aching, swollen, or tired hands and feet or athlete's foot.

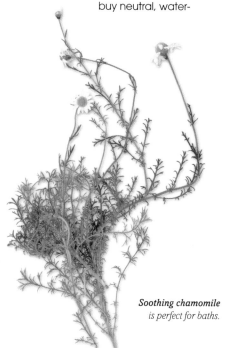

Soothing chamomile is perfect for baths.

Infuse your bath with your favourite blend of essential oils, then lie back and relax.

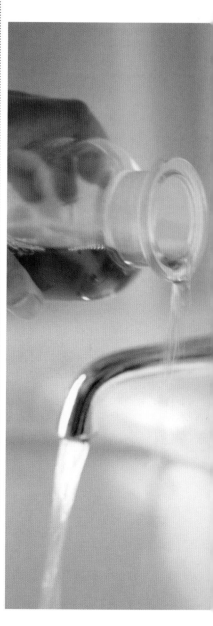

Adding calming oils to warm water soothes body and mind.

Compresses

A compress infused with therapeutic essential oils is a simple and effective way to treat local complaints such as bruises, burns and scalds, headaches, and varicose veins.

Hot or cold? Using hot or cold water can be down to preference, but some conditions do require cooling while others respond to heat.

A hot compress is ideal for complaints such as skin infections, including abscesses and boils, and muscular or joint problems, including strains, backache, rheumatism, and arthritis. For example, a hot compress with ginger, cypress, juniper, pine, and lavender essential oils is wonderfully warming and relieving for aching muscles and joints.

A cold water compress is ideal for sprains and sports injuries, especially if the area already feels hot and inflamed, and for headaches. Using essential oils such as lavender, neroli, peppermint, and eucalyptus helps to enhance the cooling process.

Making a compress Add 3–4 drops of essential oil to a shallow bowl of hot or cold water. Disperse well. Soak a flannel, wring this out well, and apply to the relevant part of the body. For a hot compress,

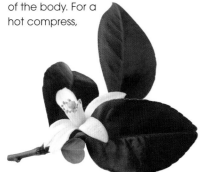

Neroli has calming properties that work well in a compress.

once the flannel is positioned, you can cover it with a towel or piece of cling film to insulate it if you wish. This also stops the water dripping onto clothes. Leave the flannel on the skin until it reaches body temperature, then repeat the whole process three times.

If you are using essential oils that can irritate the skin in a compress, it's important to always pre-dilute the essential oils in a base, or carrier, oil, such as almond or sunflower, before adding the oils to the water.

When **to use**

Try a hot compress to relieve aching and tired muscles after an exercise workout or strenuous physical activity.

A cold compress works especially well for soothing eye strain brought on by looking at computer screens for long periods of time.

Showers and saunas

Essential oils make a wonderful addition to saunas and steamy showers. Experiment with different blend combinations and aromas to suit your needs at different times. For example, if you wish to have an energizing shower to kick-start the day, choose stimulating and invigorating oils such as basil and rosemary. Or to help lift the spirits and create a sense of positivity, try uplifting oils such as bergamot, lemon, and rose.

Using oils in the shower
For a steamy aromatherapy shower, put 5–8 drops of an essential oil, or oil blend, on a warm, damp flannel, then place the flannel in the area you are having a shower, but don't use the

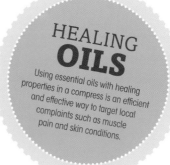

HEALING **OILS**
Using essential oils with healing properties in a compress is an efficient and effective way to target local complaints such as muscle pain and skin conditions.

flannel to wash yourself. If possible, hang the flannel at face level to enjoy the aroma fully. Make sure the shower is hot enough to produce steam. You can also add the essential oil drops to 2 tablespoons unscented shower gel.

Using oils in a sauna Add 20–40 drops of an essential oil, or oil blend, to the pitcher of water that is used to splash the coals during a sauna. Cypress, eucalyptus, and pine essential oils all work well in a sauna.

When **to use**

Adding essential oils to a sauna or shower is a great way to clear sinuses, relieve tension headaches, and to soothe irritating hay fever and allergy symptoms.

Using oils in a shower or sauna also invigorates the mind and helps you to feel calm and relaxed.

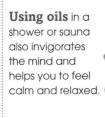

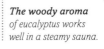

The woody aroma of eucalyptus works well in a steamy sauna.

Diffusion

This increasingly popular way to use essential oils disperses tiny molecules of the oil into the air in a fine vapour or mist. Traditionally, oil burners have been used to diffuse oils. Today, there are several types of diffuser including ultrasonic ones, vaporizers that use a small fan or warm water, electronic aromastones, and reed diffusers. Room sprays can also be used to disperse oils.

Using a diffuser, vaporizer, or oil burner To use an oil burner, pour a little warm water on the hotplate before adding the oil drops to stop the oil from burning too quickly. To use electronic diffusers or vaporizers, add the oils and use according to the manufacturer's instructions.

Making a room spray A room spray is a type of diffusion that releases a more concentrated amount of oil into the air very quickly. To make a room spray, combine 20–30 drops of essential oils with 2 tablespoons each of mineral water and vodka, and transfer the solution to a sterilized atomizer bottle.

Most essential oils can be used to fragrance a room, but citrus oils are particularly refreshing. Essential oils that have antiseptic properties, such as cedarwood, eucalyptus, lavender, and tea tree, are ideal for fumigating rooms, while lemon, lemongrass, and citronella can be used in a spray to repel insects.

When **to use**

Diffusers can deodorize or fumigate a room, or simply create a special atmosphere.

Sitting near to a burner or vaporizer is an effective way to inhale the vapours of the oils and to benefit from their therapeutic properties.

Use a room spray to change the mood in a room, either to create a feeling of calm, invigorate, or perhaps to add a little romance.

Room sprays

are also useful for disinfecting and deodorizing an area such as a sick room and for repelling insects.

Cedarwood oil can be added to a diffuser to clear stale air.

Personal scents

While some oils, such as lavender, rose otto, chamomile, jasmine, vanilla, and ylang ylang, can be worn on their own as a scent, most need diluting in a base – perfumes are usually a mixture of fragranced oils in an alcohol base. You can use a single oil or several oils in a blend to create a scent that may have different "notes". When you smell a perfume, the top notes are typically the first thing you smell, followed by mid- and then base notes (see p164).

Creating a scent Don't be afraid to experiment with blends to find your favourite scent – see page 164 for blending guidelines. Essentially, try to keep blends to no more than 4–7 oils, and try a blend for a day or so to let it settle to get a better idea of its true aroma. To make your own personal scent, see the recipe on page 184.

When **to use**

Adding essential oils to a base solution is a great way to create your own personal fragrance. You can tailor the scent to suit your unique style and preferences and to create daytime and evening perfumes.

Mouthwashes and gargles

Although essential oils should not be swallowed, you can dilute them in water or a base of aloe vera juice to make an effective mouthwash or gargle that can be used to support good oral health and hygiene.

Home-made mouthwashes are cost effective and can be tailored to your needs. They also avoid a range of synthetic ingredients that are often found in commercial mouthwashes.

Making a mouthwash To make a basic mouthwash or gargle solution, dilute 4–5 drops of essential oil (clove, fennel, ginger, lemon, mint, rosemary, and sage are all good antiseptic choices) into a tablespoon of base oil. Further dilute this blend into a tumblerful of hot water and use as needed. Do not swallow the mixture.

When **to use**

Mouthwashes and gargles are ideal for mouth ulcers, gum disease, throat infections, and to help combat bad breath.

Peppermint has a fresh, menthol aroma.

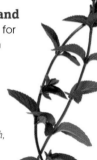

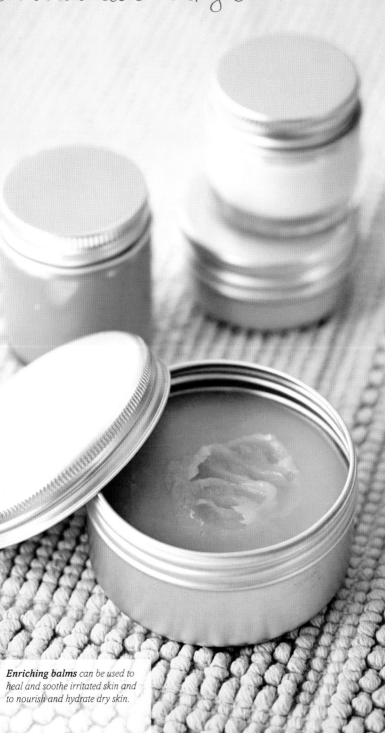

Dab a small amount of cream on irritated or itchy skin.

Enriching balms *can be used to heal and soothe irritated skin and to nourish and hydrate dry skin.*

Ointments, balms, and creams

Using oils in ointments, balms, and cream bases is an effective way to promote skin healing and to nourish skin. Ointments tend to be oil-based, while balms and creams contain extra ingredients for a creamier texture. Treat localized areas, applying a balm or ointment where needed, to encourage healing or to combat skin dryness.

When **to use**

Use for skin conditions such as eczema, psoriasis, bruising, and varicose veins, and apply to wounds to encourage healing.

Essential oils in a cream can form part of a daily skincare regime.

Use ointments with tea tree and manuka as first-aid remedies.

Hair care

Combining essential oil blends with herbal infusions, or creating conditioning hair oils by mixing essential oils with nourishing bases such as coconut oil, are great ways to enjoy a hair-care regime using natural products. See pages 202–03 for essential oil hair products that can help to restore shine and lustre to hair while avoiding the many added ingredients in commercial products.

When **to use**

Use nourishing essential oil hair treatments to revive dry and dull-looking hair.

Storing essential oils

Essential oils are **volatile** substances, which means they evaporate and deteriorate more quickly when exposed to light, air, and heat. Sunlight is especially harmful to the oils as it can cause chemical reactions that degrade them. To get the complete **therapeutic** benefits from your essential oils, store them correctly so that they remain as **fresh** as possible.

Looking after
your essential oils

Following the guidelines below will help you to maximize the life span of your essential oils and enjoy their benefits to the full.

- **Avoid storing your essential oils** in plastic containers. Plastic is not recommended as it is not totally inert, which means that over time the essential oils will interact with the plastic and may become

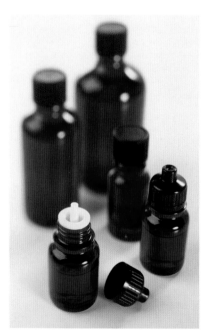

Small, dark-coloured bottles help to protect oils from the damaging effects of light and air.

contaminated by potentially toxic ingredients that leak out of the plastic.

- **Store your essential oils** and essential oil blends in sterilized glass (or stainless steel) bottles with lids that seal tightly. Bottles with dark-coloured glass are best as ultraviolet rays of light can taint oils by reacting with chemicals in the oil. Amber, dark blue, or deep violet glass bottles offer the best protection for your essential oils, keeping them as fresh as possible.

- **Store bottles in a cupboard** out of direct light and away from heat. Some oils, such as citrus ones, should be stored in the fridge (see opposite).

- **Make a note on the bottle** of the date it was opened, or label made-up blends that you've bottled with the names of the oils that were used and the date the blend was made.

- **Essential oil bottles** should have a dropper insert, which makes them harder to spill (see p36), and easier to measure out. This is also a good safety device if a child gets hold of a bottle.

Disposing of
essential oils safely

If you have essential oils that are past their best or that you no longer need, contact your local authority waste disposal department, or check their web page, for advice on how to dispose of them, and follow their recommendations.

If there is no specific advice, dispose of essential oils at your local household waste recycling centre in the same way as you would do for unused paints and solvents.

- **Keep oils away from children.** Though safe if properly diluted, essential oils are highly concentrated and can irritate the skin or the eyes if they are rubbed in, and can be toxic if taken internally (see page 36 for what to do if an oil is ingested).

- **Essential oils, like alcohol,** are flammable, so should never be left near sources of ignition, such as fires, cookers, candles, or naked flames.

Follow the storage advice to ensure oils stay as fresh as possible so that you enjoy their full benefits.

Shelf life of **essential oils**

The following chart is a useful guide to how long you should keep your essential oils before they are past their best. These guidelines are based on an oil being relatively fresh when you buy it from your supplier (check the batch number or use-by date), being opened and therefore exposed to air, and on their being stored under ideal conditions (see opposite). As such tiny amounts of essential oils are used at any one time, the oils usually come in small bottles that can be replaced as needed.

If you are in any doubt about how fresh an essential oil is, avoid using it on the skin (some oils that are non-irritant when fresh may irritate the skin when oxidized) or for therapeutic use. Instead, use the oil around the house, in a diffuser perhaps, or added to a household cleanser.

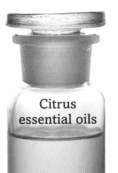

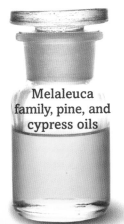

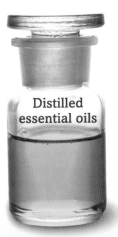

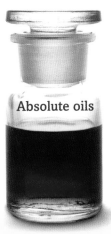

9–12 months

Citrus oils *such as grapefruit have the shortest shelf life. This is because they have a lot of the highly volatile components terpenes, which are prone to oxidization. Store in the fridge.*

12–18 months

The melaleuca family *(tea tree, niaouli) and pine and cypress essential oils have a fairly short shelf life due to relatively volatile components in their chemical composition.*

2–3 years

Most of the essential oils *that are steam-distilled have a shelf life of 2–3 years. Some resinous oils, such as sandalwood or myrrh, may last for longer than this.*

3–5 years

Absolutes*, such as rose absolute and jasmine, have the greatest longevity of all the oils and can last for up to five years.*

Shelf life of **base oils**

Base oils generally have a shorter shelf life than essential oils. Unlike essential oils, they become rancid when they go off. Your nose should tell you that something is wrong, and at this point the oil is unsuitable for use on the skin.

Store base oils in dark glass bottles too, away from light and heat.

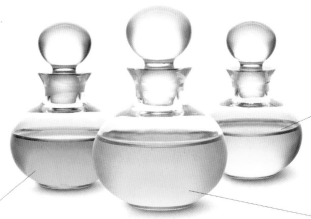

12–18 months

Most base oils *have a shelf life of 12–18 months once opened.*

2–3 years

Coconut and jojoba oils *last the longest and should keep well for 2–3 years.*

10–12 months

Borage, grapeseed, and evening primrose oils *tend to oxidize at 10–12 months.*

Using essential oils safely

As essential oils are **highly concentrated,** they need to be used sensibly and **diluted** properly. Follow advice on what to do if oils are spilt or misused, using oils on infants, and oils to avoid in pregnancy, when breastfeeding, and for some conditions.

TAKING CARE WITH OILS

Essential oils are perfectly safe if used sensibly. Before using an oil, carefully check the safety advice and make sure you follow the recommendations for dilution.

Spillage and **accidents**

Many essential oils irritate the skin if applied neat, without being diluted in a base, or carrier, oil, or other lotion. If you spill an essential oil, it can strip away varnish on furniture and stain fabrics such as carpets and bedding. Here are some tips for dealing with essential oil spillages and accidents and for cleaning diffusers and burners:

Accidentally ingesting oils Drink milk to dilute the oil and get medical advice quickly (see the box, below, for general information on ingesting essential oils).

Spilling oil on skin Quickly pour on a vegetable oil to dilute the essential oil: use sunflower, olive oil, or any other cooking or base oil. Once you've diluted the oil, gently wash the area with soapy water. If you don't have vegetable oil to hand, rinse the area with plenty of cold water.

Splashing oil in the eyes Rinse the eye with milk or, if you don't have milk, flush the area with plenty of cool water, then seek urgent medical advice.

Spills on furniture Wearing gloves, mop up spills immediately with kitchen paper, then wash the area with soapy water. If a surface is damaged, you may need to repair or re-varnish. Place bottles on saucers or tubs, not directly on furniture.

Spills on soft furnishings and bedding Apply a stain remover for oil stains and then wash with detergent.

To clean an essential oil burner or diffuser Wipe with a cloth soaked in white spirit or white vinegar, then use a cloth dipped in soapy water to get rid of the vinegary smell. Rinse out the cloth; give the diffuser or burner a final wipe to remove any soapy residues.

Medical **conditions**

Essential oils are generally safe to use with medical conditions, but there are some cases where caution is needed. There have been concerns that oils should be avoided with **hypertension,** but there is no evidence for this.
- **If you have asthma**, avoid directly inhaling vapours in a steam inhalation (use a diffuser instead) and use essential oils extremely well diluted.
- **If you have epilepsy**, avoid hyssop and wormwood oils.
- **For atopic children** (with a tendency to allergic reactions, or a family history of allergic responses), or those with hypersensitive skin, use no more than 1 per cent essential oils in a blend and do a patch test first (see opposite).
- **For all other contraindications**, check the safe usage for each oil in the A–Z section of the book (see pp38–145).

Ingesting essential oils

Never take an essential oil internally without the supervision of a suitably qualified medical practitioner. Some essential oils that are totally non-toxic when applied to the skin are highly toxic when taken internally, and there can be a risk of irritation to the throat or stomach, or even liver or nervous system damage.

Safe usage terms

In the A–Z entries of the book, individual safe usage advice is given for each oil. All the recommendations are based on the essential oil being properly diluted in a suitable base oil when used on the skin (see the table, opposite). Note that though many oils are safe for most people to use and are considered non-toxic and non-irritant in general, an individual reaction or allergy to an oil is possible. If you react to an oil, or oil blend, stop using it immediately. The following terms are used in the guidance for safe usage throughout the A–Z section:

Non-toxic An oil does not represent a hazard when used as directed and an adverse reaction is unlikely.

Non-irritant Is unlikely to cause irritation or an adverse skin reaction.

Sensitizing Repeated use may cause irritation or an adverse reaction in some individuals.

Photo-toxic May cause the skin to be more susceptible to damage on exposure to the sun's UV rays.

Pregnancy and **breastfeeding**

There are a few essential oils that should be avoided in pregnancy and when breastfeeding. They may be too stimulating in the early weeks of pregnancy, as is the case with sage, or an oil may have a level of toxicity, as is the case with basil. The skin can be hypersensitive in pregnancy, so oils such as cinnamon bark oil should be avoided. Check the A–Z entries for advice on each oil.

Essential oils for pregnancy

The following essential oils are safe to use in pregnancy and when breastfeeding. Check the botanical name on the label as different varieties of a plant may not be safe in pregnancy. Also check the safe usage advice for each oil in the A–Z entries on pages 38–145.

- *Anthemis nobilis –* **Roman chamomile**
- *Boswellia carterii/sacra –* **Frankincense**
- *Cananga odorata –* **Ylang ylang**
- *Cedrus atlantica –* **Cedarwood**
- *Citrus aurantifolia –* **Lime**
- *Citrus aurantium, Citrus aurantium amara –* **Neroli/Petitgrain**
- *Citrus aurantium bergamia –* **Bergamot (bergaptene-free)**
- *Citrus limonum –* **Lemon**
- *Citrus paradisi –* **Grapefruit**
- *Citrus reticulata –* **Mandarin**
- *Citrus sinensis –* **Orange**
- *Coriandrum sativum –* **Coriander**
- *Cupressus sempervirens –* **Cypress**
- *Cymbopogon martinii –* **Palmarosa**
- *Elettaria cardamomum –* **Cardamom**

Refreshing thyme is soothing in pregnancy.

- *Eucalyptus globulus/radiata –* **Eucalyptus**
- *Helichrysum italicum –* **Helichrysum (Immortelle)**
- *Lavandula angustifolia –* **Lavender**
- *Matricaria recutita –* **Chamomile (blue)**
- *Melaleuca quinquenervia –* **Niaouli**
- *Origanum marjorana –* **Marjoram**
- *Pelargonium graveolens –* **Geranium**
- *Piper nigrum –* **Black pepper**
- *Pogostemon cablin –* **Patchouli**
- *Rosa centifolia –* **Rose absolute**
- *Thymus vulgaris CT linalool –* **Thyme**
- *Vetiveria zizanoides –* **Vetiver**
- *Zingiber officinale –* **Ginger**

Babies and **children**

Be cautious about using oils on young infants as their skin is sensitive and very permeable and babies can struggle to deal with adverse effects. Diffusers can be the best way to use oils with infants.

Guidelines for babies and children

Premature babies and infants up to 3 months old *Essential oils aren't recommended on the skin. Use simple base oils such as olive and grapeseed.*

3–6 months old *Use only lavender or Roman chamomile. Dilute at 0.25 per cent: 2 drops of essential oil to 2 tablespoons of base oil.*

6–12 months old *Use only chamomile, Roman chamomile, lavender, mandarin, neroli or rose absolute. Dilute at 0.5 per cent: 4 drops of essential oil to 2 tablespoons of base oil.*

1–6 years old *Use only oils listed in the A–Z as non-toxic and non-irritant. Dilute at 1 per cent: 8 drops of essential oil to 2 tablespoons of base oil.*

7–15 years old *Use only oils listed as non-toxic and non-irritant. Dilute at 1.5 per cent: 12 drops of essential oil to 2 tablespoons of base oil.*

Use olive oil *to moisturize the skin of young babies.*

Doing a **patch test**

If you have sensitive skin or you have never used a particular essential oil, or blend of essential oils, before on your skin, do a patch test before using the oil the first time to check that you won't have an adverse reaction.

To do a patch test, make up the oil blend using the blending guidelines in the table, right. Apply a small amount to the inside of your elbow and wait for 24 hours. If no redness or irritation occurs, you can then try using the blend on a larger area of skin.

Blending essential oils and base oils

Use this table as a guide to essential oil and base oil quantities for oil blends.	Number of drops of essential oils for base oil quantities:			
	10ml/2tsp	*15ml/1tbsp*	*30ml/2tbsp*	*100ml/3½fl oz*
Adults with delicate skin or for a facial blend (less than 1 per cent)	2 drops	3 drops	6 drops	20 drops
Massage blend for adults with no skin sensitivities (2.5 per cent)	5 drops	7 drops	15 drops	50 drops
Bath oil or therapeutic blend for applying to a small area of the body, for example, a joint (5 per cent)	12 drops	18 drops	40 drops	130–150 drops

A–Z of
Essential Oils

Discover the unique properties of over 80 essential oils. Ordered alphabetically by their botanical names, each profile details a plant's **origin and properties**, the oil's appearance and aroma, and suggests some of the **best ways to use** each essential oil.

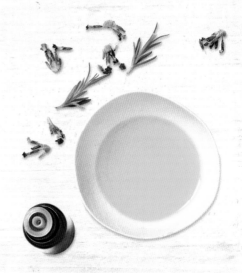

BATH OIL

FRAGRANCE

Mimosa
Acacia dealbata

Warming and **relaxing**, mimosa is a popular addition to perfumes. In skincare products, its nourishing and **soothing** properties provide a softening balm for sensitive skin, and its **calming action** helps to ease tension and lift spirits.

What is it **good for?**

Soothes skin The nourishing properties of mimosa essential oil help to soften the skin, and the oil's calming effect is useful for soothing inflamed and sensitive areas. Used as part of a daily beauty regime, mimosa oil helps to balance and tone combination skin and oily complexions.

Enhances wellbeing The deeply calming and relaxing properties of mimosa have a naturally uplifting effect on both body and mind. As well as being relaxing and soothing, the oil simultaneously energizes, and it is this ability that makes the oil a natural aphrodisiac.

Best **uses**

As a bath oil Indulge your senses and enjoy some relaxing time out by combining 4–5 drops of mimosa essential oil in 1 tablespoon base oil or full-fat milk and dispersing in a warm bath.

As a fragrance Mimosa essential oil is a good "fixative" for perfumes, helping to set the blend and make it last longer. It is often used as a "base note" in expensive scents.

Safe usage *Non-toxic and non-irritant.*

The plant

A member of the acacia family, mimosa is native to south-eastern Australia. With its cheerful, yellow, popcorn-shaped flowers, it is now widely cultivated as an ornamental plant in warm, temperate regions around the world.

The essential oil

Mimosa essential oil is an "absolute", which is solvent-extracted from the tree's flowers and twigs. The thick oil is pale yellow to brown in colour with a sweet floral scent that carries slight woody undertones.

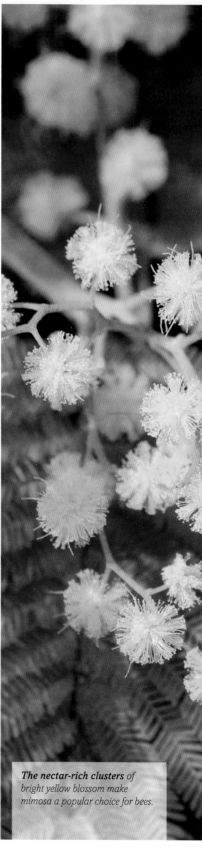

The nectar-rich clusters of bright yellow blossom make mimosa a popular choice for bees.

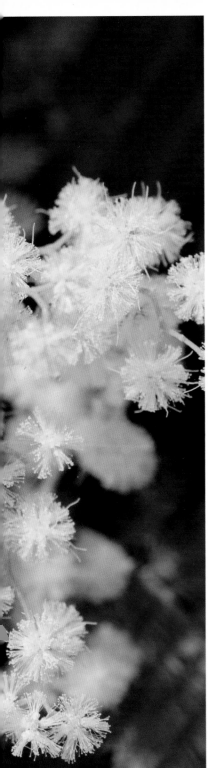

MASSAGE OIL   STEAM INHALATION

Yarrow

Achillea millefolium

Revered by the ancient Greeks and Egyptians, yarrow is derived from the Greek *hieros*, meaning **"sacred"**. Its traditional use as a **skin healer** still holds today, and its clearing properties can relieve sinus-related headaches.

What is it **good for?**

Soothes aches and pains
Massage this natural anti-inflammatory into stiff joints to reduce pain and inflammation, or try a gentle abdominal massage to ease menstrual cramps.

Eases sinus pain
Yarrow loosens congestion, relieving sinus-related headaches and breathing problems.

Heals skin
Its antiseptic properties help treat minor cuts and wounds, and its potent healing action works on scar tissue, ulcers, slow-to-heal wounds, and itchy skin complaints such as eczema.

Balances oily skin
Add a few drops of the oil to face creams or toners to balance oily skin and help keep acne under control.

Relieves stress
With its soothing action, yarrow is an effective oil for stress-related conditions, such as hypertension or insomnia.

Best **uses**

As a massage oil Mix 2–3 drops with St John's wort macerated oil and rub into sore, inflamed joints for pain relief.

In a steam inhalation To relieve the symptoms of hay fever and alleviate nasal congestion, add 2–3 drops of yarrow essential oil to a bowl of hot water, place a towel over your head, and inhale the steam deeply for 2–3 minutes.

Safe usage Non-irritant in dilution. Avoid during pregnancy and breastfeeding.

The plant

A grassland plant from the daisy family and a native of Europe and Western Asia, yarrow is now found worldwide. The oil of the Green Yarrow (Achillea nobilis) should be avoided for use in aromatherapy.

The essential oil

The herb is dried then steam-distilled to release the pale to dark blue or greeny-blue oil that has a powerful, herbaceous and slightly sweet smell, reminiscent of chamomile.

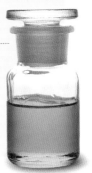

DIFFUSER

OINTMENT

STEAM INHALATION

MASSAGE OIL

COMPRESS

Buchu

Agathosma betulina

One of South Africa's best-known **medicinal** plants, buchu is a versatile essential oil that treats a wide range of ailments. Its **antiseptic, anti-inflammatory**, and detoxifying properties help to **soothe** and facilitate healing and calm digestive upsets.

What is it **good for?**

Heals skin With a potent antiseptic effect, buchu essential oil is ideal for treating skin infections.

Aids detox Buchu essential oil encourages the removal of toxins such as uric acid, which in turn relieves inflammation and sore joints. Its strong detoxifying action also helps to reduce water retention and to tackle areas of cellulite.

Eases digestive upsets Added to a massage blend, the essential oil helps to calm and soothe an irritable tummy and can also stimulate a sluggish digestion.

Acts as an insect repellent The sharp aroma of buchu oil makes this a natural insect repellent. Keep some of the oil on hand when travelling to instantly ward off pesky flies, mosquitoes, and fleas.

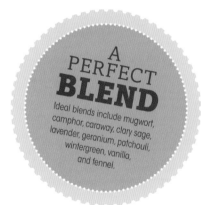

A PERFECT BLEND

Ideal blends include mugwort, camphor, caraway, clary sage, lavender, geranium, patchouli, wintergreen, vanilla, and fennel.

Best **uses**

In a diffuser Add 2–3 drops of buchu essential oil to an oil burner, vaporizer, or diffuser to help freshen stale air; or dilute in water and use in a spray bottle as an insect spray.

In an ointment Add 2–3 drops to 1 tablespoon ointment base to create an antiseptic skin treatment.

Safe usage Use very well diluted (less than 1 per cent). Avoid in pregnancy and when breastfeeding.

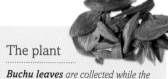

The plant

Buchu leaves are collected while the plant is flowering and fruiting, and then dried. The pungent aroma of the leaves increases as the plant dries out.

The essential oil

The golden oil is extracted from the dried leaves and flowers by steam-distillation. The oil has a sweet, medicinal aroma with hints of blackcurrant and peppermint.

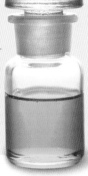

Fragonia™

Agonis fragrans

Relatively new to aromatherapy, Fragonia has a reputation for working at a deep level to restore **physical** and **emotional balance.** In particular, it's thought to help regulate the body clock and to boost immunity by encouraging efficient lymph circulation.

What is it **good for?**

Soothes aches and pains Reviving for tired joints and muscles, Fragonia also acts as a mild painkiller, helping to ease joint and muscle soreness and pain, mild toothache, and menstrual cramps.

Balances emotions The essential oil is an effective stress reliever. Deeply soothing, it helps to release emotional blockages.

Regulates body clock Its ability to help keep body systems in synch makes Fragonia essential oil an ideal remedy for overcoming the confusion and exhaustion caused by jetlag and coping with the demands of shift work.

Helps fight infection Its broad-acting antibacterial and antifungal properties help fight skin infections, and its antiviral action is a first-line defence against colds.

Strengthens immunity Fragonia aids lymph circulation and drainage, strengthening the immune system.

Best **uses**

In a steam inhalation Add 3–4 drops of the essential oil to hot water to create a steam inhalation to relieve respiratory and throat infections, break up catarrh, and fight infection.

In a massage oil Use in a massage blend to stimulate lymph circulation.

As a compress Add 3–4 drops to warm water and make a compress to relieve pain, congestion, cramping, and swelling and tenderness in the breasts.

Safe usage *Non-toxic and non-irritant.*

The plant

A native of Australia, the small shrub fragonia is commonly called "coarse tea tree" by the cut-flower industry. Although the petite white flowers are fragrant, the healing essential oil is concentrated in the branchlets and leaves.

The essential oil

Steam-distilled *from the leaves and branches, Fragonia oil is a clear to pale yellow with a similar scent to tea tree, but milder, with citrus, spicy, and floral notes.*

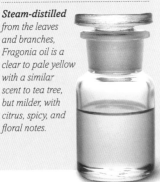

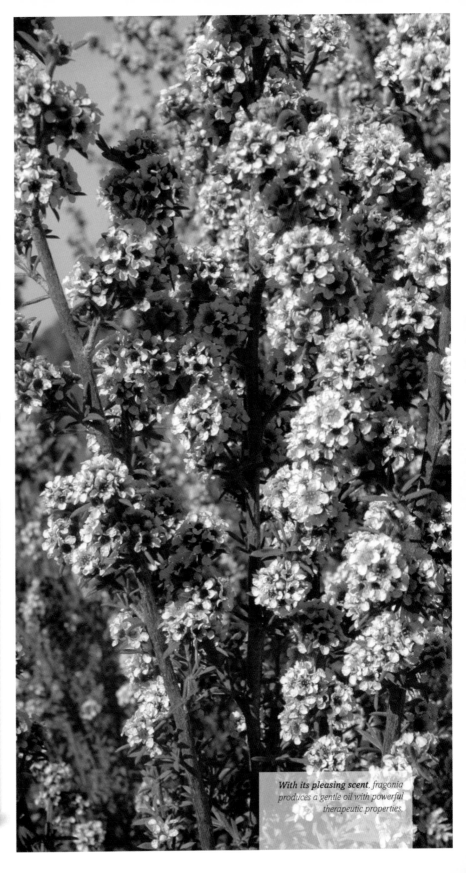

With its pleasing scent, fragonia produces a gentle oil with powerful therapeutic properties.

DIFFUSER

MASSAGE OIL

SKIN CARE

Lemon verbena

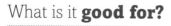
Aloysia triphylla

Behind the sunny, **uplifting** scent of lemon verbena lie some serious healing properties. It has a toning and **strengthening** effect on the nervous, digestive, respiratory, and immune systems. Its **antiseptic** action aids healing, while **anti-inflammatory** properties restore tired post-workout muscles.

A PERFECT BLEND

Ideal blending partners include lemon, elemi, neroli, lavender, rose, bergamot, cedarwood, juniper, eucalyptus and palmarosa.

What is it **good for?**

Relieves anxiety and aids focus Lemon verbena has a wonderfully calming, sedative effect. As well as easing feelings of panic, it also aids focus, concentration, and retention when studying or reading.

Acts as an aphrodisiac The soothing effect of lemon verbena on breathing and heart rates lies behind the claim that it can be an effective aphrodisiac for both sexes.

Supports immunity As well as supporting liver function, lemon verbena helps to bring down a fever by encouraging perspiration.

Fights colds and flu With its fresh citrus scent and antiseptic action, the oil relieves cold and flu symptoms, easing irritating coughs and loosening congestion in the sinuses and lungs.

Soothes aches and pains Massaging with lemon verbena after a workout tones muscles and reduces the buildup of lactic acid. The oil also encourages the repair of weak connective tissue and speeds up the healing process of joint-related

injuries. It has an anti-inflammatory effect that can help lessen the pain of arthritis and improve overall mobility.

Soothes digestion and relieves menstrual cramps A gentle massage with a lemon verbena blend eases stomach upsets and nausea. Its antispasmodic properties act on menstrual cramps, and it's thought the oil helps regulate menstrual cycles.

Best **uses**

In a diffuser Dispersed into the air, the oil helps to calm nerves, and can also be used to bolster the spirits when dealing with periods of stress, or when feeling down and depressed.

As a massage oil Lemon verbena provides skin benefits and supports health at a deeper level by lowering breathing and heart rates and boosting immunity and liver function. For a massage, blend 8–9 drops in 2 tablespoons base oil.

In a lotion Add 1–2 drops of the essential oil to 1 tablespoon lotion base to help soften and tone the skin. The oil is also useful for reducing skin puffiness and inflammation.

Safe usage *Use well diluted (less than 0.5 per cent). Avoid on sensitive skin, children under 15 years old, before exposure to the sun, and during pregnancy and breastfeeding.*

The plant

A native of Chile and Peru, *lemon verbena now grows in many tropical areas worldwide. With its pointed pale green leaves and stems bearing tubular flowers, the plant has a strong and distinct lemon aroma.*

The essential oil

The leaves and stalks *are steam-distilled for the oil, which is a yellowish-green colour. It has a fresh lemony smell described as simultaneously hot and bitter. Its extremely subtle aroma has proved difficult to reproduce synthetically.*

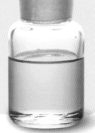

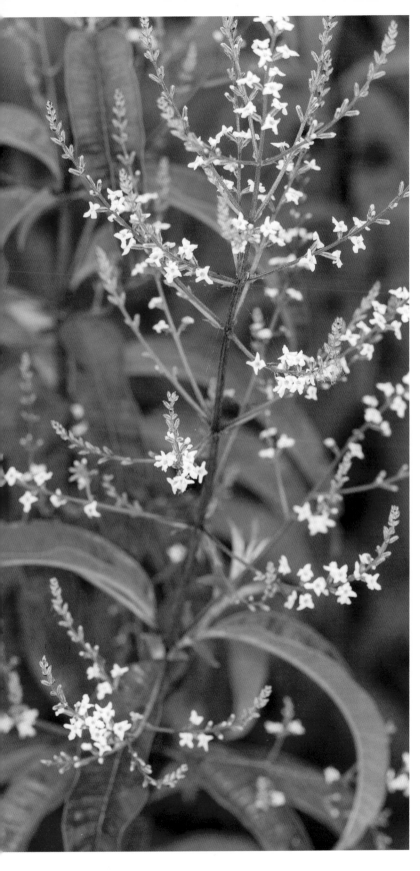

The oil's fresh, lemony aroma brings a feeling of calm and helps to enhance concentration.

This aromatic shrub *flowers in the summer months, producing stems of delicate white or pale lilac flowers.*

INHALATION

BATH OIL

MASSAGE OIL

BATH OIL

Galangal

Alpinia officinarum

This previously little-known essential oil is rapidly rising in popularity thanks to its **warming**, stimulating, and **antiseptic** properties. It can relieve nausea and motion sickness, has a natural **deodorizing** quality, and also helps fight fungal infections.

What is it **good for?**

Helps fight infection The combined antibacterial and antifungal properties of galangal essential oil make it an especially useful oil for treating skin eruptions. The oil can also be used to protect wounds, keeping them clean, and helps to bring fungal infections such as athlete's foot under control.

Eases digestion and soothes tummy upsets Warming and soothing, galangal essential oil aids digestion and the assimilation of nutrients and helps to release uncomfortable trapped wind. If you suffer from travel sickness and nausea, this is a useful remedy to carry on long journeys.

Acts as a deodorant The anti-perspirant action of galangal helps reduce body odour, to keep you feeling fresh.

Energizes and lifts mood As well as lifting fatigue and jet lag, galangal has a long history as an aphrodisiac because of its warming, stimulating aroma and ability to ease anxiety.

Best **uses**

In an inhalation To relieve travel sickness, add 2–3 drops to a tissue, keep in a plastic bag, and sniff as needed.

As a bath oil Mix 3–4 drops with 1 tablespoon base oil, full-fat milk, or bath oil. Add to your bath to heal dry, cracked skin.

Safe usage Non-toxic, non-irritant in dilution. Avoid near the face or nose of children under seven years old.

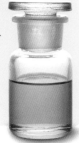

The plant

A native of Indonesia, galangal belongs to the same family as ginger and looks similar. The root (see above) is also a popular cooking ingredient and can be used like ginger.

The essential oil

The pale yellow to olive brown oil is obtained by the steam-distillation of the dried galangal root. Its aroma is reminiscent of ginger, but milder.

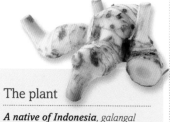

Dill

Anethum graveolens

For centuries, dill has been renowned for its impressive **healing** powers. It **stimulates** digestion, **calms** frazzled nerves, and has **antibacterial** properties that help speed the healing of wounds. It also has a mild diuretic effect that makes it a natural aid to detox.

What is it **good for?**

Supports digestion Dill has a calming, anti-inflammatory effect on the digestive tract, so has long been used as a treatment for stomach upsets and bouts of colic.

Fights infection Dill is a natural antibacterial and diuretic that can be used to relieve the symptoms of cystitis and bladder infections.

Heals skin Dill is highly effective in promoting the quick healing of cuts, grazes, and wounds, and helps to protect them from infections.

Aids restful sleep Sedating and calming on the nerves, dill essential oil helps to promote a deep sense of relaxation. This makes it a useful oil for relieving feelings of anxiety, tension, anger, and depression, and it can even ease hypertension, all of which helps to combat insomnia.

Aids detox The diuretic properties of dill essential oil aid the processes of perspiration and urination, helping to prevent a buildup of fluids and toxins.

Best **uses**

As a massage oil Add 6–8 drops of the essential oil to 2 tablespoons base oil to support a detox regime and create a state of calm.

As a bath oil Disperse 5–6 drops in 1 tablespoon base oil or full-fat milk and add to the bath. Relax in the bath and inhale the steam deeply.

Safe usage Non-toxic, non-irritant in dilution.

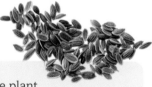

The plant

The feathery leaves of the dill plant are commonly used to flavour food. The tiny flowers eventually give way to oil-rich seeds (see above).

The essential oil

The pale yellow essential oil is extracted through steam-distillation of both the dried seeds and the whole plant. The oil has an appealing grassy aroma and blends well with lime, lemon, and other citrus oils.

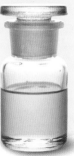

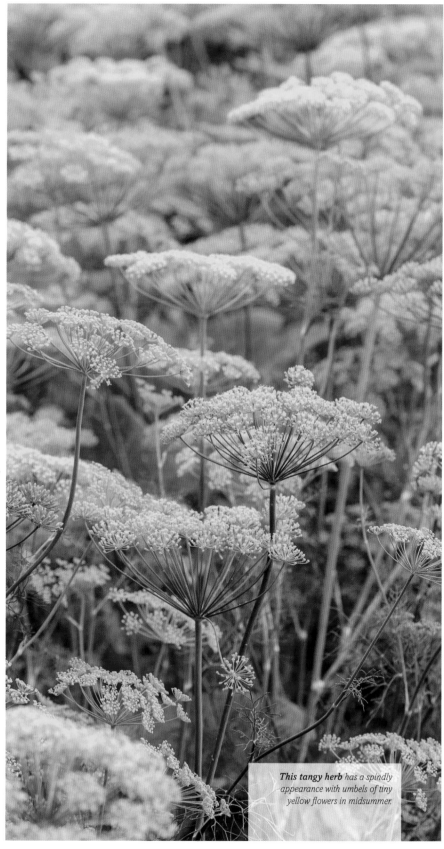

This tangy herb has a spindly appearance with umbels of tiny yellow flowers in midsummer.

MASSAGE OIL   COMPRESS

Angelica

Angelica archangelica

A **warming** oil, angelica is fondly referred to as the "oil of the angels" because its **uplifting** effect promotes calm, positivity, and restful sleep. It is also soothing and **clearing**, relaxing muscles and relieving congestion.

What is it **good for?**

Aids detox A mild diuretic, angelica also encourages perspiration, which promotes health by aiding the removal of toxins from the body.

Soothes aches and pains
Angelica's warming properties help to boost the circulation to aching joints and muscles, and provide effective relief from menstrual cramps.

Relieves congestion Used in a chest massage oil blend or added to a steam inhalation, angelica essential oil can help to break up stubborn congestion.

Enhances wellbeing Reputed to lift flagging spirits, angelica essential oil is thought to help you "discover" your true self and can be useful during periods of upheaval or in times of transition.

Best **uses**

As a massage oil Used in a blend, angelica provides a detoxifying massage that lifts the spirits and improves wellbeing. Mix 2–4 drops in 2 tablespoons base oil.

In a compress Add 2–3 drops to warm water, dip a cloth in, squeeze out, and use to ease menstrual pain.

Safe usage Non-toxic, use well diluted *(less than 1 per cent). Avoid use on skin for 12 hours prior to sun exposure.*

The plant

A native of northern Europe, the dramatic umbrella-like flowerheads of the angelica plant produce a vast number of seeds. The seed oil is considered safest for aromatherapy as it contains less of the photo-toxic chemical bergapten than is found in the root oil.

The essential oil

Both the roots and seeds can be dried and then steam-distilled to produce a pungent oil with a sweet, spicy aroma. Oil from the seed is clear, while the oil from the roots is a pale yellow.

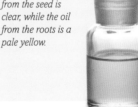

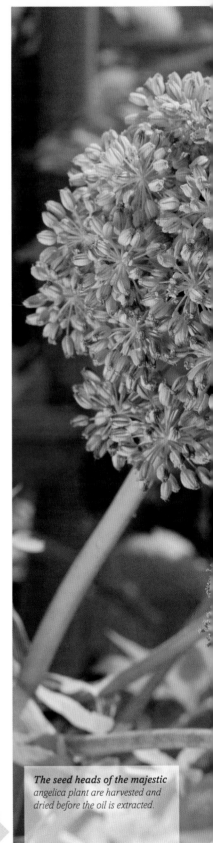

The seed heads of the majestic angelica plant are harvested and dried before the oil is extracted.

BATH OIL

DIFFUSER

Rosewood

Aniba rosaeodora

Rosewood, also called **bois de rose,** is a member of the laurel family – a relative of cinnamon and bay. A **grounding** and centring oil, it works on the mind and emotions.

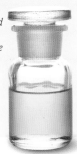

A PERFECT **BLEND**

Match rosewood with geranium, patchouli, lavender, rose, bergamot, neroli, black pepper, cinnamon, and other spicy oils

What is it **good for?**

Conditions skin This oil has tissue-regenerating properties that can help slow signs of premature ageing, making this an effective treatment for dull, dry, or mature skin. Rosewood also has a healing action on wounds, making this an excellent first-aid remedy for cuts and insect bites.

Tones and calms skin Rosewood essential oil balances the levels of oil in combination or oily complexions, so helps to control pimples, acne, and blackheads.

Acts as a hair tonic As with skin, rosewood has a balancing effect on the scalp, helping to regulate excessively dry or oily hair.

Acts as a mild pain reliever The mild analgesic action of this oil means rosewood can alleviate headaches and muscle and joint pain.

Balances emotions Thought to bring emotional stability and to create a sense of calm and empowerment, rosewood essential oil also helps you to relax and is considered an aphrodisiac.

Best **uses**

As a bath oil Add 5–6 drops to 1 tablespoon base oil or full-fat milk and enjoy a restorative, steamy soak.

In a diffuser Diffuse this spicy, woody, floral aroma to calm emotions.

Safe usage *Non-toxic and non-irritant.*

The plant

This native Brazilian tree *grows up to 40m (130ft). Now endangered, harvesting is strictly controlled. Oil from the heartwood should be avoided. A more sustainable oil from the leaves and twigs may be available.*

The essential oil

The light yellow oil *is steam-distilled from the wood chippings of the tree and has a spicy, sweet, floral aroma.*

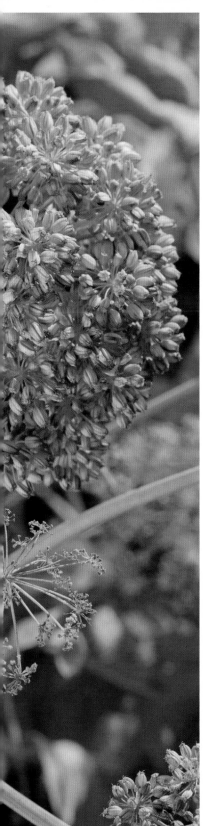

MASSAGE OIL

FOOT BATH

DIFFUSER

MASSAGE OIL

Tarragon
Artemisia dracunculus

A popular kitchen herb, tarragon also has a long history of use as a **medicinal** herb. The oil yields a warming massage, helping to **improve circulation** to the extremities, and is mildly **analgesic**. It also offers **emotional support** in times of upheaval.

What is it **good for?**

Eases digestion In a massage blend, tarragon oil stimulates appetite and has a pronounced effect on sluggish digestion, helping food move more efficiently through the digestive tract. It also helps calm flatulence, hiccups, and nervous indigestion.

Aids detox Its mild diuretic and laxative action helps to eliminate toxins.

Eases aches and pains Tarragon contains a natural anaesthetic, eugenol, also found in clove. Like clove, it is a traditional toothache remedy. It also has a warming action that helps increase circulation to muscles, joints, and extremities, eases menstrual pains, and helps regulate periods.

Acts as a deodorant The oil's spicy scent acts on body odour, inhibiting the growth of microbes on the skin, so reducing stale, unwelcome smells.

Provides emotional support Tarragon is said to ward off feelings of despair and provide emotional support in times of change by alleviating fear and feelings of being "stuck".

Best **uses**

As a massage oil Blend 1-2 drops in 2 tablespoons base oil to ease digestive discomfort and menstrual pains.

In a foot bath Add 2-3 drops to a foot bath to boost circulation, warm the body, and inhibit foot odour.

Safe usage Use extremely well diluted (less than 0.1 per cent). Avoid during pregnancy and breastfeeding, and on children under seven years old.

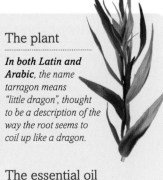

The plant

In both Latin and Arabic, the name tarragon means "little dragon", thought to be a description of the way the root seems to coil up like a dragon.

The essential oil

The oil is steam-distilled from the leaves and the flowering tops to produce a clear to pale green oil with an herbaceous aroma, somewhere between celery and aniseed.

Mugwort
Artemisia vulgaris

A **powerful** oil that should be used sparingly, mugwort can nevertheless have **profound** effects. Used in massage or simply dispersed in the air, it has a pleasant **warming** quality that stimulates circulation, clears the airways, and relaxes the mind.

What is it **good for?**

Eases aches and pains Useful for arthritis and other inflammatory joint conditions, mugwort eases stiff muscles and improves circulation.

Fights colds The oil works as a decongestant, loosening phlegm and mucus to ease bronchitis and colds.

Supports women's health With gentle massage, the oil eases cramps, relaxes abdominal tension, and encourages blood flow when periods are delayed or very light.

Provides emotional support Uplifting and relaxing, a drop on a pillow is said to bring pleasant dreams.

Best **uses**

As a diffuser Add 2-3 drops each of mugwort and lavender essential oils to a diffuser, vaporizer, or oil burner

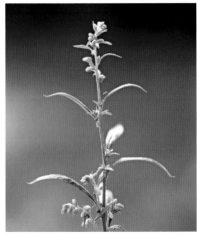

Pungent mugwort produces small clusters of white to yellow flowers in midsummer.

to produce pleasant feelings of peace and tranquillity.

As a massage oil For aching joints and muscles, massage with a warming mugwort blend for deep relief. Add 3–6 drops to 2 tablespoons base oil.

Safe usage Use well diluted (less than 1 per cent). Avoid in pregnancy and if breastfeeding, on children under seven years old, and with epilepsy.

The plant

A shrubby herb, mugwort is found in temperate regions, in meadows and on waysides. The name is derived from the Old English mucg wyrt, meaning "marsh plant". In Chinese medicine, the dried, compressed leaves (moxa) are burnt and briefly held close to the skin to provide warmth.

The essential oil

The oil is extracted by steam-distillation of leaves, buds, and the flowering tops of the mugwort tree to produce an amber oil with a sweet, almost floral, citrussy scent.

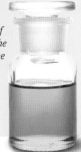

HAIR CARE

MASSAGE OIL

Birch (leaf)
Betula alba

In Scandinavia, birch leaves and twigs are bound together and used in saunas to **tone skin** and **boost circulation**. White birch oil is **stimulating** and **detoxifying**, helping the kidneys to function efficiently and promoting perspiration to hasten the removal of toxins.

What is it **good for?**

Aids detox Birch oil facilitates both perspiration and urination, which hastens the removal of toxins and impurities from the body. Added to a massage oil blend, it helps to improve a sluggish circulation.

Soothes aches and pains A natural anti-inflammatory and analgesic, birch essential oil can help to ease sore muscles and joints after a work-out and numb pain locally. These same properties also help to ease the discomfort caused by arthritis and rheumatism.

Acts as an antiseptic The antiseptic properties of birch essential oil make it a useful remedy for skin eruptions such as cold sores. The oil is also an effective healer for irritating skin conditions, such as eczema and psoriasis, but ensure it is well diluted before using.

Tones skin and hair Birch has a balancing effect on combination skin, and can soften and tighten skin, giving mature skin a youthful appearance. Used in a hair rinse, it helps promote shine and tackles stubborn dandruff.

Best **uses**

In a hair rinse Add 4–5 drops to a final rinse to combat dandruff.

As a massage oil Mix 6–10 drops with 2 tablespoons base oil for a full-body massage to help improve circulation and remove toxins.

Safe usage Use well diluted (less than 2 per cent). Avoid in pregnancy and if breastfeeding; on children under 15 years old; if on anticoagulants or sensitive to salicylates.

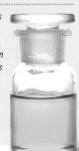

The plant

European white birch or silver birch is native to the northern hemisphere. The distinctive papery bark can be distilled into a highly antiseptic birch tar oil, unsuitable for aromatherapy. The young leaves produce the milder white birch oil.

The essential oil

The oil, which has a slightly spicy, woody aroma, is steam-distilled from the leaf buds and is pale yellow in colour.

OINTMENT

SKIN CARE

DIFFUSER

MASSAGE OIL

Frankincense (Olibanum)

Boswellia carterii, B. sacra, B. frereana, et al

This is an important oil for **toning** and **invigorating** the complexion, particularly for mature or sun-damaged skin. Frankincense can be used as both an antiseptic and anti-inflammatory, and its distinct aroma helps to **soothe** and **calm** frayed nerves, making it useful for treating anxiety.

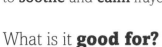

A PERFECT **BLEND**

Natural blending partners include citrus and spice oils, basil, cedarwood, chamomile, myrrh, neroli, pine, sandalwood, and vetiver.

What is it **good for?**

Soothes aches and pains The potent anti-inflammatory action of frankincense has been found to ease arthritis and rheumatic pain.

Tones skin The oil helps to close pores and tone skin. Its rejuvenating qualities make it an excellent choice for mature skins, helping to minimize wrinkles and fine lines and reduce the appearance of blemishes and long-term sun damage.

Acts as an antiseptic Diluted, frankincense oil can be used topically to heal wounds and skin ulcers.

Fights colds Frankincense essential oil helps to soothe the mucous membranes, calming and deepening breathing, and easing coughs, bronchitis, and laryngitis.

Relieves anxiety This calming oil lifts the spirits, increases energy and focus, and aids meditation, ideal when feeling stressed, tired, or overwhelmed.

Best **uses**

In an ointment The powerful anti-inflammatory properties of frankincense make it an effective ointment to use on sore joints, helping to reduce pain and increase movement.

As a toner Make a facial toner by adding 2 tablespoons aloe vera juice to 6 tablespoons water and 4 drops of frankincense.

In a diffuser Add 3–4 drops to a diffuser, vaporizer, or oil burner.

In a massage oil Add a few drops of the oil to a base oil for a soothing and toning massage.

Safe usage Non-toxic, non-irritant in dilution.

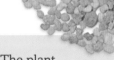

The plant

Frankincense trees grow wild in north-east Africa and Oman. They produce an aromatic sap that, when dried, is called the "pearl of the desert", and is traditionally burned as incense.

The essential oil

The rich fragrant oil is steam-distilled from the tree resin (above). It produces a pale yellow or greenish oil with a sweet, spicy, resinous odour.

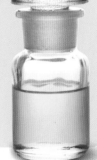

Frankincense promotes feelings of positivity, enhancing wellbeing.

SKIN CARE

HAIR CARE

FRAGRANCE

MASSAGE OIL

BATH OIL

Ylang ylang

Cananga odorata

With its **exotic**, highly floral aroma, ylang ylang is **uplifting** and **arousing**, and at the same time eases feelings of anxiety. A key constituent of the traditional hair preparation, macassar oil, its **balancing** properties make it suitable for all skin types.

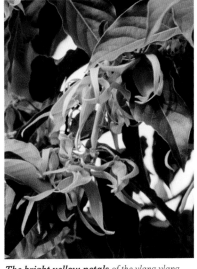

The bright yellow petals of the ylang ylang yield an exceptionally floral essential oil.

What is it **good for?**

Improves complexion Ylang ylang has a balancing action on the secretion of sebum, helping to regulate its production, making it an ideal skin cleanser for both oily and dry skin types. It is a particularly effective tonic for acne-prone complexions.

Tones skin With its stimulating effect, ylang ylang helps to improve the structure and appearance of tired or sagging skin, restoring a youthful glow.

Nourishes hair The essential oil has a long history as a treatment for dry hair. It nourishes and stimulates the scalp, and conditions dry, brittle hair. It is even reputed to promote hair growth.

Aids relaxation Stimulating and calming, ylang ylang essential oil is well placed for increasing feelings of wellbeing. Its calming properties have demonstrable effects, helping to lower blood pressure and breathing rates, in turn reducing feelings of anxiety.

Acts as an aphrodisiac The arousing aroma of ylang ylang and its renowned relaxing effect make this oil a popular aphrodisiac, as it helps to release inhibitions and ease tension, while arousing the olfactory senses. Traditionally, petals were scattered on the beds of newlyweds to help shed inhibitions and dispel anxiety.

Treats depression The sedating and calming properties of ylang ylang make it a useful support in the treatment of depression and tension.

Best **uses**

As a skin toner Add 1–2 drops of the oil to 2 teaspoons witch hazel and 3 tablespoons water. Dab on skin with a cotton ball.

As a hair tonic For a dry scalp, add 1–2 drops to 1 teaspoon olive oil and massage into the scalp before bed. Brush through with a natural-bristle brush, and wash out in the morning.

As a perfume The essential oil can be used neat as a simple perfume. Or you can mix 1–2 drops in a teaspoon of a base oil, such as apricot kernel, and apply it to the pulse points.

In a massage oil For a skin-toning and relaxing massage, add 1–2 drops of ylang ylang oil to a base oil blend.

As a bath oil Add 1–2 drops of the oil to 1 tablespoon base oil or full-fat milk and disperse in the bath.

Safe usage *Non-toxic and non-irritant. As it has a powerful odour, use well diluted, unless using neat as a perfume.*

The plant

A native of Asia, ylang ylang means "flower of flowers"; the waxy petals have been used in medicines and skin creams for millenia. Now grown mainly in Madagascar and the Comoros, it is a base of high-end oriental scents and a key ingredient in Chanel No.5.

The essential oil

The pale yellow oil is steam- or water-distilled from the flowers to create an oil with an intensely sweet, exotic floral scent. The scent can be overpowering, so use sparingly at first to discover how strong you like it.

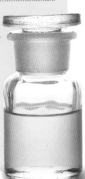

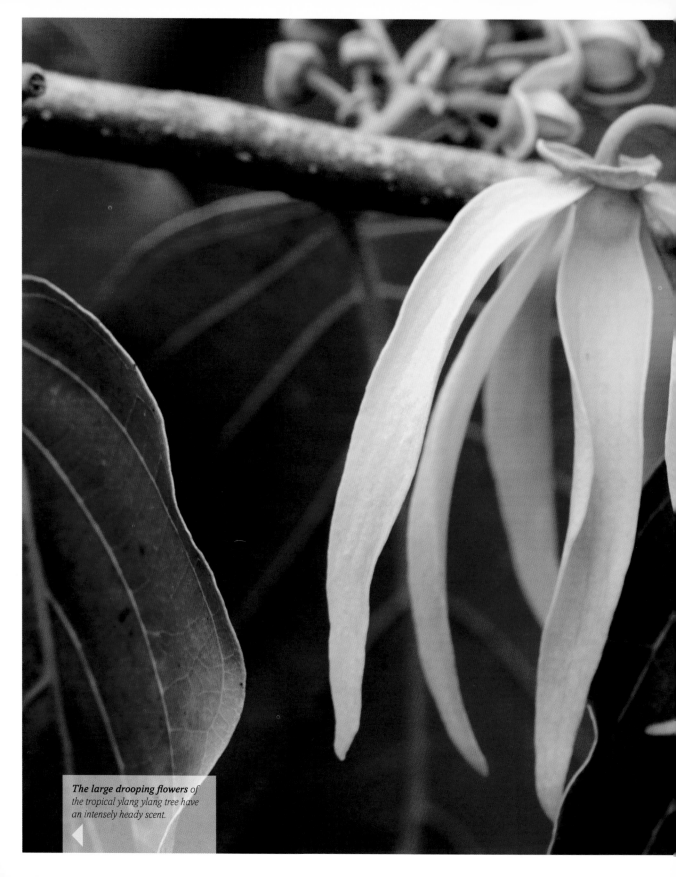

The large drooping flowers of the tropical ylang ylang tree have an intensely heady scent.

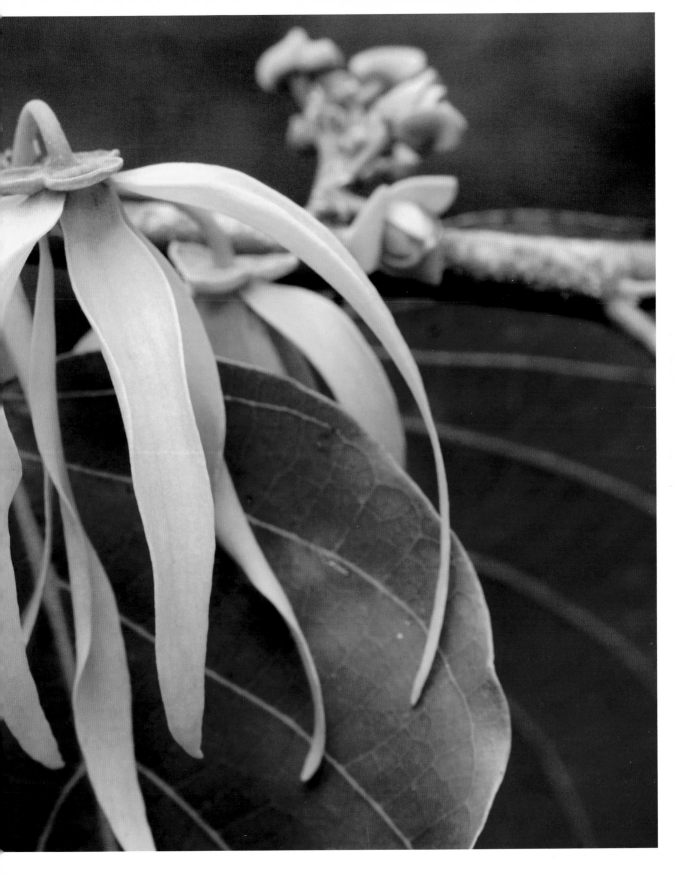

SKIN CARE

STEAM
INHALATION

MASSAGE OIL

SKIN CARE

Elemi

Canarium luzonicum

Elemi has a long history in skin care, traditionally used in **healing** skin salves in the Middle East and Europe. Today, its ability to **tone** and **firm** skin makes it a favourite ingredient in high-end beauty products. It also helps to relieve congestion in the lungs.

What is it **good for?**

Combats signs of ageing Elemi is ideal for dry or sun-damaged skin. It accelerates skin-cell renewal and supports collagen synthesis, helping to prevent sagging and the appearance of premature fine lines. In skin-care products, elemi helps to harmonize both dry and oily skin types.

Heals skin The healing properties of elemi can help to reduce scarring, and its effective antiseptic action helps prevent infection in cuts and wounds.

Eases respiratory problems With expectorant and antiviral properties, a few drops of the oil added to a steam inhalation brings relief to respiratory problems such as chest infections, catarrh, sinusitis, and bronchitis.

Lifts moods Calming and uplifting, this a good oil to choose when stressed, or suffering from nervous exhaustion.

Best **uses**

In a cream Add 2–4 drops of elemi essential oil to 2 tablespoons unscented cream or lotion base for a revitalizing skin treatment to apply before bedtime as part of an evening skincare regime.

In an inhalation Add 3–4 drops to a bowl of hot water and inhale for welcome relief from the symptoms of hay fever, as well as to ease the congestion that leads to coughs and sinus-related headaches.

Safe usage Non-toxic, use well diluted (less than 0.5 per cent).

The plant

A relative of frankincense and myrrh, the elemi tree is native to the tropical forests of the Philippines and neighbouring nations. The name means "above and below" in Arabic, suggesting that it was valued both spiritually and physically.

The essential oil

Steam-distilled from the resin of the elemi tree, the essential oil is pale yellow and has a distinctive sharp, citrussy, pine aroma.

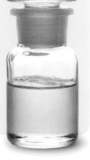

The honey-coloured resin produces the oil.

Caraway

Carum carvi

This **warming** essential oil works on both mind and body, **relieving** mental strain and emotional fatigue. It also supports the digestive and urinary systems, helps **clear** the respiratory system, and can be used to treat stubborn skin and scalp conditions.

What is it **good for?**

Soothes nerves Caraway oil is a natural tonic for frayed nerves, calming the mind and soothing mental fatigue. It also settles nervous digestion, colic, flatulence, and gastric spasms.

Helps fight infection Its expectorant action means that caraway can help to clear bronchitis, bronchial asthma, and irritating coughs. It also helps to soothe sore throats and laryngitis, supports the healthy function of the urinary system, and helps to flush out toxins.

Heals and soothes skin The tissue-regenerating qualities of caraway essential oil can be harnessed to help disperse bruises, reduce boils, and clean infected wounds. The oil is used to combat oily skin, help clear acne and flaky scalps, and relieve itching.

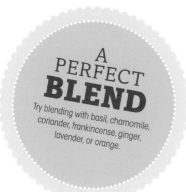

A
PERFECT
BLEND
Try blending with basil, chamomile,
coriander, frankincense, ginger,
lavender, or orange.

Best **uses**

As a massage oil Blend 3–6 drops
with 2 tablespoons base oil for a
soothing massage to relieve
abdominal discomfort.

In a cream Add 3–6 drops to 2
tablespoons base cream and use
to relieve dry, itchy skin and scalp.

Safe usage Non-toxic. Use well
diluted (less than
1 per cent).

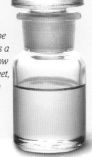

The plant

A native of south-eastern Europe,
caraway now grows in the wild and
is cultivated all over Europe and
temperate Asia. A member of the
Umbelliferae family, it is related
to cumin, fennel, and dill.

The essential oil

Caraway oil
is extracted by
steam-distillation
from the dried ripe
seeds. It produces a
clear to pale yellow
oil that has a sweet,
spicy aroma with
a hint of pepper.

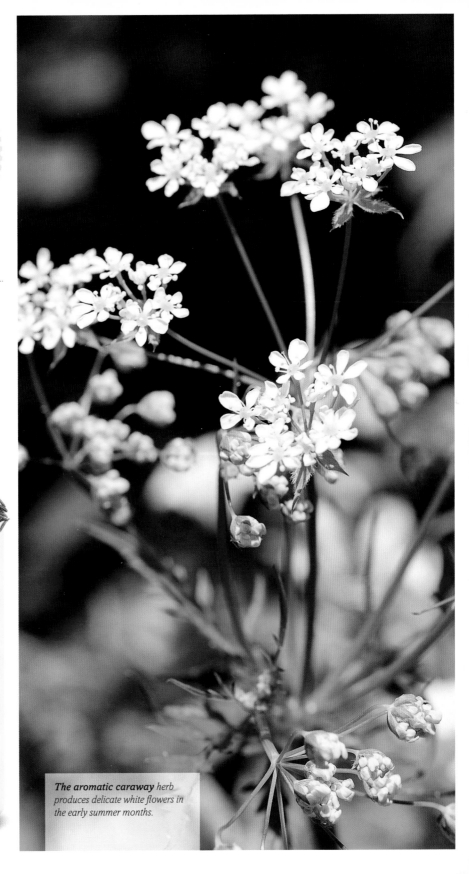

The aromatic caraway herb
produces delicate white flowers in
the early summer months.

HAIR CARE

FRAGRANCE

OINTMENT
MASSAGE OIL

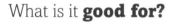

Cedarwood
Cedrus atlantica

A long-established essential oil, cedarwood has an impressive range of benefits. Both **antiseptic** and **astringent**, it balances and tones complexions and facilitates healing in infections and skin eruptions. Its **uplifting** aroma makes it a perfect pick-me-up, helping to release tension and lift feelings of lethargy.

A PERFECT BLEND

Blends well with rose, black pepper, bergamot, jasmine, neroli, juniper, cypress, clary sage, frankincense, and mimosa.

What is it **good for?**

Soothes skin Cedarwood contains the highest level of the anti-inflammatory substances known as sesquiterpenes of any essential oil. This makes it helpful for easing itchy, irritated skin, especially in cases of acne, dandruff, or athlete's foot.

Relieves pain Cedarwood essential oil has a warming, regenerative effect, making it a useful treatment for chronic degenerative conditions, such as arthritis.

Tones and heals skin The astringent properties in this essential oil can help to balance oily or acne-prone skin and make it an effective tonic for oily hair. It also promotes healing of wounds and skin ulcers.

Supports women's health The stimulating effect of cedarwood can help regulate the menstrual cycle and is a useful antiseptic treatment for unwanted vaginal discharges.

Aids detox Cedarwood helps to stimulate the flow of lymph, reduce water retention, and aid the removal of toxins from the body.

Fights colds and coughs Used as an inhalation or in a diffuser, the oil can help break up excessive catarrh, and soothe coughs and bronchitis.

Lifts moods Grounding and calming, cedarwood can combat feelings of negativity. Its uplifting qualities treat nervous tension, anxiety, depression, and tiredness, as well as aid focus. For men, it is considered an aphrodisiac.

Best **uses**

As a hair tonic Add 10–20 drops to a bottle of unscented shampoo or conditioner to combat dandruff.

As a room fragrance Use 3–4 drops in a diffuser, vaporizer, or oil burner to cleanse the air and lift anxiety, depression, and feelings of exhaustion.

In an ointment Add 12–16 drops to 2 tablespoons base oil or an ointment base and apply several times a day to provide fast relief and healing for itchy, irritated skin conditions.

As a massage oil Add 12–18 drops cedarwood essential oil to 2 tablespoons base oil for an uplifting and skin-soothing massage.

Safe usage Non-toxic, non-irritant in dilution.

The plant

The sacred Cedars of Lebanon in the Atlas Mountains are large imposing trees that can live for up to 2,000 years. As a symbol of protection and power, they have been so highly prized and sought after over the years that they are becoming an endangered species, so ensure the oil you buy is harvested sustainably.

The essential oil

The tree bark is the source of a thick, pale, yellow to amber essential oil with a sweet, mild, balsamic–woody odour that becomes gradually more woody while the oil dries out.

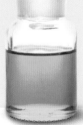

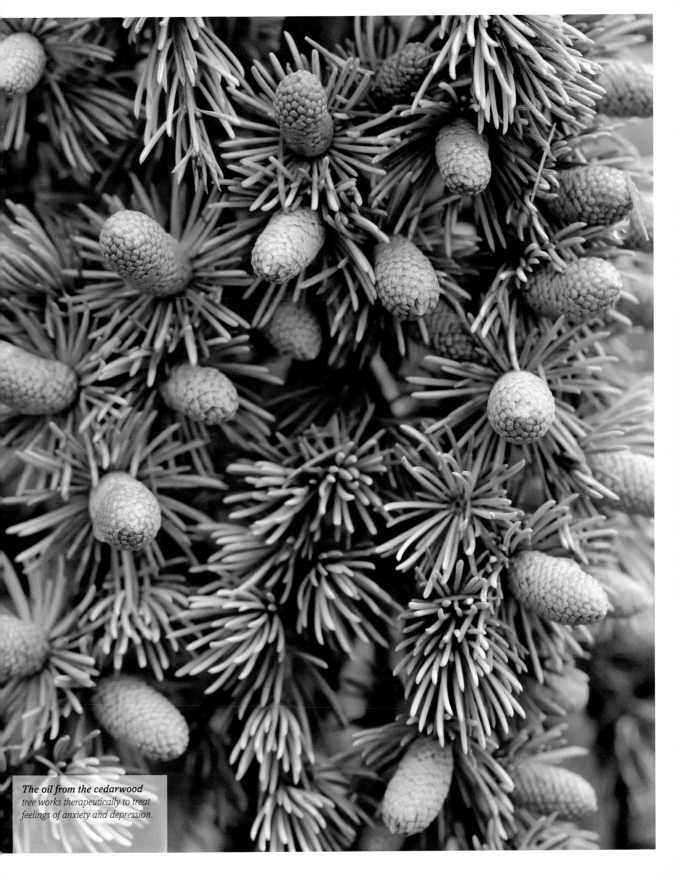

The oil from the cedarwood tree works therapeutically to treat feelings of anxiety and depression.

MASSAGE OIL   OINTMENT

FOOT BATH   DIFFUSER

Camphor

Cinnamomum camphora

With its **medicinal** aroma, camphor is a very useful oil. It has a dual action on skin, at first **cooling** then deeply **warming**, and stimulates the circulation, metabolism, and digestion. It's an effective pain reliever and also helps to clear the head and calm the mind.

What is it **good for?**

Improves circulation The stimulating effect of camphor essential oil helps to boost a sluggish circulation and digestion, and also balances the metabolic rate.

Soothes aches and pains A natural anaesthetic, camphor can provide relief from nerve pain and inflammation. It is also an effective antispasmodic and eases cramps and muscle spasms.

Fights colds and flu Camphor helps clear blocked sinuses and respiratory complaints, making breathing easier.

Best **uses**

As a massage oil If you are chilly or achy, add 2–4 drops to 2 tablespoons base oil for a warming massage that instils a sense of wellbeing.

In an ointment Add 2–4 drops to 2 tablespoons ointment base for a rub to relieve pain and sore muscles.

Safe usage *A strong oil, use well diluted and use only "white" camphor essential oil.*

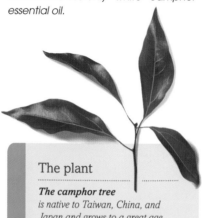

The plant

The camphor tree *is native to Taiwan, China, and Japan and grows to a great age. It must be at least 50 years old to produce the oil, which is present in all parts of the plant.*

Ho Sho, or Ho Leaf, *oil is distilled from the leaves of the camphor tree and is a much milder oil than the oil from the rest of the plant, and is soothing for the skin and mind. It is non-toxic and non-irritant in dilution.*

The essential oil

When the wood, *branches, and leaves of the camphor plant are steam-distilled, they produce a brown oil that must be distilled twice more before it becomes the clear oil , known as "white camphor" that is safe to use in aromatherapy.*

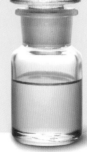

Cinnamon

Cinnamomum zeylanicum

This spicy, **warming** oil was used by the ancient Egyptians as an aromatic foot massage. It is used in very small amounts in cosmetics for its antiseptic properties, and its **energizing** and **stimulating** aroma makes it ideal for lifting flagging spirits.

What is it **good for?**

Soothes aches and pains Cinnamon is warming if you feel particularly chilly, as it helps to boost circulation to the extremities. It's especially effective for reviving and soothing sore joints aggravated by cold, damp weather.

Aids digestion Massaged over the abdomen, cinnamon oil can stimulate circulation, improve sluggish digestion, and relieve constipation. It also has an antispasmodic action that helps to calm stomach cramps and spasms.

Acts as an antiseptic Cinnamon is effective against a broad range of bacteria, viruses, and parasites, especially lice and scabies.

Balances emotions An uplifting room scent, the oil can help to counter exhaustion and depression.

BATH OIL

MASSAGE OIL

Best **uses**

As a foot bath Warm cold feet by adding 1–2 drops of cinnamon oil to a relaxing foot bath.

In a diffuser Add 1–2 drops to a diffuser to disinfect air in a sick room or to get rid of unpleasant smells.

Safe usage *Use very well diluted (less than 0.5 per cent), and use only cinnamon leaf oil on the skin (not cinnamon bark).*

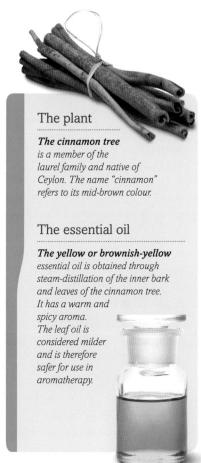

The plant

The cinnamon tree *is a member of the laurel family and native of Ceylon. The name "cinnamon" refers to its mid-brown colour.*

The essential oil

The yellow or brownish-yellow *essential oil is obtained through steam-distillation of the inner bark and leaves of the cinnamon tree. It has a warm and spicy aroma. The leaf oil is considered milder and is therefore safer for use in aromatherapy.*

Cistus

Cistus ladaniferus

Derived from the flowering plant also known as rock rose, Rose of Sharon, and labdanum, **fragrant** cistus has powerful **skin-toning** and **healing** properties. It is a useful immune stimulant, and its antiseptic properties fight infection. It also helps centre the mind.

What is it **good for?**

Aids detox Used in massage oils, blended with a favourite base oil, cistus helps to encourage effective lymphatic drainage, improves circulation, and boosts immunity.

Heals skin Known for its healing properties, cistus oil can help to speed up tissue healing in wounds. Its astringent properties also make it useful for treating bleeding gums, bruises, and mouth ulcers.

Tones skin Rich in antioxidants, cistus essential oil is beneficial for your skin and brightens tired-looking complexions. A good astringent, it can help tighten and tone mature skin.

Acts as an antiseptic Cistus oil has an effective antiviral action that is especially useful in the treatment of respiratory congestion caused by colds and flu and other infections.

Helps balance emotions The oil has a centring effect that facilitiates meditation and contemplation. Its earthy aroma stimulates the senses and strengthens emotions after loss.

Best **uses**

As a bath oil Add 4–6 drops to 1 tablespoon base oil or full-fat milk for a refreshing, toning soak.

In a massage oil Add 8–12 drops to 2 tablespoons base oil for a toning and detoxifying massage that helps eliminate a build-up of toxins.

Safe usage *Non-toxic, non-irritant in dilution.*

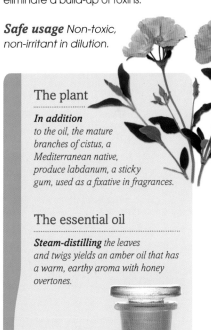

The plant

In addition *to the oil, the mature branches of cistus, a Mediterranean native, produce labdanum, a sticky gum, used as a fixative in fragrances.*

The essential oil

Steam-distilling *the leaves and twigs yields an amber oil that has a warm, earthy aroma with honey overtones.*

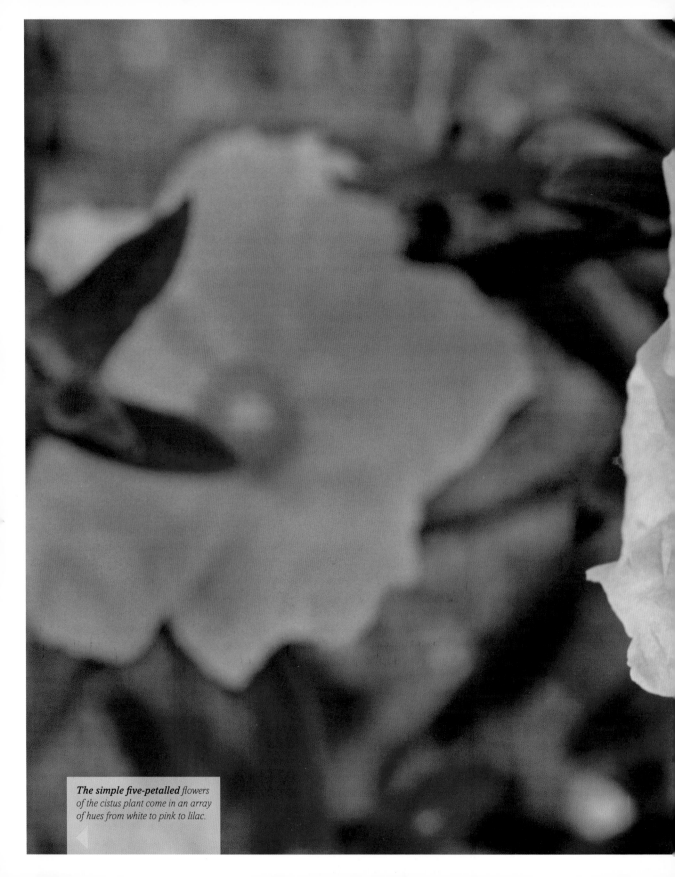

The simple five-petalled flowers *of the cistus plant come in an array of hues from white to pink to lilac.*

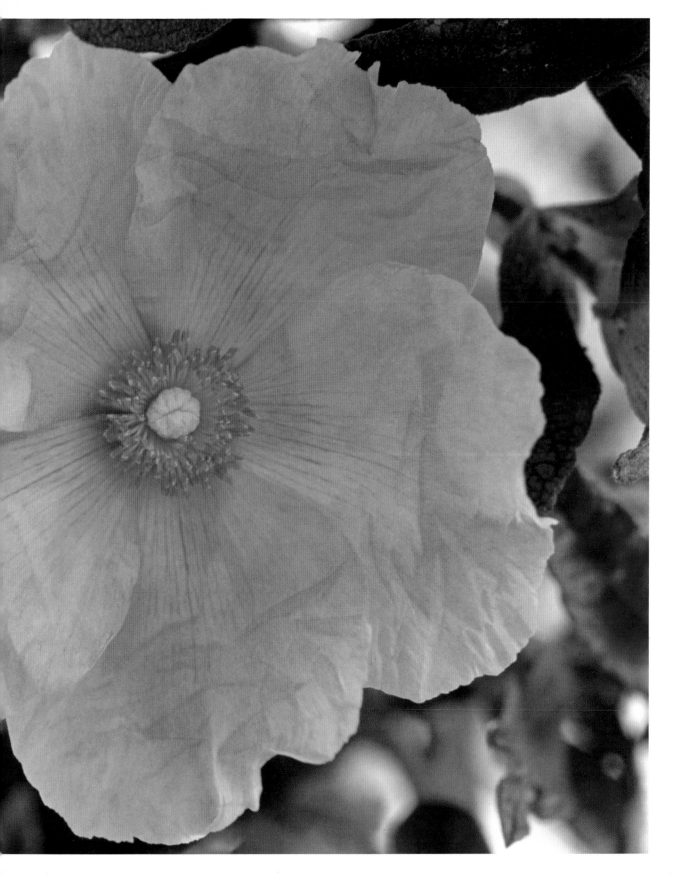

SKIN CARE   DIFFUSER

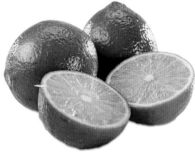

DIFFUSER   SKIN CARE   FRAGRANCE

Lime

Citrus aurantifolia

Stimulating and **refreshing,** lime can be relied on for its **cleansing** properties, and its fresh aroma calms and clears the mind. Like its relatives, grapefruit and lemon, it is a key oil for reducing water retention and puffiness. It also balances oily skin and hair.

What is it **good for?**

Aids detox Lime's strong detoxifying action helps tackle cellulite and the puffiness linked to water retention. As with grapefruit oil, inhaling lime oil has been shown to help weight loss by boosting the metabolism.

Balances oily skin and hair Lime has a toning effect that helps clear oily and acne-prone complexions. Added to a hair rinse, it conditions and removes excess oil to refresh the scalp. Treat dandruff by mixing lime juice in water and use it as a final rinse.

Has a cooling effect Lime oil "turns down the heat", helping to calm cold-related fevers. It also boosts the immune system, and eases bronchitis, coughs, sinusitis, and asthma.

Acts as an antiseptic The oil's soothing and antiseptic properties help to heal cold sores, insect bites,

and cuts. Treat cuts by putting two drops of the oil in a cold compress and pressing on the affected area.

A stress reliever The refreshing and stimulating scent relieves stress, exhaustion, and anxiety, and its ability to calm promotes creativity and focus.

Best **uses**

As a lotion Added to a skin cream or lotion, lime essential oil clears and brightens dull, congested skin.

In a diffuser Add 1–3 drops to a diffuser, vaporizer, or oil burner to lift the spirits and keep the mind sharp.

Safe usage Non-toxic, use very well diluted (less than 1 per cent). Avoid use on skin 12 hours prior to sun exposure.

The plant

The lime tree, grown widely in tropical and subtropical areas, produces an acidic green fruit that is a popular food and drink flavouring.

The essential oil

Lime oil, which is cold-pressed from the rind of the fruit, has a sharp citrus scent, and is either pale yellow or light olive in colour.

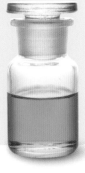

Neroli

Citrus aurantium

The blossom of the bitter, or Seville, orange tree is the source of a **calming,** refreshing, and uplifting oil that has long been considered a treatment for anxiety and depression. It is intense, yet **refreshing** and light, and a component of Eau de Cologne.

What is it **good for?**

Relieves stress Neroli has a long history as a remedy for anxiety. Its power to balance and revive makes it a first choice in cases of acute shock. It alleviates the effects of chronic stress on the adrenal, circulatory, and digestive systems.

Hydrates and tones skin Mixed in an oil-based elixir or cream, the oil balances moisture levels in the skin, helping to reduce fine lines caused by dehydration. Its gentle toning action makes it ideal for fine skin, helping to maintain elasticity, and for oily and acne-prone skin.

Promotes healing The oil's antiseptic and antibacterial properties speed the healing of cuts and wounds.

Improves digestion A gentle massage with a neroli blend soothes stomach cramps and diarrhoea.

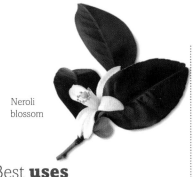

Neroli blossom

SKIN CARE   MASSAGE OIL

Best **uses**

In a diffuser If you have anxiety, add 3–4 drops of calming neroli to a diffuser, vaporizer, or oil burner.

As a skin toner Make a simple toning facial spritz by combining 2 teaspoons aloe vera juice with 6 tablespoons water and 4 drops of neroli in a spray bottle.

As a perfume Neroli has sufficient complexity to be worn neat as a scent in its own right, a trait it shares with rose and jasmine.

Safe usage Non-toxic and non-irritant.

The plant

This species of orange tree is native to China, but has been cultivated for hundreds of years in the countries bordering the Mediterranean. It takes at least 450kg (1000lb) of orange blossom flowers to make just 450g (1lb) of neroli oil.

The essential oil

With delicate blossoms, the best-quality oil is water- rather than steam-distilled. The pale yellow oil darkens with age, and its sweet floral smell is powerful yet refreshing.

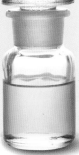

Petitgrain

Citrus aurantium amara

Another **beneficial** oil from the bitter orange tree – the other being neroli from the flowers. One of its most valuable properties is its **balancing** and toning effect on oily skin and hair. The relaxing aroma of petitgrain helps calm body and mind.

What is it **good for?**

Tones skin and hair Added to lotions and toners, petitgrain balances greasy skin by inhibiting the over-production of oil, helping to brighten and lift a dull complexion. Added to a rinse, it helps manage greasy hair.

Acts as an antiseptic Petitgrain oil helps to calm acne outbreaks and other skin eruptions. Its antiseptic action keeps wounds clean while they go through the healing process.

Acts as a deodorant Its astringent properties help to regulate perspiration, and its antibacterial action helps to control unwelcome body odour.

Calms body and mind Petitgrain's woody aroma has a relaxing sedative effect on body and mind. It counters nervous exhaustion and stress-related conditions, especially anger and panic, and helps to calm a rapid heartbeat.

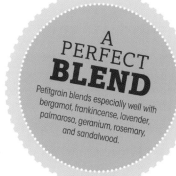

A
PERFECT
BLEND

Petitgrain blends especially well with bergamot, frankincense, lavender, palmarosa, geranium, rosemary, and sandalwood.

Best **uses**

As an acne treatment To control oily skin and to help clear up existing pimples and acne outbreaks, add 2–4 drops to a skin toner or lotion.

Massage oil A gentle massage with a petitgrain oil blend restores calm and balance when you are feeling angry or anxious. Add 12–18 drops to 2 tablespoons base oil.

Safe usage Non-toxic, non-irritant in dilution.

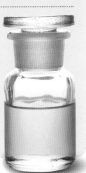

The plant

In the past, the oil was extracted from the cherry-sized unripe oranges, hence the name "petitgrain", meaning "little grains".

The essential oil

Petitgrain oil is extracted from the green twigs and leaves to produce a pale yellow to amber oil whose floral aroma has woody and green undertones.

MASSAGE OIL

COMPRESS

Bergamot

Citrus aurantium bergamia

An aromatherapy favourite, this oil has a balancing effect on body and mind. Soothing and **cooling,** bergamot is ideal for dry or itchy skin conditions, and its fruity aroma helps to **elevate** a low mood, enhancing wellbeing.

What is it **good for?**

Soothes skin Bergamot essential oil is useful for balancing combination and oily skin and improving skin tone. Its strong soothing effects help to calm dry, itchy skin, and its natural healing properties can reduce the appearance of scars over time.

Enhances wellbeing The sweet aroma of bergamot acts as an antidepressant by balancing mood and easing anxiety. It is a popular ingredient in colognes.

Cools fevers Bergamot has a cooling action that can help to bring down fevers.

Acts as an antiseptic The oil has antibacterial and antiviral properties. Dab, diluted, on cold sores (it is active against the herpes virus) and pimples.

Best **uses**

As a massage oil To promote feelings of relaxation and help ensure a restful sleep, make a refreshing blend by mixing 2–4 drops with 2 tablespoons base oil and use to massage your feet before bedtime.

In a compress Add 2–3 drops to cool water and add to a compress, then apply directly to the skin to help relieve heat stroke or a fever.

Safe usage Non-toxic, non-irritant in dilution. Ensure you buy bergaptene-free (also called Bergamot FCF), otherwise it is photo-toxic.

The plant

Named after the Italian city of Bergamo, these oranges are very sour, but with a deeply scented rind. The familiar aroma is used, among other things, as an ingredient in Earl Grey tea and Eau de Cologne.

The essential oil

The rind of the bergamot fruit is cold-pressed to produce either a light yellow or pale green oil which carries an extremely rich, sweet, fruity smell.

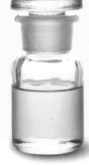

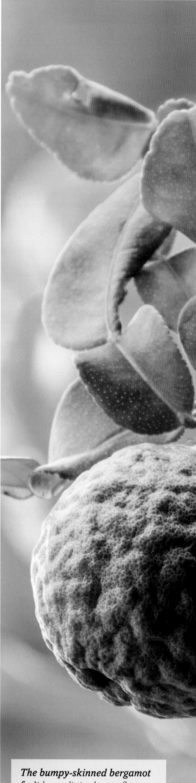

The bumpy-skinned bergamot fruit has a distinctly sour flavour with fresh floral overtones.

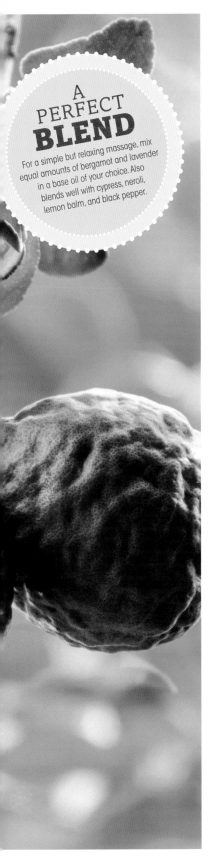

MASSAGE OIL

COMPRESS

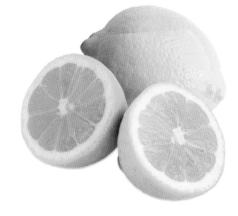

A PERFECT BLEND

For a simple but relaxing massage, mix equal amounts of bergamot and lavender in a base oil of your choice. Also blends well with cypress, neroli, lemon balm, and black pepper.

Lemon

Citrus limonum

Fresh and **invigorating**, lemon stimulates the senses and clears the mind. **Detoxifying** and **toning**, the oil lends itself naturally to massage blends and skin products, and its citrus aroma and antiseptic properties make it a natural deodorizer.

What is it **good for?**

Tones skin Lemon boosts circulation, helping to reduce varicose veins and prevent chilblains. It cleanses oil-prone skin and hair, and tones, helping to ward off wrinkles and "spider" veins.

Acts as an antiseptic Lemon acts as an antiseptic, stimulating the defences against bacteria and viruses and killing germs. Use in a compress for boils and skin eruptions, or apply neat to warts and verrucas.

Aids detox A lemon oil massage supports the liver, aids lymphatic cleansing, and reduces cellulite and fluid retention.

Eases digestion It stimulates the digestive system, helping to combat obesity and loss of appetite.

Lifts moods A cheerful, deodorizing scent, lemon is great for busy days when you need mental focus and positivity.

Best **uses**

As a massage oil Add 8–12 drops to 2 tablespoons base oil for a detoxifying body massage.

In a compress Dilute 5–6 drops of lemon oil in almond oil or calendula tincture, and add to water to use as a compress to sooth skin eruptions.

Safe usage Non-toxic, use well diluted (less than 2 per cent). Avoid using for 12 hours prior to sun exposure.

The plant

The lemon tree is native to India, but arrived in Europe with the Crusaders in the 12th century. As well as being a natural remedy, the rind is used in baking and cooking, and the essential oil, expressed from the rind of the fruit, has a long history of use in perfumery.

The essential oil

The clear oil with its fresh, citrus smell, is pressed from the peel of the lemon fruit.

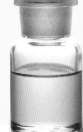

MASSAGE OIL

FRAGRANCE

BATH OIL

DIFFUSER

MASSAGE OIL

Grapefruit
Citrus paradisi

Grapefruit has an **energizing** and stimulating effect on body and mind. It makes an **uplifting** room spray, and in a massage blend boosts circulation, aids detox, and reduces water retention. Gently antiseptic and astringent, it is useful for controlling oily skin and hair.

What is it **good for?**

Aids detox The oil aids lymphatic drainage, helps boost metabolism, and assists weight loss. Massaged into skin, its diuretic and cleansing properties combat cellulite and water retention, and it stimulates, boosting circulation.

Tones skin and scalp The oil's gently antiseptic and astringent effects make it ideal for oily complexions, open pores, and acne, as well as oily hair. It helps to tone and tighten skin.

Combats tiredness With its fresh, zesty scent, grapefruit oil can help lift emotions and is revitalizing if you are suffering from mental exhaustion or are recovering from a late night.

Soothes aches and pains Add a few drops of the oil to a favourite base oil and use as a massage blend to help provide relief from muscle and joint pain, and tension headaches.

Acts as an air freshener Its uplifting, zesty aroma can help eliminate unpleasant odours in kitchens and bathrooms.

Best **uses**

As a massage oil Add 6–8 drops to 2 tablespoons base oil to cleanse skin.

In a room spray Clear stale air by adding 8–10 drops to water in a spray bottle. Shake well before use.

In a bath oil Add 5–6 drops to 1 tablespoon base oil or full-fat milk and disperse in a bath.

Safe usage Non-toxic, non-irritant in dilution (less than 3 per cent). Avoid using 12 hours prior to sun exposure.

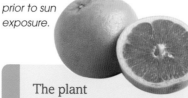

The plant

Unlike other citrus fruits, *grapefruit originates from the Caribbean, and not Southeast Asia. Its name comes from the grape-like cluster in which the fruits grow.*

The essential oil

The oil, *which is cold-pressed from the peel of the fruit, can be yellow, pale green, or pale orange, with a zesty, sweet, citrussy smell.*

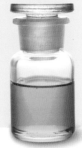

Mandarin
Citrus reticulata, Citrus nobilis

Mandarin (also known as tangerine) has **antiseptic** and anti-fungal properties, similar to other citrus fruits. It has a tonic effect on the digestive system, nourishes the skin, and its sweet, **cheerful** aroma is almost instantly **uplifting**.

What is it **good for?**

Tones skin Mandarin essential oil nurtures skin. It can help reduce the appearance of stretch marks and tone areas of flabbiness.

Aids detox In a massage oil, mandarin encourages lymphatic drainage and helps improve circulation. Its diuretic action helps combat water retention and cellulite.

Heals skin This stimulating oil helps regenerate skin cells. Its antiseptic and gently astringent properties make it useful for combating oily skin and outbreaks of acne.

Aids digestion Mandarin has a tonic effect on the digestive system. It helps food move along the digestive tract and eases indigestion and constipation, especially if these are stress-related. If you feel nauseous, it can calm your stomach.

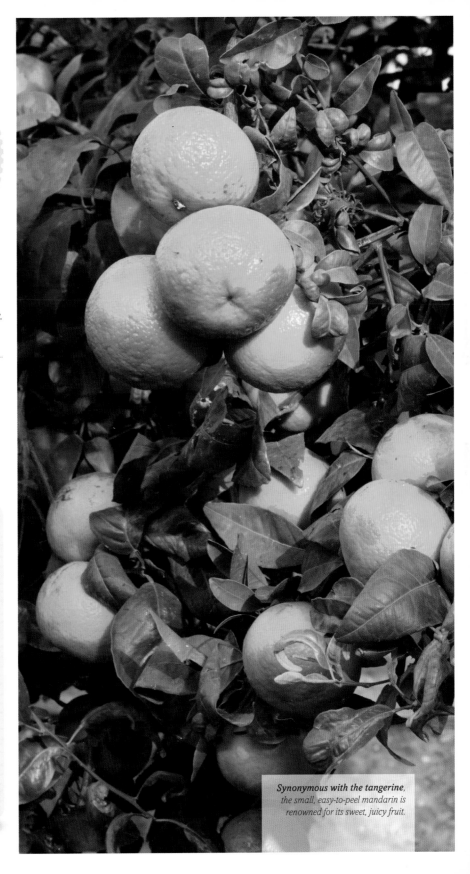

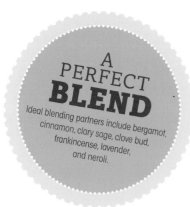

Enhances wellbeing A gentle, relaxing yet uplifting oil, mandarin is especially good for calming restless children, and is safe to use in pregnancy.

Best **uses**

In a diffuser Add 3–4 drops to a diffuser to freshen air or calm nerves.

In a massage oil Add 2–3 drops to a base oil for a soothing massage.

Safe usage Non-toxic, non-irritatant in dilution.

The plant

A native of China and the Far East, the mandarin tree was introduced to Europe in the nineteenth century. From Europe, the tree was shipped to the United States, where it was renamed tangerine.

The essential oil

An orange or amber colour with a tangy sweet, floral aroma, the oil is cold-pressed from the rind of the fruit.

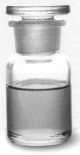

Synonymous with the tangerine, the small, easy-to-peel mandarin is renowned for its sweet, juicy fruit.

BATH OIL   MASSAGE OIL   DIFFUSER

Orange
Citrus sinensis

Sometimes called sweet orange, this **versatile** oil is widely used for its **uplifting** and **detoxifying** effects. It is also **calming**, it may help ease tense muscles, and its **rejuvenating** properties help skin maintain a youthful appearance. Cheering and familiar, its aroma acts as a reviving tonic.

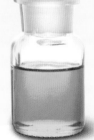

A PERFECT BLEND
Orange marries well with lemon, sandalwood, vetiver, frankincense, cinnamon, ginger, black pepper, clary sage, and clove essential oils.

What is it **good for?**

Aids detox Orange essential oil has a detoxifying and cleansing effect throughout the body. Used as part of a massage blend, the oil helps to improve the circulation, stimulates the lymphatic system, and supports the action of the bladder and kidneys, facilitating the removal of toxins and waste from the body.

Tones skin Used in skincare products, orange essential oil helps to promote the production of collagen and supports the skin's natural repair process. The oil has inherent healing properties that are attributed to the aromatic compound limonene, also an effective antiseptic.

Revitalizes and brightens skin
Orange essential oil has toning and slightly astringent properties that can help to clarify oily-looking skin and revitalize a dull or tired-looking complexion.

Boosts immunity Orange supports the immune system, and its cooling and refreshing properties can also help to relieve the symptoms of a feverish cold or flu virus.

Improves digestion As with other citrus oils, orange calms the digestive system, helping food to move efficiently through the gut, and in turn relieves constipation and trapped wind, and eases indigestion.

Relieves anxiety Orange essential oil has a sweet, uplifting scent that can calm nervous tension, lift feelings of depression, and promote restful sleep in cases of insomnia.

Best **uses**

As a bath oil Enjoy a relaxing bath that smoothes and tones skin by blending 6–8 drops in 1 tablespoon base oil or full-fat milk and dispersing in a warm bath.

As a massage oil To relieve nausea and indigestion if you have over-indulged and to release trapped wind, add 4–6 drops to 1 tablespoon base oil and massage the abdomen.

In a diffuser Used in a diffuser or room spray, the oil can help clear the air and mind. Its disinfectant action is useful in sick rooms, while its calming aroma can aid restful sleep for both adults and children.

Safe usage Non-toxic, non-irritant in dilution.

The plant

Like most citrus trees, the sweet orange tree originated in China. Today, however, most of the commercial production of orange essential oil takes place in Brazil, the USA, and Cyprus.

The essential oil

Orange oil is cold-pressed from the rind of the fruit. A fine oil, it is a pale orange-greenish colour with the same sweet, fresh, and fruity smell you get when you peel an orange.

Sweet-smelling citrus oil is reviving and uplifting, enhancing feelings of wellbeing.

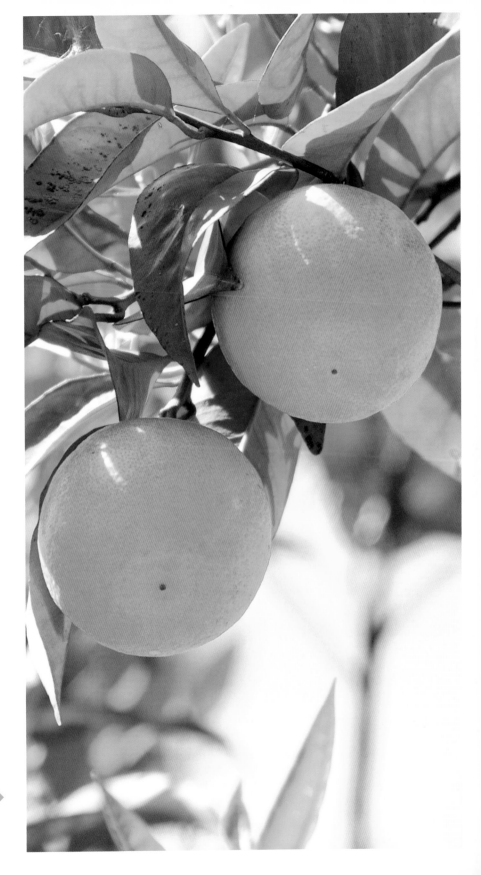

The sweet orange tree *grows abundantly in warm, temperate climates around the world.*

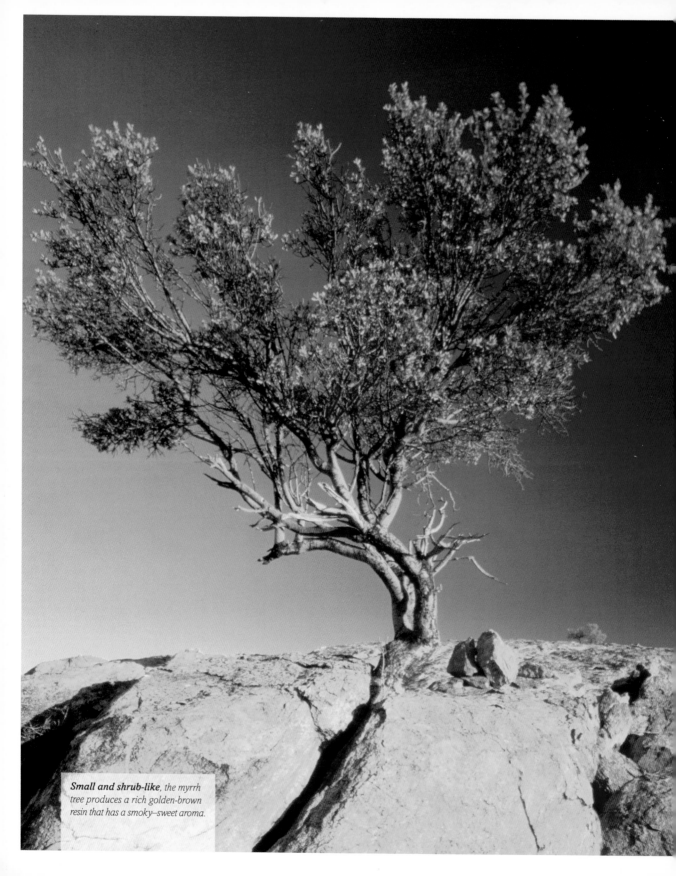

Small and shrub-like, the myrrh tree produces a rich golden-brown resin that has a smoky–sweet aroma.

SKIN CARE   MOUTHWASH

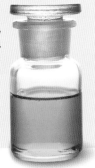

A PERFECT BLEND

Make a spicy blend by combining with oils such as cedarwood, cypress, frankincense, lemon, patchouli, and sandalwood.

Myrrh

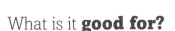

Commiphora myrrha, C. molmol

The **antiseptic** properties of myrrh make it a popular remedy for healing cuts and wounds. As a well-established **anti-ageing** treatment, it is added to skincare products to help prevent the premature appearance of fine lines. A grounding and centring oil, it both stimulates and **fortifies** the emotions.

What is it **good for?**

Heals skin Myrrh has an established history treating various types of skin eruptions, such as acne, athlete's foot, weeping eczema, and cold sores. Its healing properties make it useful for cuts, burns, and wounds. A non-irritating oil, myrrh can be applied neat to skin.

Tones skin Its ability to preserve skin tone helps delay wrinkles and other signs of ageing. It is also ideal for healing chapped and broken skin.

Cares for teeth and gums As part of a mouthwash, the antiseptic properties of myrrh help tackle infection and inflammation, soothing ulcers, sore throats, bleeding gums, bad breath, and oral thrush.

For coughs and colds Myrrh makes an excellent expectorant, particularly when coughs and colds produce thick, white mucus. Try using myrrh in a steam inhalation to ease chronic lung conditions, coughs, colds, and bronchitis.

Enhances wellbeing The aromatherapeutic properties of myrrh are purported to help strengthen confidence in overcoming difficulties and to enhance focus and provide a strong sense of purpose.

Best **uses**

As a skin toner Add 2–4 drops of myrrh essential oil to 2 tablespoons facial lotion or toner to improve skin tone and quality, especially for mature and sun-damaged skin.

In a mouthwash Add 1–2 drops of the oil to water for a mouthwash to fight gum disease and bad breath.

Safe usage *Non-irritant in dilution. Only use extremely well diluted (less than 0.2 per cent) in pregnancy and when breastfeeding.*

The plant

The myrrh tree *belongs to a family of small spiky shrubs and bushes native to the Middle East, North Africa, and northern India. The resin is gathered by making incisions in the tree that allow it to flow freely.*

The essential oil

Dried lumps of resin *are steam-distilled to produce the essential oil, which is pale orange to amber in colour.*

Strengthening and healing, myrrh has a rejuvenating effect on skin.

MASSAGE OIL

MOUTHWASH

Coriander

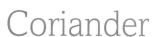
Coriandrum sativum

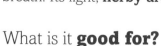

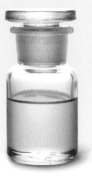

This highly **aromatic** oil has a long history in traditional medicine, especially in Ayurvedic and Chinese medicines. Its **antiseptic** action helps clear pimples and fungal infections, and when used in a mouthwash, the oil freshens breath. Its light, **herby aroma** energizes and is a natural tonic for flagging spirits.

A PERFECT BLEND

Coriander essential oil blends well with bergamot, ginger, lemon, neroli, jasmine, cinnamon, clary sage, and other spicy oils.

What is it **good for?**

Relieves pain Coriander has a warming effect that helps stimulate circulation and relieve stiffness and pain in muscles and joints. The oil's analgesic properties help relieve general headaches and localized neuralgia pain, and can ease menstrual cramps.

Acts as an antiseptic Coriander essential oil is useful for dealing with occasional spots, pimples, and fungal infections. The oil's strong antiseptic and deodorizing effect also makes it especially helpful for dealing with the bacteria that cause smelly feet, bad breath, and gum disease.

Enhances wellbeing Used as a room spray, coriander's soothing herbal aroma has an energizing effect that helps lift apathy and feelings of nervous exhaustion.

Best **uses**

As a massage oil Add 6–12 drops to 2 tablespoons base oil for a warming and deodorizing massage.

In a mouthwash Mix 1–2 drops of the essential oil in a teaspoon of glycerine or calendula tincture and add to water before using as a gargle or mouthwash to treat gum infections.

Safe usage *Non-toxic and non-irritant.*

The plant

Both the leaves and seeds *of the coriander plant produce useful oils. When the oil is distilled from the leaves it is known as cilantro essential oil. The leaves are also a popular culinary ingredient.*

The essential oil

Steam-distillation *of the crushed ripe seeds produces a clear to pale yellow oil with a sweet, spicy, slightly fruity, warm herbaceous scent that is warming, uplifting, and calming.*

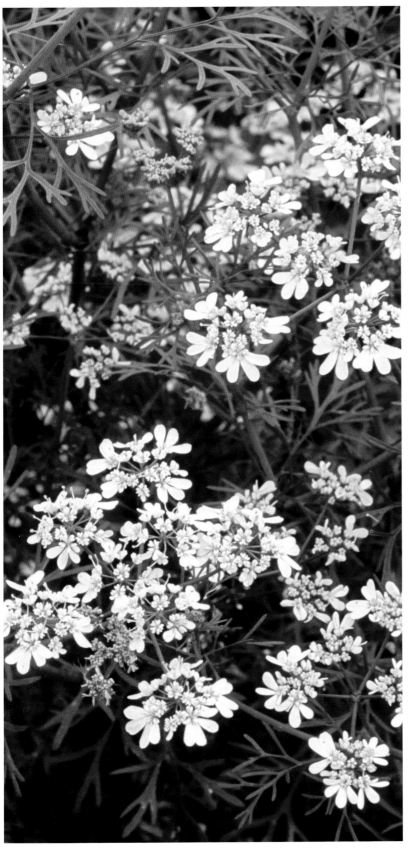

Warming coriander makes a gently stimulating and soothing oil, perfect for lifting the spirits.

The seeds produced *from the flowering coriander plant are used to make the aromatic essential oil.*

MASSAGE OIL

COMPRESS

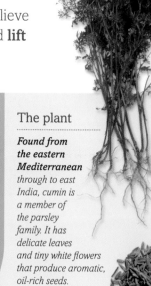

Cumin

Cuminum cyminum

The use of cumin can be traced back to the Ancient Egyptians and Assyrians. This **warming** essential oil helps to **relax** muscles and relieve aching joints. It stimulates circulation and helps **calm** the nerves and **lift** the spirits. It is also a useful antiseptic that can support healing.

What is it **good for?**

Aids detox The detoxifying action of cumin makes this a useful massage oil for fighting stubborn cellulite. Cumin also supports liver function, aiding the removal of toxins.

Boosts circulation Cumin has a tonifying effect on the body. It helps to boost the general circulation and can also be useful for helping to control high blood pressure.

Eases pain and digestive discomfort Cumin helps to fortify the digestive tract, relieving nausea, bloating, and constipation. It brings relief to mild headaches.

Heals skin Added to skin preparations, cumin essential oil has an antiseptic action that helps to heal dry or cracked skin, reduce bruising, and control acne, eczema, and psoriasis. It also revitalizes mature and tired-looking skin.

Fights fatigue The stimulating aroma provides a welcome lift if you feel lethargic, weak, or unable to focus.

Best **uses**

As a massage oil Add 2–4 drops to 2 tablespoons base oil for a massage to relieve joint and muscle pain.

In a compress Add 2–3 drops to some glycerine or almond oil, add to cool water, and use as a compress to relieve itchy skin and bruises.

Safe usage Dilute very well (less than 0.5 per cent). Avoid using for 12 hours prior to sun exposure.

The plant

Found from the eastern Mediterranean *through to east India, cumin is a member of the parsley family. It has delicate leaves and tiny white flowers that produce aromatic, oil-rich seeds.*

The essential oil

The crushed seeds *of the cumin plant are steam-distilled to produce a pale yellow oil that darkens with age. The oil has a pungent spicy–woody aroma that is musky and sensual as well as stimulating.*

This relaxing oil is ideal for easing and soothing muscular pains.

COMPRESS

MASSAGE OIL

FRAGRANCE

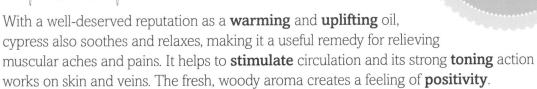

A PERFECT BLEND

Clary sage, bergamot, lemon, lavender, ginger, juniper, pine, and geranium essential oils are all natural blending partners for cypress

Cypress

Cupressus sempervirens

With a well-deserved reputation as a **warming** and **uplifting** oil, cypress also soothes and relaxes, making it a useful remedy for relieving muscular aches and pains. It helps to **stimulate** circulation and its strong **toning** action works on skin and veins. The fresh, woody aroma creates a feeling of **positivity**.

What is it **good for?**

Improves circulation Cypress oil has a powerful toning action on the veins and helps to regulate blood flow. This makes it especially useful for treating spider veins, varicose veins, and troublesome haemorrhoids.

Tones skin The oil's balancing properties make it ideal for evening out oily and puffy complexions and also for toning areas of loose skin, for example, after weight loss.

Aids detox Strongly astringent, cypress oil is useful in combating water retention and cellulite. It also supports healthy circulation and helps flush out toxins.

Acts as a deodorant Its astringent quality makes the oil an effective antiperspirant and deodorizer. Added to a foot bath, the oil helps control perspiration and foot odour.

Supports women's health The soothing action of cypress helps ease menstrual discomfort and cramping.

Soothes aches and pains Diluted in a base oil and massaged over affected areas, cypress can relieve rheumatism and osteoarthritis, as well as general muscle and joint pain. It can help control spasms, relieve menstrual cramps, and may be used for injury rehabilitation.

Heals wounds A popular ingredient in antiseptic lotions and creams, cypress essential oil has antiseptic properties that help heal wounds. Its astringent properties can slow bleeding, such as nosebleeds.

Calms nerves Refreshing and mentally toning, cypress oil helps to ease stress-induced nervous strain and tension and to lift weariness.

Best **uses**

As a compress To stem nosebleeds, apply 4–5 drops to a cold compress. Keeping your head level, gently press your nostrils together with the compress.

As a massage oil Dilute 16–20 drops in 2 tablespoons base oil for a warming massage to relieve rheumatism, arthritis, menstrual cramps, and varicose veins.

As a cologne The masculine notes suit men's colognes and aftershaves.

Many women also enjoy using this essential oil as an alternative to heavy floral scents.

Safe usage Non-toxic, non-irritant in dilution.

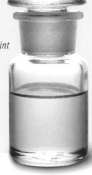

The plant

This coniferous evergreen tree can grow up to to 35m (115ft) tall and live for more than 1000 years. A native of the Mediterranean regions, cypress has long been an important ingredient in incense for ritual uses as well as being a source of the therapeutic healing oil.

The essential oil

The clear to very pale yellow oil has a woody, nutty aroma with a hint of spice. It is produced by steam-distilling the fresh leaves and cones.

SKIN CARE

DIFFUSER

FIRST AID

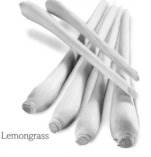
Lemongrass

BATH OIL

MASSAGE OIL

DIFFUSER

Lemongrass

Cymbopogon citratus, C. flexuosus

This essential oil works on body and mind to **refresh** and **stimulate**. It has antiseptic and astringent effects that work on oily or acne-prone skin. Lemongrass is **deodorizing**, **antibacterial**, and makes an effective **insect repellent**.

What is it **good for?**

Acts as an antiseptic Its astringent and antiseptic effects cleanse skin: a few drops in a facial steam work on open or blocked pores. Its antiseptic properties and fresh scent also help control sweating and the bacteria that cause body odour, and it relieves acne, eczema, and athlete's foot.

Acts as an insect repellent Lemongrass is one of the key active ingredients in natural insect repellents.

Aids digestion Lemongrass is a natural appetite stimulant. It is also a good remedy for gastric infections.

Eases aches and pains Diluted in a blend, a lemongrass massage strengthens muscle tone and slack tissues, ideal for a pre-sport massage or to treat aching muscles or muscle strain. It can also soothe headaches.

Enhances wellbeing Lemongrass calms and fortifies nerves and eases depression and stress.

Best **uses**

As a toner Add 4–8 drops to 2 tablespoons witch hazel or a light lotion to refresh and tone skin.

In a diffuser Disperse into a room to raise spirits and lift exhaustion.

As an insect repellent Dilute 10–12 drops in a small spray bottle of witch hazel. Or mix 4–8 drops with 2 tablespoons lotion to dab on skin.

Safe usage Use only very well diluted (less than 0.5 per cent). Avoid use on hypersensitive skin and on children less than seven years old.

The plant

Lemongrass is a native of India. Its oil is used in cosmetics and scents. There are two main types: West Indian (Cymbopogon citratus) and East Indian (Cymbopogon flexuosus), both with similar properties. After distilling the oil, the grass is used as cattle feed.

The essential oil

The essential oil is produced by steam-distillation of the chopped grass. The liquid is pale yellow to amber in colour, and has a fresh, herbaceous, lemony aroma.

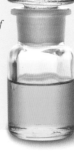

Palmarosa

Cymbopogon martinii

Palmarosa comes from a wild grass native to India. The pleasant floral aroma has hints of rose. Its **balancing** action makes it a popular skincare product: it **hydrates** dry skin, **rejuvenates** tired or mature skin, and helps controls sebum secretions in oily skin.

What is it **good for?**

Nourishes and tones skin Palmarosa hydrates and balances. By stimulating cell regeneration and controlling sebum, it helps keep skin supple and elastic and improves the appearance of scar tissue and stretch marks. A natural toner, the oil helps to reduce the appearance of wrinkles and fine lines and to brighten tired complexions. In a facial steam, it can unclog pores and tone sagging skin.

Aids recuperation A gentle tonic, the oil helps to hasten recovery after illness. It aids digestion and boosts poor appetite. Diluted and massaged over the abdomen, it may also relieve symptoms of diarrhoea.

Acts as an antiseptic Its antiseptic properties are specifically active against the bacteria that cause acne. It can also treat athlete's foot, dermatitis, and minor skin infections.

Enhances wellbeing A palmarosa massage helps relieve stress, anxiety, and tension, and is a mild aphrodisiac, countering strong negative emotions that interfere with sexual fulfilment.

Best **uses**

As a bath oil Mix 4–6 drops with 1 tablespoon base oil or full-fat milk for a fortifying bath when you are tired, recuperating, or have a digestive upset.

As a massage oil Add 16–24 drops to 2 tablespoons base oil to tone skin.

In a diffuser Diffuse to freshen air, fight fatigue, and focus the mind.

Safe usage Non-toxic, non-irritant in dilution (less than 5 per cent).

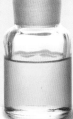

The plant

Also called *Indian or Turkish geranium, palmarosa grass is a relative of lemongrass, but has a floral, rather than citrus, scent. Native to India, it is now cultivated in Indonesia, East Africa, the Comoro Islands, and Brazil.*

The essential oil

The thin, pale yellow *essential oil can be steam- or water-distilled from the fresh or dried grass. It has a sweet floral aroma with a subtle hint of rose.*

DIFFUSER

SKIN CARE

Citronella
Cymbopogon nardus

Best known as an **insect repellent** used in a variety of candles, potpourri, and lotions, citronella has other important uses. As a room scent it helps to **clear** and **refresh** the mind, and its antiseptic properties make it effective in deodorants.

What is it **good for?**

Tones skin The toning properties of citronella help balance skin that is prone to oiliness.

Acts as an insect repellent This popular insect repellent is a very useful holiday companion. Carry a citronella-infused tissue to help keep annoying bugs at bay.

Freshens and clears air The antiseptic properties of citronella help to clear the air of viruses, which is especially useful during the cold and flu season or to clear the air in a sickroom. Its antiseptic effect also makes it a useful ingredient in deodorants.

Enhances focus Citronella essential oil can lift the emotions when you feel downcast and also helps you to keep a clear head and maintain focus.

A PERFECT BLEND

Try blending citronella essential oil with bergamot and other citrus oils. It also blends well with geranium, lavender, pine, and peppermint.

Best **uses**

In a diffuser Add 2–3 drops to a diffuser or to water for a room spray to make an effective insect repellent.

In a lotion For a foot lotion to combat odours, add 3–6 drops to 2 tablespoons unscented lotion base.

Safe usage Non-irritant in dilution (less than 15 per cent). Avoid using on hypersensitive skin.

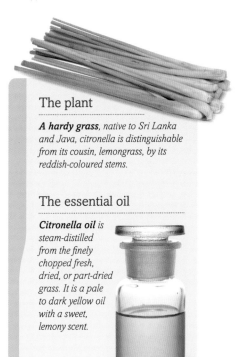

The plant

A hardy grass, *native to Sri Lanka and Java, citronella is distinguishable from its cousin, lemongrass, by its reddish-coloured stems.*

The essential oil

Citronella oil *is steam-distilled from the finely chopped fresh, dried, or part-dried grass. It is a pale to dark yellow oil with a sweet, lemony scent.*

DIFFUSER

SKIN CARE

Carrot seed

Daucus carota

This unusual oil has a **rejuvenating** effect on many body systems. A **grounding** oil, it can relieve feelings of stress and lift exhaustion. It also has a mild diuretic action that helps to eliminate toxins, and its **healing properties** can be harnessed to **revitalize** problem complexions and nourish dry and mature skin.

What is it **good for?**

Aids detox The mild diuretic effects of carrot essential oil help to reduce excess fluid retention. This detoxifying oil also supports the efficient functioning of the liver, and strengthens the digestive system.

Relieves stress The earthy aroma of carrot essential oil is grounding and calming, helping to relieve feelings of stress, and give the body stamina to fight feelings of exhaustion and general lethargy.

Soothes aching muscles As part of a massage oil blend or diluted in the bath, carrot seed oil is deeply warming, helping to ease aches and pains and boost the circulation.

Repairs skin Highly valued in cosmetics, carrot essential oil is added to face and body creams to nourish, tighten, revitalize, tone, and rejuvenate tired-looking skin. Its calming properties also make it suitable for itchy and irritated skin.

Best **uses**

In a diffuser Add 3–4 drops of carrot seed oil to a diffuser, vaporizer, or oil burner to impart a very subtle, grounding aroma to the air.

In a cream Add 6–8 drops of carrot seed essential oil to 2 tablespoons cream or lotion base and use to help soften dry skin, and also to encourage healthy cell growth and skin rejuvenation.

Safe usage Use in dilutions of less than 2 per cent. Avoid using during pregnancy or while breastfeeding.

The plant

Wild carrot, also known as "Queen Anne's lace" is a European native that has hairy leaves and delicate white lacy flowers with purple centres that spread out in a distinctive umbrella shape. Though wild carrot bears little resemblance to the commerical root vegetable, it does share the same aroma.

The essential oil

Steam-distilling the dried seeds of the wild carrot plant produces a yellow–brown oil that has a fairly viscous texture. The oil has an understated, mildly sweet, dry, and distinctly earthy aroma with some noticeable herbaceous undertones.

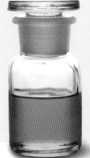

With its subtle aroma, this oil holds potent healing properties.

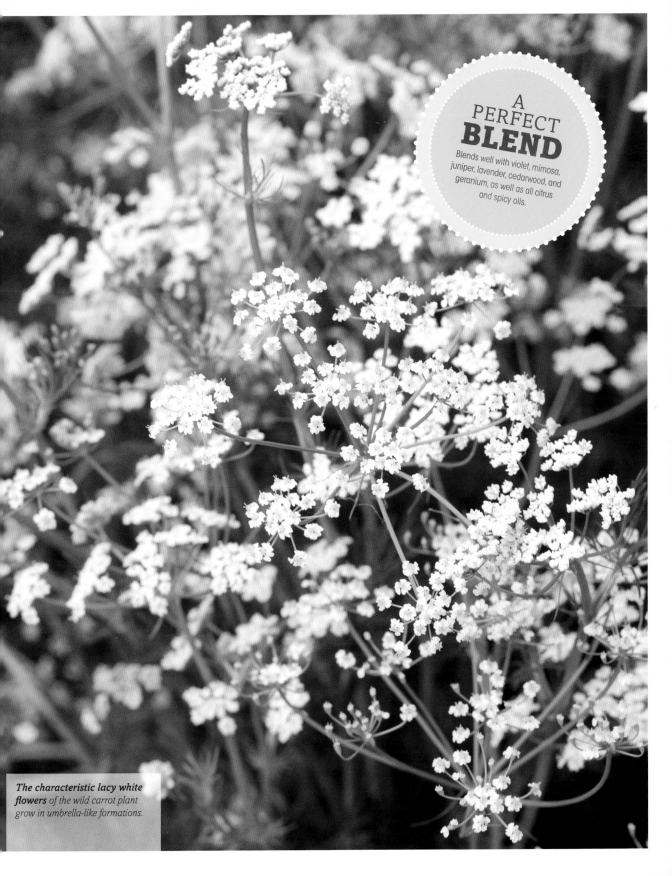

The characteristic lacy white flowers of the wild carrot plant grow in umbrella-like formations.

MASSAGE OIL

MOUTHWASH

Cardamom

Elettaria cardamomum

A natural **diuretic** and digestive stimulant, cardamom **boosts** the metabolism and helps the body to metabolize fat efficiently. It is also an effective **antiseptic**, making it a popular component of natural mouthwashes and deodorants.

What is it **good for?**

Acts as a deodorant Cardamom essential oil is a good addition to deodorants, helping to eliminate the bacteria that cause body odour.

Cares for teeth and gums Its antiseptic properties are useful for treating bad breath and for helping heal sore, bleeding gums.

Aids detox Diluted with a base oil, cardamom makes a stimulating massage blend, helping to boost circulation. Its mild diuretic action also helps facilitate the removal of toxins.

Soothes digestive upsets Cardamom has a calming action ideal for an upset stomach and nausea. It also relieves heartburn.

Combats tiredness The oil relieves stress and is refreshing, helping combat fatigue. A reputed aphrodisiac, especially if you are overtired.

Best **uses**

As a massage oil Add 6–8 drops to 2 tablespoons base oil for a refreshing, detoxifying full-body massage.

In a mouthwash Mix 1–2 drops in a teaspoon of glycerine or calendula tincture; add to water for a mouthwash.

Safe Usage Non-toxic and non-irritant. Avoid using in children under seven years old.

The plant

A native of India, cardamom seeds and pods have been used for centuries as a culinary spice and a healing remedy. Cardamom is also used in traditional Chinese medicine.

The essential oil

The essential oil is extracted by steam-distillation from the seeds and produces a colourless to pale yellow oil that has a sweet–spicy aroma with woody notes.

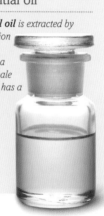

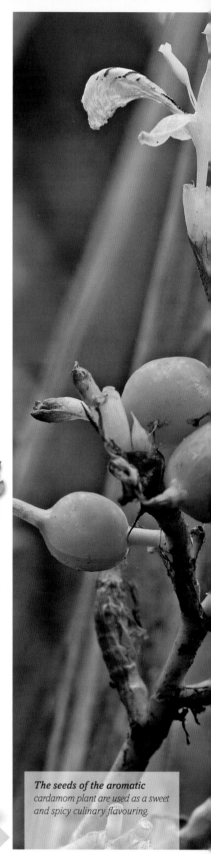

The seeds of the aromatic cardamom plant are used as a sweet and spicy culinary flavouring.

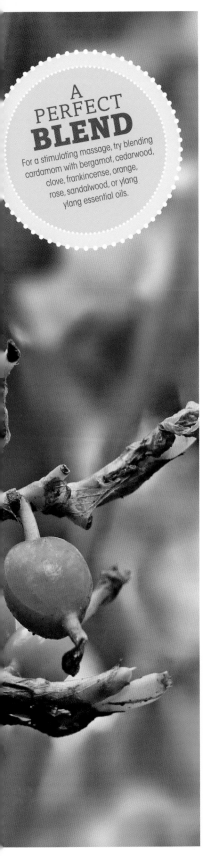

MASSAGE OIL   STEAM   DIFFUSER
               INHALATION

A PERFECT BLEND

For a stimulating massage, try blending cardamom with bergamot, cedarwood, clove, frankincense, orange, rose, sandalwood, or ylang ylang essential oils.

Eucalyptus

Eucalyptus globulus

This **warming** and **antiseptic** oil is great for relieving aches and pains as well as healing mouth ulcers and insect bites and stings. The oil **tones** and balances the skin, and its sharp aroma helps **increase concentration** and lift feelings of depression.

What is it **good for?**

Acts as an antiseptic Dab onto skin to heal bacterial and fungal infections and wounds and soothe bites. In a bath, it can relieve cystitis. The oil makes a good sick-room spray.

Tones skin A facial steam with a few drops of the oil helps to cleanse and tone oily or acne-prone skin.

Eases aches and pains Add the oil to a base oil or an ointment to warm and loosen tight muscles and joints.

Improves focus Eucalyptus refreshes the mind, banishing headaches and improving concentration.

Best **uses**

As a massage oil Blend 2–3 drops in an ointment to rub on the chest to clear sinuses and aid sleep when congested.

In an inhalation Add 6–8 drops to hot water and use as a facial steam to unclog pores, cleanse and tone, and leave you clear-headed and refreshed.

In a diffuser Diffuse 3–4 drops to combat tiredness.

Safe usage Non-toxic externally; non-irritant in dilution (less than 20 per cent). Avoid near nose or face on children under seven years old.

The plant

The blue gum eucalyptus, a tree native to Australia, is the most widely cultivated of hundreds of species of eucalyptus.

Several other varieties are used in aromatherapy, notably the slightly gentler Eucalyptus radiata and the more cooling Eucalyptus citronella.

The essential oil

This oil is steam-distilled from the leaves of the tree. It has a clear to pale yellow hue and has a strong, camphorous, woody smell.

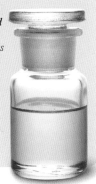

MASSAGE OIL

MOUTHWASH

Fennel (sweet)
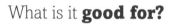
Foeniculum vulgare

With a long history as a sacred and medicinal herb, fennel is a **cooling** and **cleansing** essential oil. Its main action is to **unblock**, where it works on both body and mind, easing constipation and other complaints and providing the courage to express held-in emotions.

What is it **good for?**

Aids detox Fennel has a diuretic effect and helps to stimulate circulation. Diluted in a base oil, it provides a good detoxifying massage that helps tackle stubborn cellulite.

Cares for teeth and gums Well diluted, fennel essential oil can be gargled in a mouthwash to help fight the bacteria that causes tooth decay and bad breath.

Soothes digestion Fennel has unblocking properties. A massage blend containing fennel helps relieve flatulence, bloating, digestive cramps, and constipation. The oil also stimulates appetite, and eases nervous indigestion brought on by a rushed meal or emotional upset.

Fights colds A mild expectorant, fennel essential oil helps loosen phlegmy coughs. Blend with a base oil for a chest rub, or add to a diffuser, vaporizer, or oil burner.

Best **uses**

As a massage oil For indigestion, blend 4–6 drops of fennel essential oil in 1 tablespoon light base oil and gently massage the abdomen in a clockwise direction.

In a mouthwash Mix 1–2 drops in a teaspoon of glycerine or calendula tincture and add to water to use as a mouthwash.

Safe usage Dilute well before use (less than 2 per cent). Avoid during pregnancy and if breastfeeding. Not suitable for children under seven years old..

A PERFECT **BLEND**
To relieve indigestion, blend with ginger, nutmeg, and peppermint oils. Also blends well with geranium, lavender, marjoram, and rose.

The plant

The fennel plant *grows up to 2m (6ft) high. Its green feathery leaves and golden yellow flowers attract insects and bees and eventually produce the oil-rich seeds.*

The essential oil

The essential oil *is steam-distilled from crushed fennel seeds. It is pale yellow with a sweet–spicy smell that is reminiscent of aniseed.*

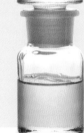

COMPRESS

DIFFUSER

OINTMENT

Wintergreen

Gaultheria procumbens, G. fragrantissima

A pungent **medicinal** oil, wintergreen should be used sparingly. Its strong minty aroma can clear the head and even small amounts applied topically can provide **pain relief**.

What is it **good for?**

Relieves pain The oil is a popular ingredient in muscle ointments and rubs. It contains a natural aspirin-like analgesic that can help to relieve pain locally. Used in a compress, the oil can alleviate headaches, muscle cramps, joint pain, and tendonitis, and can also bring some relief to pain caused by chronic conditions such as arthritis and rheumatism.

Aids digestion Once absorbed through the skin, the oil can stimulate the digestive process by triggering the release of digestive juices.

Tones skin and hair Arguably too strong for use on the face, when well-diluted, wintergreen's astringent and antiseptic action can help to treat acne on the body. Its antifungal properties also help prevent dandruff and can work to clear athlete's foot.

Clears the head A few drops of wintergreen essential oil in a vaporizer or diffuser aids breathing and helps relieve stress and tension.

Best **uses**

In a compress Blend 3 drops each of wintergreen and lavender oils for an effective hot or cold compress to relieve localized aches and pains.

In a diffuser Used in a diffuser, vaporizer, or oil burner, the oil opens up the nasal and respiratory passages.

In an ointment Add 1–2 drops to an ointment base to relieve pain locally.

Safe usage Dilute well before use (less than 2 per cent). Avoid during pregnancy and if breastfeeding. Not suitable for young children. Avoid if on anticoagulant medication and if sensitive to aspirin.

The plant

A shrubby evergreen, wintergreen is native to North America. It has glossy, green, oval leaves and abundant white blooms in the summer, which turn into bright red berries during the winter, often lasting through to spring. The berries were used traditionally in herbal medicine to help relieve muscular aches and pains.

The essential oil

Steam-distilled from the chopped-up leaves, wintergreen essential oil has a sweet, fresh, and pleasant minty aroma. The oil is pale yellow or pinkish yellow in colour. Wintergreen blends well with other minty oils, such as peppermint, and also complements bergamot, basil, lavender, and lemongrass essential oils.

This essential oil has strong anti-bacterial and antifungal effects.

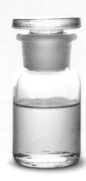

FIRST AID

COMPRESS

STEAM INHALATION

DIFFUSER

SKIN CARE

Helichrysum (Immortelle)

Helichrysum italicum

Also known as immortelle, or **"everlasting" oil**, this is a fantastic, **regenerative** oil that **cools** and soothes the skin. Its antiseptic and **anti-inflammatory** properties help heal scars and skin eruptions. Deeply **de-stressing**, it's perfect for relieving anxiety, nervous exhaustion, and feelings of depression.

What is it **good for?**

Enhances wellbeing The oil's therapeutic properties help treat tension, depression, exhaustion, and other stress-related conditions. Uplifting, it curbs negativity and promotes a feeling of safety, helping to heal old emotional wounds.

Relieves pain An effective anti-inflammatory, this is a good choice for joint pain, arthritic conditions, and general strains and sprains.

Heals wounds and fights infections Helichrysum can be applied in a cream to wounds to help reduce swelling, disinfect, and promote healing through tissue regeneration. It has demonstrated antibacterial properties.

Heals and protects skin The anti-inflammatory and regenerative properties of helichrysum oil make it useful for treating skin problems such as acne, dermatitis, bruises, boils, and abscesses. It can also help to fade scars, stretch marks, and blemishes. The oil's antioxidant properties protect the skin from harmful free radicals that cause premature skin ageing.

Soothes skin The oil's calming action helps soothe allergic skin breakouts and numbness and tingling in nerve-related conditions.

Boosts circulation The oil stimulates circulation. It can also help to control blood pressure and provide relief from conditions such as varicose veins.

Relieves coughs and colds The oil has an antispasmodic effect that relieves asthma and persistent coughs. It may act as a decongestant in cases of sinusitis and catarrh, especially when these are allergy- or stress-related.

Best **uses**

As first aid The oil can be applied in a cream as an effective emergency treatment for burns, grazes or cuts.

As a compress Add 6–8 drops to a cool compress and hold over skin flare-ups and bruises.

As an inhalation Add 8–10 drops to a steam inhalation to help clear blocked sinuses.

In a diffuser Add 3–4 drops to a diffuser to create a calming ambience.

As a skin toner Added to facial spritzers, toners, or lotions, helichrysum essential oil leaves skin feeling fresh and toned and helps to reduce the appearance of fine lines and skin blemishes.

Safe usage Use well diluted (less than 0.5 per cent).

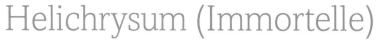

A PERFECT **BLEND**

For a balancing aroma, try blending with chamomile, geranium and lavender oils. Also blends well with rose, rosewood, clary sage, bergamot, and other citrus oils.

The plant

A Mediterranean herb, helichrysum's small, cheerful flowers are popular with florists. Part of the sunflower family, the oil's names, "everlasting" and "immortelle", come from the reputation of the flowers for retaining their brilliant colour even when dried.

The essential oil

This watery yellow essential oil that occasionally has a tinge of red is steam-distilled from the flowers. It has a distinctive straw-like aroma with hints of fruit, tea, and honey.

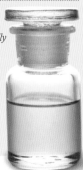

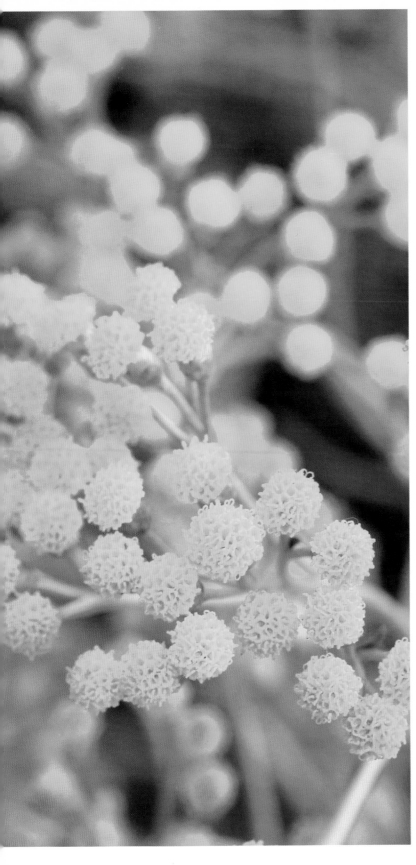

This cooling and soothing oil nourishes, rejuvenates, and heals skin.

This fragrant evergreen shrub produces clusters of bright yellow flowers in the summer months.

STEAM
INHALATION

MOUTHWASH

Star anise

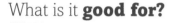

Illicium verum

Star anise has been in use since ancient times in Europe, the Middle East, and Asia, favoured for both its **therapeutic benefits** and distinctive flavour. With its sharp aroma, the essential oil acts as a mild **pain reliever** and also makes an effective **antiseptic**.

What is it **good for?**

Relieves aches and pains Star anise has pain-relieving properties that provide localized relief from muscular aches and pains, and help to ease rheumatism and arthritis.

Acts as an antiseptic The essential oil has a strong antibacterial action. It also has potent antifungal properties that can help heal skin infections such as athlete's foot, and it can be used to treat head lice and mites.

Acts as a deodorant Star anise is often added to soaps to combat body odour, and the oil makes a natural breath freshener.

Tones skin Its skin-balancing properties are useful for calming oily and combination skin.

Promotes restful sleep The oil has a sedative action that helps to calm, slowing the heart rate and aiding sleep, making it especially useful for anxiety-related sleep problems.

Best **uses**

In an inhalation Add 3–4 drops of star anise oil to a steam inhalation to provide temporary relief from bronchitis, cold, and flu symptoms.

In a mouthwash Add 1–2 drops to a teaspoon of glycerine or calendula tincture. Add to a glass of water and rinse in the mouth to fight the germs that cause bad breath. Do not swallow.

Safe usage Use well diluted (less than 1 per cent). Avoid during pregnancy and if breastfeeding. Not suitable for children under seven years old.

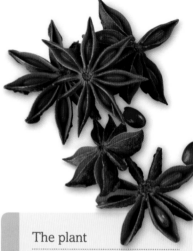

A PERFECT **BLEND**

Star anise blends well with vetiver, palmarosa, orange, and other citrus oils, as well as neroli, frankincense, lavender, ylang ylang, and tea tree.

The plant

An evergreen tree from China and Vietnam, star anise produces distinctive star-shaped fruits that are commonly used in Asian cooking as well as in traditional medicine.

The essential oil

The pale yellow oil has an aroma similar to black liquorice and is steam-distilled from the fresh and partly-dried fruits.

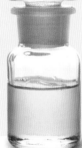

FRAGRANCE   SKIN CARE

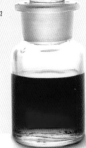

Jasmine

Jasminum officinale

The heady aroma of jasmine is highly prized by perfumers. The essential oil is one of the most **uplifting**, and its deeply **relaxing** effects account for its reputation as an aphrodisiac.

What is it **good for?**

Soothes skin Added to skin lotions, the oil can be a calming treatment for sensitive and inflamed skin that feels hot to the touch.

Tones skin Naturally toning, jasmine improves skin elasticity. Diluted in a massage blend and used regularly, it can help to fade stretch marks and scars.

Enhances wellbeing The warm, floral aroma of jasmine has a powerfully uplifting effect, helping to increase feelings of alertness, relieve tension, stress, and anxiety, and disperse feelings of negativity. It is traditionally regarded as an aphrodisiac for men and women.

Fights coughs and colds

A few drops of jasmine oil added to a steam inhalation can help to soothe irritating coughs and hoarseness and relieve laryngitis.

Best **uses**

As a perfume Jasmine oil can be applied neat as a perfume, creating a sense of relaxation and imbuing the wearer with a feeling of enjoyment.

As a toner Make a simple facial toner by adding 2–3 drops of jasmine absolute to a teaspoon of glycerine or witch hazel, then add to water. Soak a piece of cotton wool in the solution and apply to the skin.

Safe usage Non-toxic and non-irritant.

The plant

A native of northwest India, the name "jasmine" is derived from the Persian "yasmin", which means "fragrant flower". The waxy flowers are esteemed in perfumery for their exotic, intensely floral aroma.

The essential oil

The flowers are too delicate to be steam-distilled so solvent extraction is used to create a thick orange–brown oil known as an absolute.

Fresh and floral, the sweet aroma of jasmine is instantly uplifting.

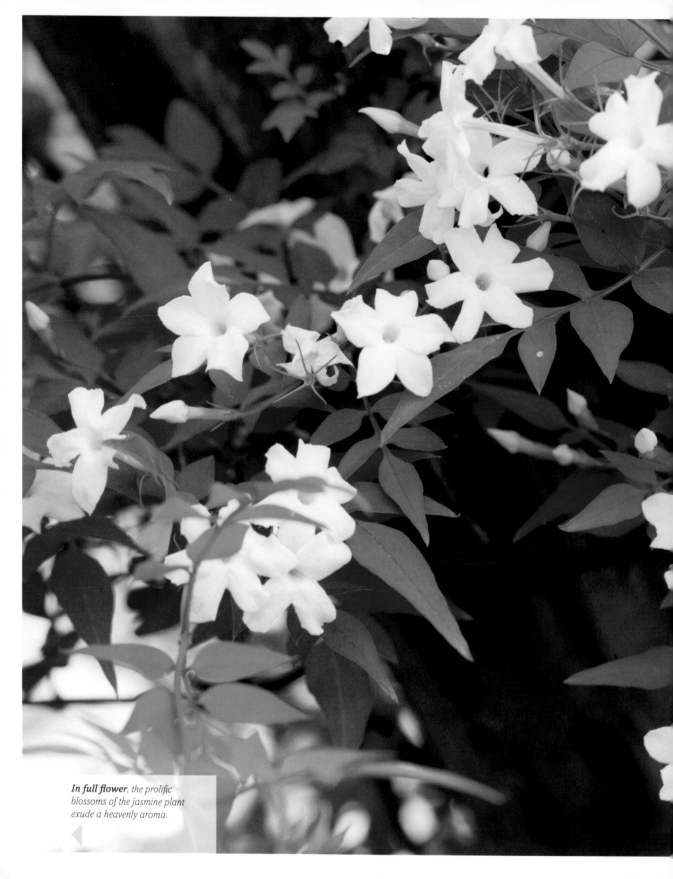

In full flower, *the prolific blossoms of the jasmine plant exude a heavenly aroma.*

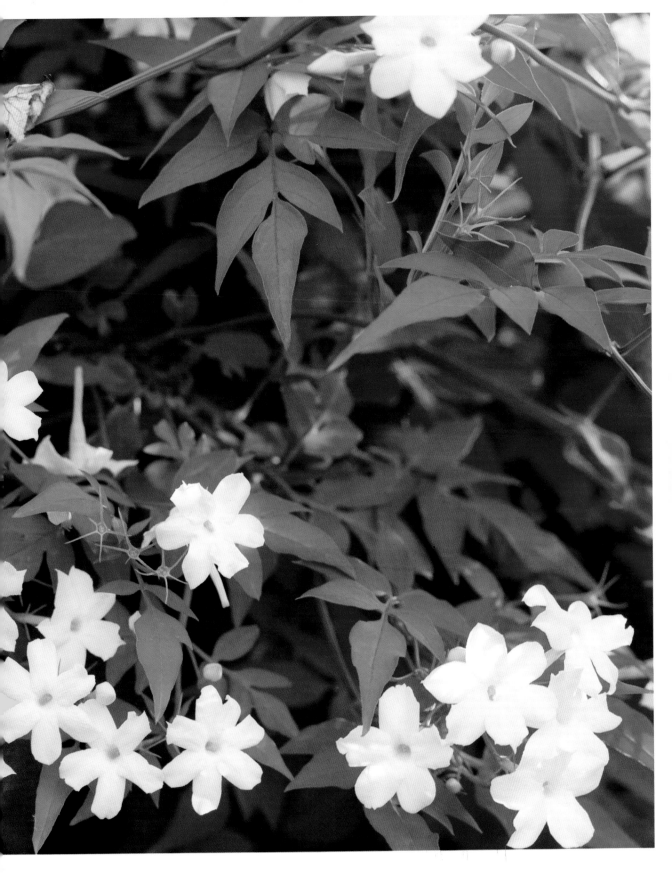

MASSAGE OIL

DIFFUSER

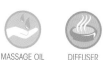
COMPRESS

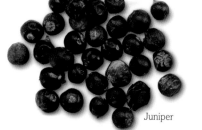
Juniper

STEAM INHALATION

MASSAGE OIL

Juniper

Juniperus communis

A distinctive, crisp-smelling oil that stimulates and **strengthens** the nerves and **bolsters spirits**. It has a mild diuretic effect that helps relieve water retention, a **warming** action that **soothes** aching muscles and joints, and a toning and **balancing** effect on the skin.

What is it **good for?**

Tones skin and hair Juniper oil is stimulating, astringent, and detoxifying. It helps to unblock pores, and balances oily skin and skin prone to blackheads and acne. Diluted, it can be applied to eczema and psoriasis, and in a hair rinse it helps treat dandruff.

Aids detox Juniper's purifying action reduces water retention. As a diuretic, it helps to dispel toxins, making it useful for gout, rheumatism, and arthritis.

Treats urinary infections A few drops in a warm, shallow bath can ease symptoms of cystitis. Try as a massage or compress on the lower back to ease kidney stone discomfort.

Eases aches and pains Juniper essential oil soothes rheumatic and arthritic pain. Its tonic effect helps regulate the menstrual cycle and can ease cramps.

Relieves varicose veins Its gentle astringent action can help to shrink varicose veins and haemorrhoids.

Relieves anxiety Juniper eases tension and mental exhaustion. It is reputed to dispel negative emotions such as insecurity, loneliness, and guilt.

Best **uses**

As a massage oil Add 6–8 drops to 2 tablespoons base oil to enjoy the benefits of this oil in a massage.

In a room freshener Add 2–3 drops to a diffuser or spray to clear stale air.

In a compress In a cool compress the oil can soothe skin eruptions.

Safe usage Non-toxic, non-irritant in dilution.

The plant

Evergreen juniper trees produce seed cones called berries. While oil can be distilled from the needles and twigs, the sweetest oil comes from the berries.

The essential oil

Steam-distilled from the berries, the colourless or pale yellow oil has a fresh, warm, woody, herbaceous smell. If it smells like a cocktail, that's because the berries also flavour gin.

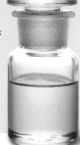

Bay laurel

Laurus nobilis

The same bay leaves that flavour cooking can, when distilled in an essential oil, produce a remedy that is **warming** and **pain-relieving** and that can lift spirits and **relax** the mind. The oil is an effective **antiseptic**, especially useful in the cold and flu season.

What is it **good for?**

Soothes aches and pains With a mild analgesic action, bay laurel can relieve sore muscles and lower back ache and ease tension headaches and migraines.

Fights cold and flu symptoms An effective expectorant and decongestant, bay laurel essential oil is an excellent choice for treating congested lungs and blocked sinuses and for disinfecting sick rooms.

Acts as a sedative Try putting a drop or two of the essential oil on your pillow or a tissue before bedtime to promote relaxation and aid a restful night's sleep.

Enhances wellbeing Bay laurel has long been associated with peace, wisdom, and inner confidence, and is thought to help you to maintain courage and focus when dealing with challenges in life.

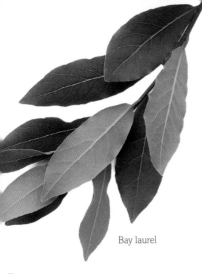

Bay laurel

Best **uses**

In an inhalation Add 3–5 drops to a steam inhalation to ease sinus congestion, breathing, and coughs.

Massage Dilute 1–2 drops of the oil in a teaspoon of base oil and massage into the temples to relieve headaches.

Safe usage Use well diluted (less than 0.5 per cent). Not suitable for hypersensitive skin or for children under seven years old.

The plant

The tree, *with its familiar deep green, sword-like leaves, originates from Asia Minor, but is established throughout the Mediterranean. Both the fruits and leaves are used medicinally and as food flavourings.*

The essential oil

The leaves are steam-distilled to produce a clear oil with a spicy, floral aroma, popular in colognes and aftershaves.

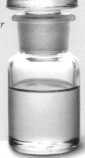

BATH OIL   MASSAGE OIL

Lavender
Lavandula angustifolia

A versatile and popular essential oil, lavender has a **calming** fragrance and is particularly renowned for its ability to relax and promote restful sleep. Its **rejuvenating** and **soothing** effects make it an effective skin treatment and a good skin healer.

What is it **good for?**

Soothes skin Lavender oil has a softening and conditioning effect on the skin. Try adding to creams, base oils, and bath preparations.

Heals skin Lavender is regenerative, making it useful for wounds and mouth ulcers. Applied neat, the oil makes an effective first-aid remedy for cuts, burns, bites, and stings. Its healing effects can ease acne, eczema, acne rosacea, and psoriasis, and reduce scarring.

Promotes restful sleep Deeply relaxing, lavender helps reduce stress levels and anxiety and is a popular remedy for promoting restful sleep.

Acts as a painkiller Mild analgesic properties make lavender a good treatment for headaches and migraine, as well as muscular and nerve pain. As an anti-spasmodic, it eases menstrual cramps.

Acts as an antiseptic It keeps wounds, ulcers, and sores clean. In a shallow bath, its antibacterial and anti-inflammatory properties make it excellent for infections such as cystitis.

Freshens the air It makes an ideal deodorizing and antiseptic room spray.

Best **uses**

As a bath oil Add 8–12 drops to 1 tablespoon base oil or full-fat milk and disperse in a relaxing bedtime bath.

As a massage oil Add 12–20 drops to 2 tablespoons base oil.

Safe usage Non-toxic and non-irritant. Can be used neat on small areas.

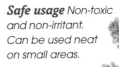

The plant

Lavandula augustifolia is commonly used for essential oils. **Lavandin** *or spike lavender is a hybrid with a medicinal aroma and antiseptic and tonic properties.*

The essential oil

Colourless or pale yellow, lavender oil has a floral, slightly harsh, sweet aroma. Some oils have synthetic compounds. Check the label for the name Lavandula angustifolia.

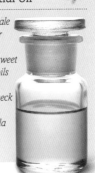

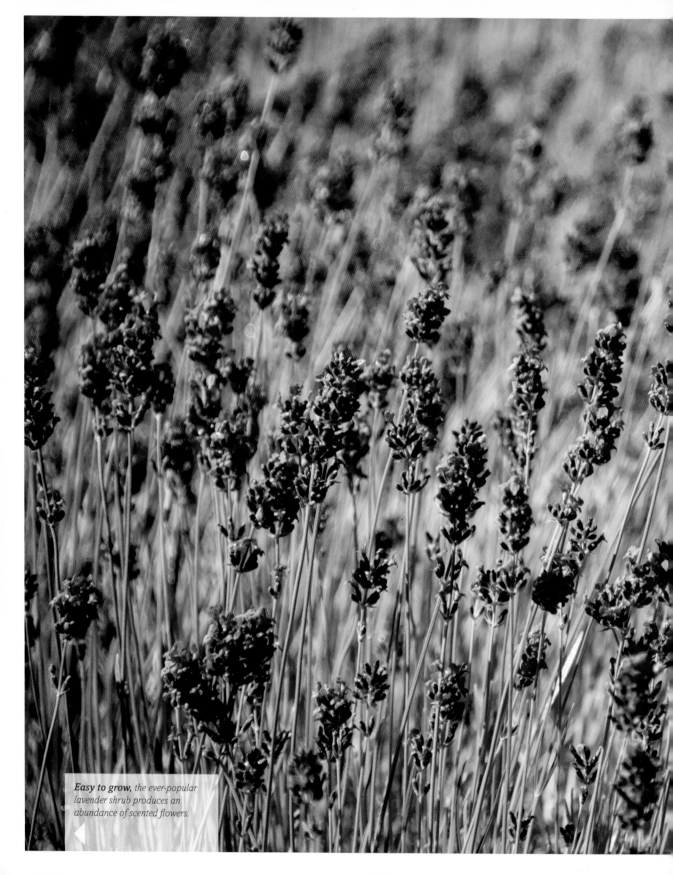

Easy to grow, *the ever-popular lavender shrub produces an abundance of scented flowers.*

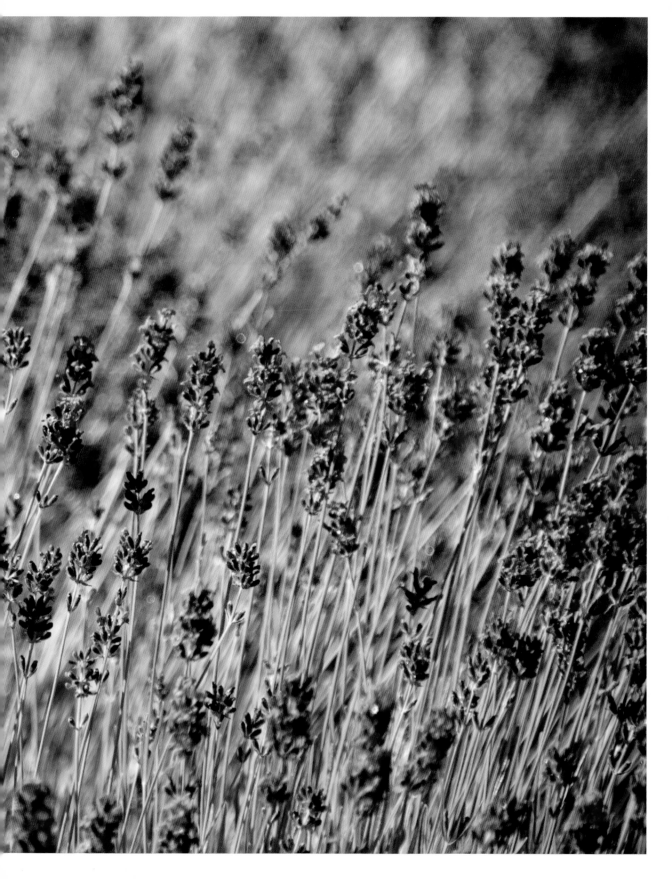

HAIR CARE

FIRST AID

Manuka

Leptospermum scoparium

Strongly **antiseptic**, manuka is ideal for use on cuts and wounds. It also contains a natural **antihistamine** that can bring welcome relief to hay fever sufferers. A sharp, **earthy aroma** clears the mind and dispels anxious or angry feelings.

What is it **good for?**

Heals skin The powerful antiseptic action of manuka speeds the healing of cuts and abrasions, as well as insect bites and stings. The oil is also strongly antifungal and can be added to ointments to treat athlete's foot, and to hair rinses to treat dandruff.

Fights colds and flu Added to a steam inhalation, manuka oil's antibacterial action makes it a good remedy for colds and coughs.

Acts as a deodorant Well diluted, manuka can control perspiration and the bacteria that cause body odour.

Soothes aches and pains An anti-inflammatory, the oil relieves joint and muscle pain and stomach cramps.

Soothes allergies Manuka contains a natural antihistamine that can calm reactions to pollen, dust, and irritants of the respiratory tract and the skin.

Enhances wellbeing If you suffer from anxiety or feelings of anger, use the oil to ground yourself, promote calm and relaxation, and help clear emotional and mental blockages.

Best **uses**

In a hair rinse Add 3–5 drops to warm water and use as a final rinse to balance excessively dry or oily hair.

As first aid Add 6–12 drops to 2 tablespoons of ointment and use to kill bacteria and speed the healing of cuts.

Safe usage Non-toxic, non-irritant in dilution.

The plant

Manuka is a shrubby tree*, native to New Zealand. Its copious pink, dark-red or white flowers attract the bees, but it's the understated leaves that produce the aromatic essential oil.*

The essential oil

Steam-distilled *from the leaves and twigs, the yellow to light brown oil has a sharp, earthy aroma with honey-like and herbaceous undertones.*

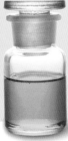

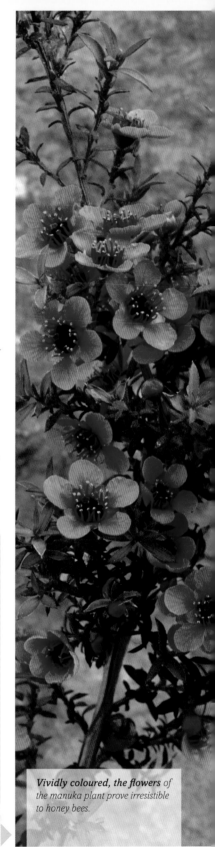

Vividly coloured, the flowers of the manuka plant prove irresistible to honey bees.

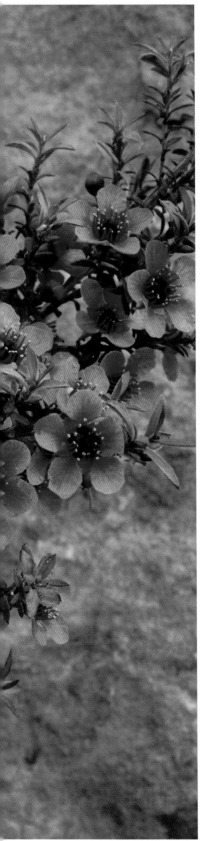

MASSAGE OIL   SKIN CARE

Litsea
Litsea cubeba

Also known as May chang, litsea is a warming, refreshing, uplifting oil that helps to calm and **soothe** frayed nerves. Its antiseptic and **skin-balancing** properties are particularly valued in skincare preparations.

What is it **good for?**

Tones skin Astringent and anti-inflammatory, litsea helps control acne and assists healing in existing breakouts, and also balances oily and combination skins.

Aids digestion The oil stimulates digestion and eases nausea. A good remedy for those with a poor appetite.

Acts as a deodorant In a body spray or footbath, the oil helps control perspiration and the bacteria that lead to body odour.

Relieves stress Litsea helps lift depression and calms the rapid heartbeat that comes with panic or stress, enabling you to think more constructively about a situation.

Soothes aches and pains The oil has a warming effect that boosts circulation and reduces inflammation in sore, tired muscles.

Best **uses**

As a massage oil A gentle massage with a litsea oil blend leaves you feeling warm, relaxed, calm, and balanced.

As a toner Add to a toner to leave skin feeling clean and refreshed.

Safe usage Use well diluted (less than 0.5 per cent). Not suitable for children under seven years old or for hypersensitive skin.

The plant

Litsea is also called Mountain, or Chinese, pepper, because its berries resemble peppercorns. All the parts of the plant contain oil, but it is the hard berries that yield the highest quality. In spite of its lemony scent, it is a relative of cinnamon and other fragrant members of the laurel family.

The essential oil

The fruit are steam-distilled to produce a yellow oil with a complex and refined lemony scent.

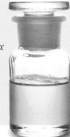

BATH OIL   MASSAGE OIL   COMPRESS   SKIN CARE

Chamomile (blue)

Matricaria recutita

Popular as a herbal tea, chamomile essential oil makes an effective skin treatment thanks to its **calming** and **toning** properties. It has a strong **anti-inflammatory** action that penetrates the skin's layers to **soothe** and repair, useful for skin conditions such as eczema, and for healing.

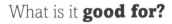

What is it **good for?**

Soothes skin A deeply soothing and calming oil, chamomile has anti-inflammatory properties that make it ideal for treating allergic skin conditions and sensitive skin and scalps. It helps to relieve the itchy, inflamed skin caused by rashes, cracked nipples, and conditions such as chicken pox. Its efficacy in treating eczema rivals treatments such as hydrocortisone.

Heals and cleanses skin A repairing oil, chamomile helps heal scratches and wounds, and also has been shown to promote faster tissue regeneration than corticosteroids. Its mildy astringent properties help to clean blocked pores.

Acts as a mild pain-reliever The anti-inflammatories present in chamomile, bisabolol and apigenin, work in a similar way to painkillers such as ibuprofen, providing effective mild pain relief and helping ease conditions such as arthritis.

Soothes digestion Chamomile is a natural soother and a popular remedy for calming digestive upsets. It can be used to treat a range of digestive complaints such as indigestion, peptic ulcers, and bouts of colic.

Strengthens immunity Use chamomile as a first line of defence against viruses and infection. It boosts immunity by stimulating leucocyte (white blood cell) production.

Promotes restful sleep Chamomile helps to calm irritability, nervousness, and tension headaches, helping promote relaxation and sleep.

Best **uses**

As a bath oil Mix 8–10 drops with 1 tablespoon base oil or full-fat milk and disperse in a warm bath to relax muscles and help calm anxiety.

In a massage oil Add 16–24 drops to 2 tablespoons base oil for a gentle massage to ease insomnia, back pain, stomach upsets, and period pains, to boost immunity, and to lift depression.

In a compress Add a few drops of chamomile essential oil to a wet, squeezed out cloth to make a cool compress that can help heal sores and calm allergic skin reactions.

In a skin cream Add 8–16 drops to 2 tablespoons cream for a skin cream.

Safe usage Non-toxic, non-irritant in dilution.

A PERFECT BLEND

Chamomile blends well with the essential oils of bergamot, clary sage, lavender, geranium, jasmine, tea tree, grapefruit, rose, lemon, and ylang ylang.

The plant

Also known as German chamomile, the plant, which has delicate feathery leaves and simple daisy-like white flowers on single stems, is cultivated widely throughout central and northern Europe.

Roman chamomile (Anthemis nobilis) is a milder, sweeter oil with similar anti-inflammatory properties that is particularly suitable for infants and children.

The essential oil

A deep ink-blue viscous liquid, the oil is steam-distilled from the flowers. The heavy, herbaceous sweet smell has a fruity note. Roman chamomile makes a paler oil.

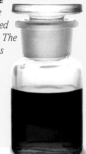

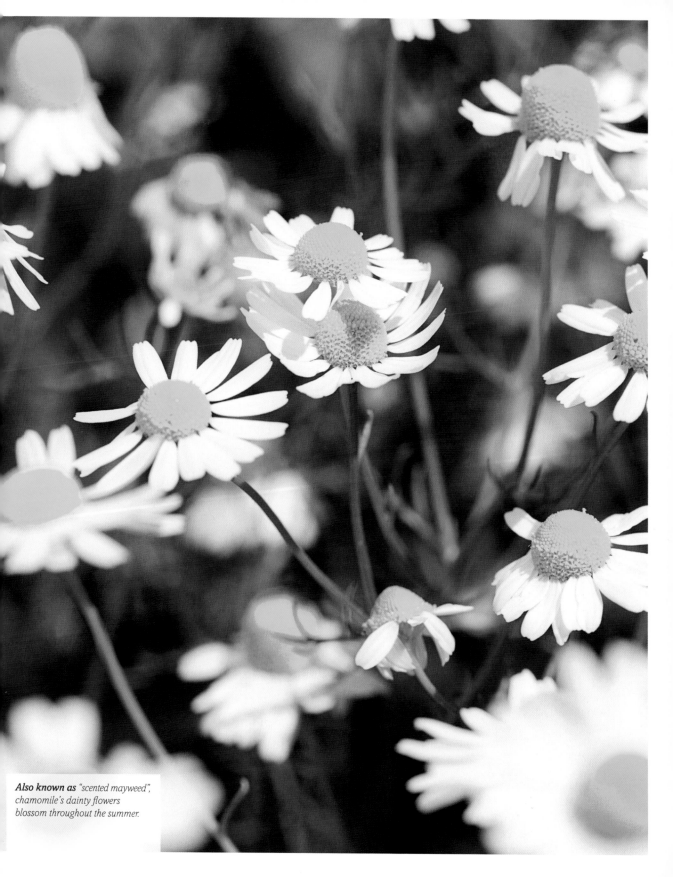

FIRST AID

FOOT BATH

Tea tree

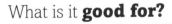
Melaleuca alternifolia

A PERFECT BLEND
Try blending tea tree with clove, eucalyptus, lavender, lemon, pine, rosemary, or thyme essential oils.

Best known for its powerful **antiseptic** properties, tea tree essential oil is a great all-rounder to keep in your first-aid kit, ready to use on wounds and sores. Studies show it is effective against a range of bacteria and fungi that can lead to infection. It also has a strong **deodorizing** action that can combat body odour.

What is it **good for?**

Boosts immunity Tea tree has immune-stimulating properties that help the body to fight off infection. A massage with a tea tree blend can aid recovery during convalescence.

Fights skin infections The oil acts as a barrier against bacteria, viruses, and fungi. It can be added to an ointment to help treat athlete's foot and ringworm, or can be dabbed on neat to cold sores, warts, and verrucas.

Heals cuts, scrapes, and bruises Tea tree promotes the formation of scar tissue to aid healing.

Helps to control acne A popular ingredient in skin remedies, the oil can be applied to pimples as an immediate treatment.

Acts as a hair tonic A tea tree scalp massage can help bring dandruff under control, and used in a rinse, tea tree can restore the balance of oils to combat greasy hair.

Mouth and gum care Use well diluted to treat bad breath, mouth ulcers, and gum infections.

Fights body odour A natural deodorizer, tea tree can be added to baths, body sprays, or creams to combat body or foot odour.

Fights cold and flu symptoms This antiseptic is effective in warding off colds and flu. Once a cold has set in, a steam inhalation with the oil eases congestion and breathing.

Eases urinary tract infections Tea tree can help to fight cystitis and other genital infections, including thrush, herpes, warts, pruritus, and trichomonas.

Best **uses**

As first aid Use tea tree essential oil in a dilution of 10 per cent (1 part tea tree to 10 parts witch hazel) to rinse and clean infected wounds and sores.

In a foot bath For tired, hot, smelly feet, or for athlete's foot, add 20 drops of tea tree oil to a small basin of warm water and soak feet for 15 minutes. Dry thoroughly.

Safe usage *Non-irritant in dilutions of less than 10 per cent. Non-toxic externally.*

The plant

A hardy tree, native to New South Wales in Australia, tea tree was an important medicine in Aboriginal tribes. Similar to the cypress in appearance, it has needle-like leaves with white flowerheads.

Two close relatives also produce essential oils: niaouli, also native to Australia, is primarily used to treat skin complaints and respiratory illnesses, and cajuput, native to Indonesia and the Philippines, is used to treat respiratory conditions.

The essential oil

Steam-distilled from the leaves of the tree, the essential oil is a clear liquid with a medicinal scent reminiscent of eucalyptus.

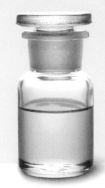

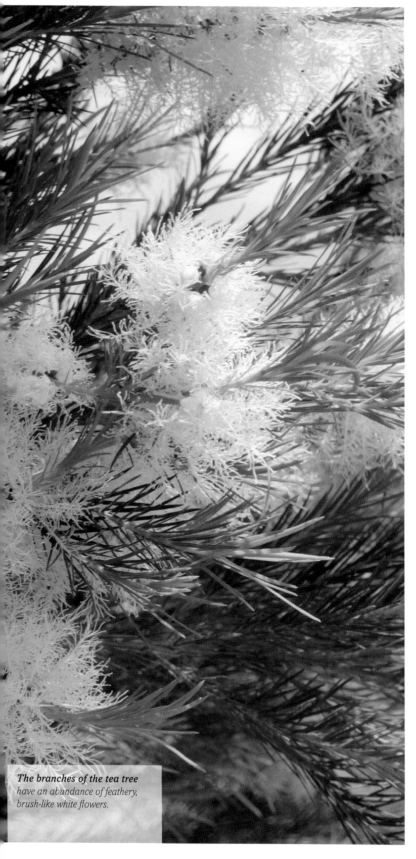

This healing essential oil, commonly used for its antiseptic effect, has a distinctive medicinal scent.

The branches of the tea tree have an abundance of feathery, brush-like white flowers.

MASSAGE OIL

DIFFUSER

Cajuput

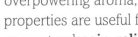
Melaleuca cajuputi

A member of the tea tree family, cajuput has a **milder** and less overpowering aroma, but many of the same benefits. Its **antiseptic** properties are useful for fighting respiratory and urinary infections, and, as a natural **pain-reliever**, it can ease headaches and muscle and joint pains.

What is it **good for?**

Acts as an antiseptic Its broad antiseptic properties make cajuput useful for fighting cold and flu viruses, bacterial urinary tract infections, and fungal infections, such as athlete's foot. Diluted, the oil can also be applied to cuts and wounds to keep these clean and infection-free.

Acts as a decongestant Cajuput makes an excellent decongestant and expectorant that helps to clear blocked sinuses and congested lungs.

Acts as a pain reliever Cajuput has soothing analgesic properties that can provide local pain relief from tension headaches and muscle and joint aches and pains.

Tones skin The oil helps to brighten oily or combination skin and keeps the bacteria that cause acne at bay.

Aids detox By promoting sweating, cajuput aids the removal of toxins from the body and also provides a pleasant cooling sensation that is especially helpful for soothing fevers.

Aids focus Cajuput helps to clear the mind and to fight mental exhaustion and apathy.

Best **uses**

As a massage oil Dilute cajuput essential oil in a massage oil blend and massage into achy, painful areas.

In a diffuser Add a few drops of the oil to a diffuser, vaporizer, or oil burner to relieve sinusitis and a blocked nose and to clear germs in the air. Or add a few drops to a steam inhalation.

Safe usage Non-irritant, non-toxic externally. Avoid use near the nose of children under seven years old.

This relatively mild oil has many therapeutic benefits.

A PERFECT BLEND

Good blending partners for cajuput include angelica, bergamot, geranium, lavender, clary sage, geranium, pine, rosemary, and ylang ylang.

The plant

Also called white tea tree, cajuput is a native of Malaysia now found throughout Southeast Asia and parts of Australia. From the Malaysian "kayu-puti" (white wood), its name describes its white bark. The oil is concentrated in its pointed leaves.

The essential oil

The clear to pale yellow essential oil is steam-distilled from the fresh leaves and twigs. Cajuput has a penetrating, slightly sweet aroma with hints of camphor.

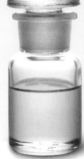

BATH OIL

FIRST AID

MASSAGE OIL

STEAM INHALATION

Niaouli

Melaleuca viridiflora, M. quinquenervia

Chiefly a **disinfectant** and astringent, niaouli helps to fight a range of infections. **Stimulating** the body and mind, it increases concentration, clears the head, and lifts the spirits. Think of niaouli as a gentler version of tea tree – suitable even for sensitive skin.

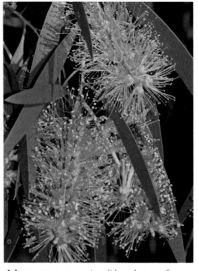

A large evergreen, niaouli has clusters of yellow flowers amid distinctive pointed leaves.

What is it **good for?**

Heals wounds Niaouli's disinfectant properties make it valuable for cleaning wounds, cuts, and applying to ulcers. Use it to help calm acne and balance oily skin.

Reduces the appearance of scars Niaouli encourages tissue regeneration, which in turn helps to minimize the appearance of scars, including the marks left by acne, pimples, or chickenpox.

Fights cold and flu symptoms A decongestant and expectorant, the oil helps to break up congestion in the lungs, bronchi, and nasal passages. Its antiviral and immune-boosting properties make it an important oil in the treatment of colds and flu.

Aids detox Niaouli stimulates the release of digestive juices as well as the circulation of blood and lymph, aiding the absorption of nutrients and encouraging the healthy excretion of waste and toxins.

Acts as a pain reliever An effective analgesic, niaouli can provide localized pain relief by numbing sensitive areas. It's useful for headaches, migraines, muscle and joint pain, and pain due to sprains.

Aids focus The sharp aroma of niaouli essential oil clears unwanted thoughts from the mind and enhances focus. This quality makes it a useful aid to meditation and helpful for concentration.

Best **uses**

As a bath oil If you feel as though you might be coming down with a cold virus, add a few drops to a bath oil blend to help fight the infection.

As first aid Dilute a few drops in a tumblerful of water and use as an antiseptic wash for cuts and other minor skin irritations.

As a massage oil Add to a base oil and use for an all-over body massage to strengthen the whole body, or use specifically, for example to help fight an infection, relieve pain, or stimulate a sluggish circulation.

In a steam inhalation Add 2–3 drops to a steam inhalation (or add to a diffuser or vaporizer) and inhale for several minutes to help you fight cold and flu symptoms, bronchitis, whooping cough, sinusitis, catarrh, and other respiratory conditions.

Safe usage *Non-toxic and non-irritant.*

The plant

A popular tree for planting on streets and in parks, niaouli has fluffy spikes of flowers and a papery bark that periodically peels. It is native to New Caledonia, Papua New Guinea, and Australia and belongs to the same family as tea tree and cajuput.

The essential oil

Niaouli oil is extracted *from the young leaves and twigs by steam-distillation. It has a mildly sweet, fresh, camphorous smell and its colour varies from clear to a pale yellowy-green hue.*

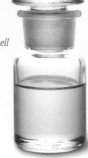

SKIN CARE

MASSAGE OIL

Lemon balm

Melissa officinalis
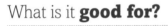

Lemon balm, also known as melissa, is often added to **skincare** products because of its calming, **anti-inflammatory** action on irritated skin. Its antiseptic effect makes it useful to have on hand for treating bee and wasp stings, and its cheerful **"feel-good"** aroma ensures it is a popular choice in aromatherapy.

What is it **good for?**

Soothes skin Lemon balm helps to calm inflamed skin and allergic skin conditions. It can be used, well diluted, to treat skin ulcers and eczema, especially when stress-related, and to reduce redness and irritation from insect bites and stings, and sunburn.

Tones skin With a stimulating action on the circulation, the oil brightens dull-looking complexions and has a tightening and toning effect on the skin. Lemon balm is exceptionally high in the antioxidants that help fight ageing caused by free radical damage.

Heals skin This antibacterial oil can be useful for treating acne and other skin eruptions such as cold sores.

Relieves headaches Uplifting and soothing, lemon balm can be a useful remedy for headaches and migraines, especially when a headache is associated with stress and held-in tension in the neck and shoulders.

Acts as an antiseptic Lemon balm has an antiviral action that works on the cold sore virus. If used at the first sign of a cold sore, it can limit its impact.

Aids digestion Added to a gentle abdominal massage blend, the essential oil can help relieve wind, colic, and dyspepsia, and is also useful for treating feelings of nausea.

Eases breathing Lemon balm has a mild antihistamine effect, helpful for hay fever and asthma. It also calms anxiety-induced respiratory problems.

Reduces anxiety A sedative action makes lemon balm especially useful in cases of panic. It can calm a racing heartbeat and help lower blood pressure. The oil makes a soothing massage when you feel overwhelmed.

Cools fevers A cooling action makes lemon balm useful for relieving heat exhaustion and soothing fevers.

Best **uses**

As a skin toner To hydrate skin, add 20 drops of lemon balm to 1 tablespoon witch hazel, or 1 teaspoon glycerine. Add to 3 tablespoons water and put in a spray bottle for a cooling spray.

In a massage oil Use 2–3 drops in 1 tablespoon base oil for a massage oil that counters the effects

of over-indugence, such as indigestion trapped wind, and nausea.

Safe usage *Non-toxic externally. Sensitization possible. Use well diluted (less than 1 per cent).*

The plant

A native of central and southern Europe, lemon balm is a member of the mint family. Its leaves are a similar shape to mint, but when you rub them between your fingers, they release a tart sweet smell, like lemons.

The essential oil

This pale yellow oil with a pleasant lemony, fresh, sweet, and herbaceous smell can be steam-distilled from the fresh leaves and flowers. Because the plant yields very little oil, lemon balm is often adulterated with other lemon-scented essential oils. Pure lemon balm oil is very expensive.

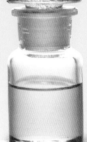

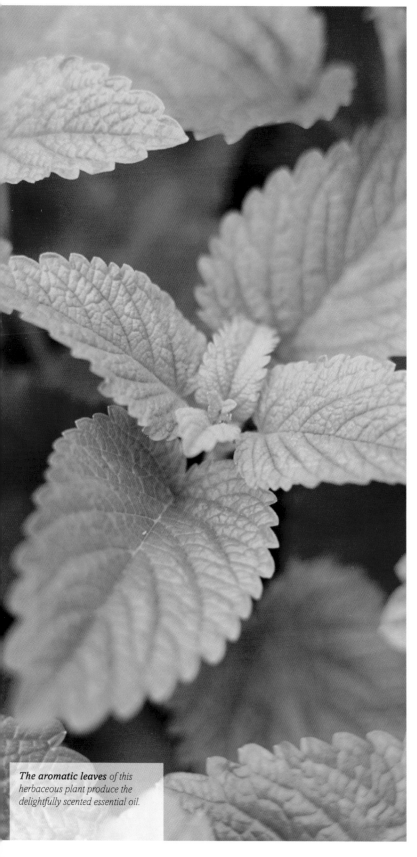

The aromatic leaves of this herbaceous plant produce the delightfully scented essential oil.

A calming oil, lemon balm is helpful for soothing insect bites or patches of irritated skin.

MASSAGE OIL

STEAM INHALATION

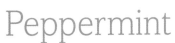

Peppermint

Mentha piperita

Applied to the skin, peppermint feels initially cooling and **refreshing,** then gently warming. Its **stimulating** and analgesic properties make it an effective remedy for neuralgia and muscular pains and headaches. It's also a first-class **antiseptic**, and a popular addition to all types of beauty products.

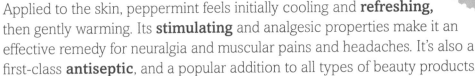
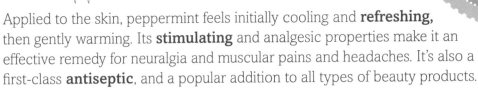

A PERFECT **BLEND**

Try blending peppermint essential oil with eucalyptus, lavender, lemon, pine or rosemary essential oils.

What is it **good for?**

Fights odour Peppermint is an effective body deodorant. Used in toothpaste, mouthwashes, and other dental preparations, its antiseptic and deodorizing properties can also help combat bad breath.

Soothes skin Diluted peppermint oil has cooling and toning effects on the skin and can be particularly soothing for skin that is irritated after excessive exposure to the elements. It can also be used to relieve hives and other allergic skin reactions.

Acts as an antiseptic Its antiseptic and antiviral properties make this a useful oil for treating cold sores, even for resistant strains of the herpes virus that causes them, and for products such as lip balms and hand creams.

Eases digestive upsets A tummy massage with a peppermint blend can ease indigestion and flatulence, calm nausea and travel sickness, and improve a sluggish digestion.

Fights cold symptoms The oil acts as an expectorant to help alleviate coughs and clear sinuses.

Soothes bites and stings Peppermint essential oil makes an effective insect repellent, and it can also be used to help soothe mosquito bites and other skin irritations.

Relieves headaches Peppermint oil has long been recognized as a safe and effective treatment for tension headaches.

Best **uses**

As a massage oil Add 1–2 drops of peppermint essential oil to 1 tablespoon base oil and gently massage the abdomen in a clockwise motion to help bring relief to symptoms of indigestion, constipation, and nausea.

In an inhalation Add 3–4 drops of peppermint essential oil to a steam inhalation (not suitable for children or those suffering with asthma) or to a diffuser, vaporizer, or oil burner, and use as a decongestant to help clear sinuses and congested lungs.

Safe usage Use well diluted (less than 2 per cent). Avoid use in cardiac fibrillation and near the nose in children under seven years old.

The plant

This popular herb is actually a hybrid of Mentha aquatica (water mint) and Mentha spicata (spearmint). It has been used as a medicinal herb for thousands of years, particularly as an infusion for digestive disorders, though in modern times it is mostly used in the flavouring and toothpaste industries. The essential oil is extracted from the flowering herb.

The essential oil

Peppermint essential oil is steam-distilled from the flowering herb. The thin, almost watery oil has a fresh, sharp, strongly menthol aroma with a sweet-smelling undertone and it is a clear to pale yellow in colour.

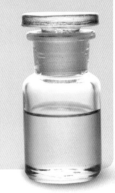

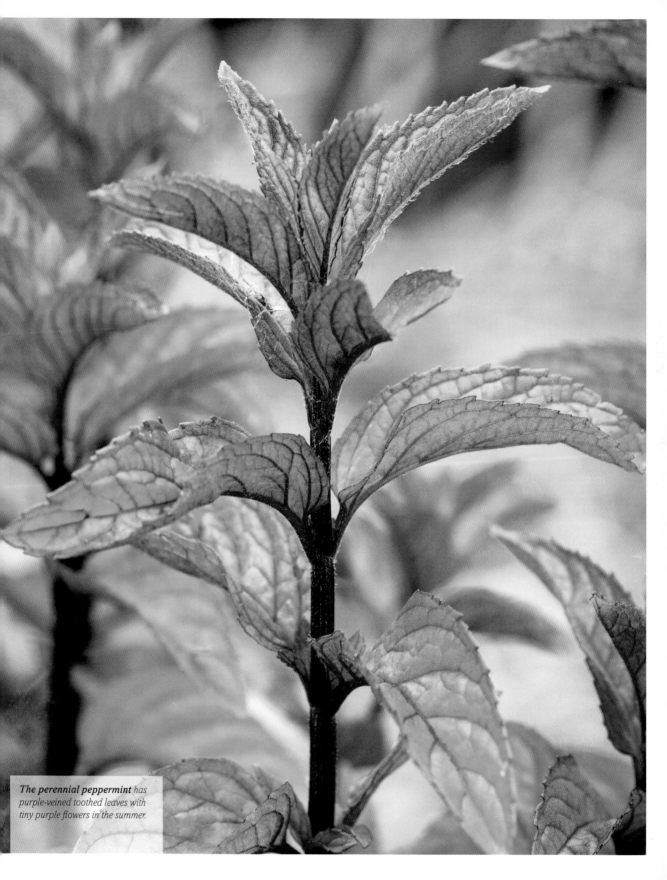

The perennial peppermint has purple-veined toothed leaves with tiny purple flowers in the summer.

MOUTHWASH

BATH OIL

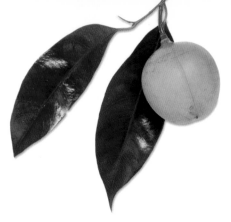

Nutmeg
Myristica fragrans

This **warming** oil with anti-inflammatory properties is useful for relieving muscle and joint pain. It helps **balance** the nervous system, **stimulating** or **calming** as needed, and also has a **detox** action that can improve digestion.

What is it **good for?**

Tooth and gum health Used well diluted as a mouthwash, nutmeg oil has an antiseptic and deodorant action that attacks the bacteria that cause bad breath and tooth decay.

Eases aches and pains A warming massage with a nutmeg oil blend can relieve inflammation and muscle pain, and boost circulation. Its mild analgesic action gives localized pain relief.

Aids sleep A well-known sedative, nutmeg helps relieve stress and can improve the quality of sleep.

Enhances wellbeing When suffering from anxiety or exhaustion, nutmeg can lift the spirits and help you regain focus.

Eases digestion Nutmeg stimulates appetite and digestion, reducing wind and soothing upsets.

Best **uses**

In a mouthwash Dilute 2–3 drops of the essential oil in 1 teaspoon of glycerin or calendula tincture and add to half a cupful of water. Do not swallow.

As a bath oil Add 5–6 drops to 1 tablespoon base oil or full-fat milk and disperse in a bath to relieve muscle aches and indigestion, and aid sleep.

Safe usage Use well diluted (less than 1 per cent).

The plant

A native of the Banda Islands of Indonesia, the evergreen nutmeg tree produces a fruit similar to a peach. This fruit is the source of two spices: nutmeg and mace. Nutmeg (the spice and oil), comes from the seed itself, while mace comes from the covering of the seed.

The essential oil

Nutmeg essential oil is obtained by steam-distilling the dried seeds of the nutmeg. This produces a clear oil with a sharp, spicy, musky aroma. West Indian nutmeg is milder and more suitable for aromatherapy than East Indian.

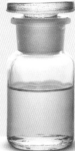

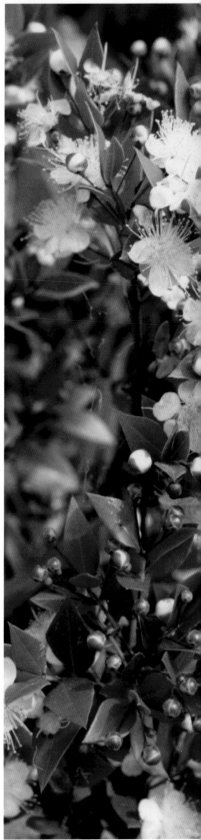

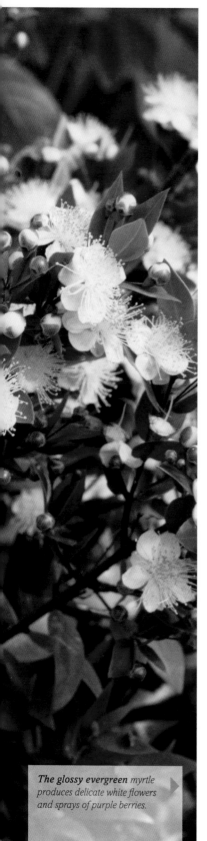

The glossy evergreen myrtle produces delicate white flowers and sprays of purple berries.

DIFFUSER

Myrtle

Myrtus communis

Myrtle oil gained its popularity because of its **antimicrobial,** astringent, antiseptic, anti-inflammatory, expectorant, decongestant, and **stimulant** properties. Today, the oil is commonly used for skin health and respiratory ailments.

What is it **good for?**

Tones skin Its astringent properties work on oily skin, open pores, and sagging skin, as welll as on spider veins and haemorrhoids.

Relieves congestion A mild expectorant, myrtle can ease asthma, coughs, and bronchitis. Its anti-inflammatory properties also calm respiratory inflammation caused by allergic reactions.

Acts as an antiseptic The oil can be applied to wounds, spots, and boils, and has been shown to inhibit the growth of several types of bacteria including *Escherichia coli, Staphylococcus aureus, Bacillus subtilis, Salmonella,* and *Listeria.*

Acts as a mild sedative Myrtle calms nerves and its sedative action can relieve depression and insomnia.

Supports the thyroid Myrtle's balancing action helps it to regulate over- and under-active thyroid glands.

Acts as an insect repellent Used in a room spray or diffuser, the oil can help to ward off insects.

Best **uses**

In a diffuser Add 4–5 drops to a diffuser, vaporizer, or oil burner (or add to a steam inhalation) to help clear sinus congestion.

Safe usage Use well diluted (less than 1.5 per cent).

The plant

Myrtle is an evergreen shrub with fragrant white or pink flowers. Native to North Africa, it is commonly found in the southern Mediterranean region. It belongs to the same plant family as tea tree and eucalyptus, and has similar medicinal characteristics.

The essential oil

Myrtle oil is steam-distilled from the leaves. It is a pale yellow to green oil with a stimulating, slightly camphorous aroma somewhere between eucalyptus and frankincense.

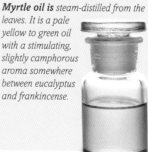

COMPRESS

DIFFUSER

BATH OIL

MASSAGE OIL

Basil

Ocimum basilicum

The name basil comes from the Greek word **"basilikon phuton"** meaning "king". Basil is highly valued in traditional Ayurvedic medicine as a protector of both mental and physical **wellbeing.** Its crisp aroma clears and refreshes the mind and helps to **calm** anxiety.

What is it **good for?**

Enhances wellbeing Basil balances, revives, and strengthens to help combat exhaustion, anxiety, or depression.

Tones and balances skin The oil refreshes skin and helps to control acne.

Supports women's health Basil can help stimulate scanty or delayed periods caused by debility and stress.

Eases digestion Soothing basil can relieve indigestion. Its antiseptic action also helps treat intestinal infections.

Fights cold symptoms The oil helps clear sinuses and soothe coughs.

Eases aches and pains Basil can ease gout and rheumatic pain.

Acts as an insect repellent Its insecticidal properties repel insects. It also relieves the irritation of insect bites.

Best **uses**

In a compress Add a few drops to warm water and make a compress with a cloth to ease pain and congestion.

In a diffuser Add 3–4 drops to a diffuser, vaporizer, or oil burner to clear headaches and refresh the mind.

Safe usage Potentially toxic over time. Dilute extremely well (less than 0.5 per cent) and do not use for prolonged periods. Avoid in pregnancy, when breasfeeding, and in children under 15 years old.

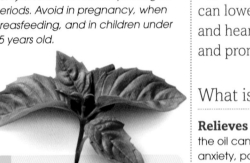

The plant

Originally from tropical Asia and the Pacific Islands, basil is now cultivated worldwide. The flowers range from white to pink in colour, and are popular with bees and other garden pollinators.

The essential oil

The oil is steam-distilled from the leaves and the flowering tops of the plant. It has a sweet, spicy, fresh and slightly balsamic odour, and is clear to pale yellow in colour.

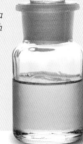

Marjoram

Origanum majorana

This aromatic, **warming,** and **relaxing** oil is known for its ability to aid digestion and relieve stomach and menstrual cramping. It has a gently **sedative** effect that can lower blood pressure and heart rate, ease anxiety, and promote restful sleep.

What is it **good for?**

Relieves anxiety A gentle sedative, the oil can treat nervous tension, anxiety, panic attacks, and insomnia.

Improves circulation The oil has a toning effect on circulation that makes it useful for treating high blood pressure.

Eases cold and flu symptoms The oil's warming decongestant action can fight off chills and help clear sinus and lung congestion.

Acts as a painkiller The oil's analgesic action can ease tension headaches and migraines. Massage into muscles, joints, and tender areas for local relief from muscle pains, sprains, strains, rheumatism, and arthritis.

Supports women's health Its warming action relieves period pains and pre-menstrual symptoms such as anxiety, weariness, and irritability.

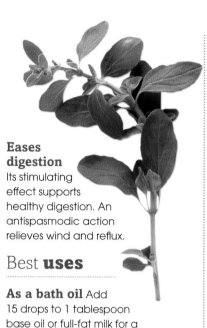

Eases digestion

Its stimulating effect supports healthy digestion. An antispasmodic action relieves wind and reflux.

Best **uses**

As a bath oil Add 15 drops to 1 tablespoon base oil or full-fat milk for a reviving soak.

In a massage oil For abdominal pain, add 10 drops to 1 tablespoon base oil and massage the tummy in a clockwise direction.

Safe usage *Non-toxic, non-irritant in dilution.*

The plant

Mediterranean sweet marjoram *has a long history of use as a medicinal herb.*

Spanish marjoram *(Thymus masticina) has some similar properties, but is harsher and should be avoided in children under seven years old.*

The essential oil

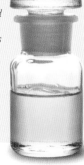

The essential oil*, steam-distilled from the dried flowering herb, is a pale yellow or pale amber hue with a warm, spicy, slightly camphorous smell.*

HAND WASH

DIFFUSER

Oregano

Origanum vulgare

Prized for centuries for its **healing** qualities, oregano has a powerful **antibacterial** action. The essential oil is traditionally used to treat complaints as diverse as indigestion and diarrhoea, insect bites, earaches, rheumatism, and coughs.

What is it **good for?**

Has an antibacterial action

Oregano contains compounds that have been shown to inhibit the growth of bacteria such as *Pseudomonas aeruginosa* and *Staphylococcus aureus*. The oil can also help to relieve urinary tract infections.

Helps fight fungal infections

The essential oil has been shown to inhibit the growth of *Candida albicans*, the fungus that causes oral thrush, canker sores, skin rashes, and athlete's foot, and also inhibits the fungi that cause nail infections.

Relieves menstrual cramps

Its analgesic action can ease menstrual cramps and other abdominal pains.

Clears sinuses

A few drops of the oil on a tissue or in a steam inhalation can help to clear blocked sinuses and loosen phlegm.

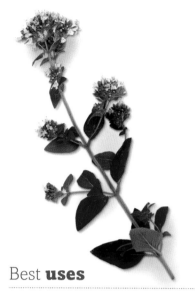

Best **uses**

As an antibacterial wash Add 8–10 drops to an unscented liquid soap for an antibacterial handwash.

In a diffuser Add 2–4 drops to a diffuser to ease congestion.

Safe usage *Dilute well before use (less than 1 per cent). Avoid using in pregnancy, when breastfeeding, and in children under seven years old.*

The plant

A member of the mint family*, this aromatic, culinary herb, sometimes called wild marjoram, originates from hilly, Greek countryside, but is now grown around the world.*

The essential oil

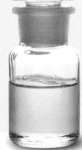

The pale yellow oil *is produced by steam-distillation of the fresh oregano leaves. It has a spicy, peppery aroma with a hint of camphor.*

BATH OIL

DIFFUSER

Geranium
Pelargonium graveolens

A **cheerful** oil, appreciated by both adults and children, geranium essential oil has a balancing, cooling, and **reviving** effect on skin, especially when it is weather-damaged or irritated. The oil is also a mild diuretic, making it a useful aid to **detox**, and it can help to soothe urinary tract infections.

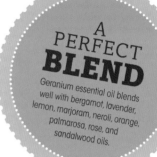

A PERFECT BLEND

Geranium essential oil blends well with bergamot, lavender, lemon, marjoram, neroli, orange, palmarosa, rose, and sandalwood oils.

What is it **good for?**

Aids detox The oil's gentle diuretic effect helps the body to eliminate excess water and reduce puffiness.

Balances emotions Both calming and uplifting, geranium makes a natural antidepressant. It can reduce restlessness and help to treat anxiety in children and adults.

Acts as a painkiller Geranium has mild analgesic properties that can relieve the pain of neuralgia and conditions such as shingles.

Tones the scalp Geranium oil helps to balance the secretion of sebum on the scalp, making it a useful treatment for flaky dandruff.

Tones skin This balancing oil is suitable for all skin types. Its antiseptic and anti-inflammatory properties help to control acne, and it is cooling for dry, inflamed skin. Its reviving effect helps to reduce the appearance of wrinkles, scars, and blemishes.

Supports women's health Geranium's cooling and balancing properties can relieve menopausal symptoms such as hot flushes and vaginal dryness. The oil can also soothe painful urinary tract infections.

Best **uses**

As a bath oil To relieve cystitis or pruritis, add 5 drops of geranium and 5 drops of lavender to 1 tablespoon base oil or full-fat milk and disperse in a shallow bath.

In a diffuser To ease anxiety and lift the spirits, add 5 drops of geranium and 5 drops of orange to a diffuser, vaporizer, or oil burner.

Safe usage *Non-toxic, non-irritant in dilution. Sensitization possible.*

The plant

A native of South Africa originally, geranium is now grown mainly in Réunion, China, and Egypt. Of the 700 different varieties of the Pelargonium plant, only 10 can be used to make the essential oil. Plants are harvested shortly after flowering to capture the highest concentrations of the oil, which comes from the plant's leaves, and not from the flowers as many assume.

The essential oil

The green to amber-coloured essential oil has a powerful, sweet, floral aroma with distinct minty undertones. Once the plant has been harvested, the oil is steam-distilled from the glands found in the leaves and from the green stems of the plant.

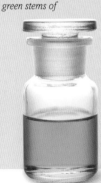

This balancing oil keeps emotions on an even keel.

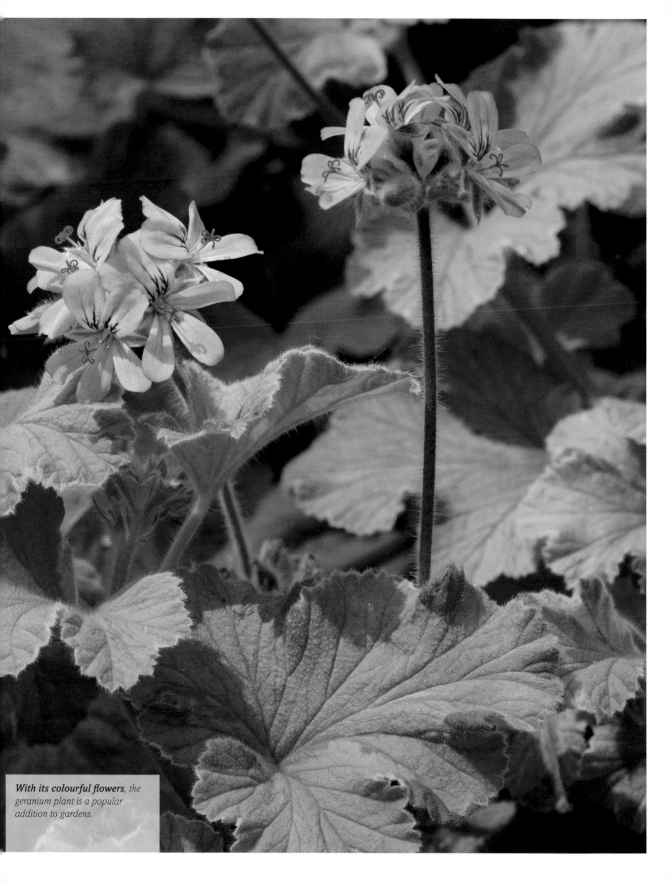

With its colourful flowers, the geranium plant is a popular addition to gardens.

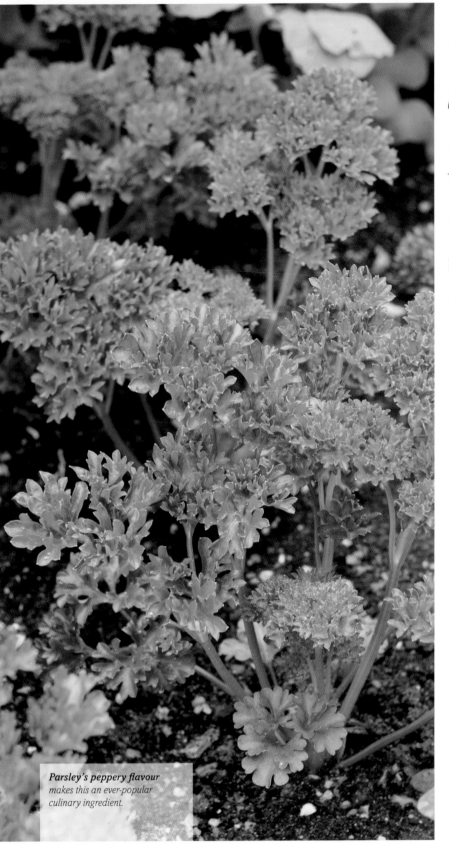

Parsley's peppery flavour makes this an ever-popular culinary ingredient.

This well-known herb has a multitude of therapeutic benefits that are present in its essential oil.

SKIN CARE   BATH OIL

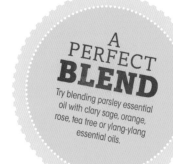

A PERFECT **BLEND**

Try blending parsley essential oil with clary sage, orange, rose, tea tree or ylang-ylang essential oils.

Parsley seed

Petroselinum crispum

More than just a garnish on your plate, parsley produces an essential oil that is **antibacterial** and has valuable **detoxing** properties that can help to reduce water retention and strengthen digestion. Its **spicy** aroma is much prized as an ingredient in soaps and perfumes – in particular, men's colognes.

What is it **good for?**

Boosts circulation The oil has a strengthening effect on blood vessels, making it useful for toning varicose veins and slowing down the spread of broken facial capillaries.

Tones skin Its antibacterial and antifungal properties help to treat pimples, acne, and skin infections, as well as disinfect pores.

Stimulates hair growth Diluted in a scalp massage, parsley essential oil encourages hair growth.

Has an antibacterial action Parsley oil helps to inhibit and kill microbes, protecting against various infections and diseases.

Acts as a painkiller By helping to boost the circulation and in turn prevent the accumulation of uric acid in the muscles and joints, parsley can act as a mild pain reliever for sufferers of arthritis and rheumatism.

Aids detox Parsley essential oil supports the healthy function of the kidneys and bladder. It has a diuretic action that can help to reduce fluid retention, and is also a mild laxative. It has an overall strengthening and tonic effect on the digestive system.

Aids digestion Like the fresh herb, the essential oil has carminative properties that can help relieve and treat indigestion, nausea, flatulence, vomiting, and stomach aches.

Calms the mind Parsley is a great de-stresser as it soothes the nerves and has a grounding and calming effect on the mind and emotions.

Enhances wellbeing The aromatherapeutic properties of parsley are purported to help strengthen confidence in overcoming difficulties and to enhance focus and provide a strong sense of purpose.

Best **uses**

As a facial elixir To help combat spider veins, mix 1 tablespoon base oil, 1 drop of parsley essential oil and 2 drops of rose essential oil. Massage very gently into the affected areas.

As a bath oil Add 6–9 drops of parsley essential oil to 1 tablespoon base oil or full-fat milk and add to a warm bath for a soothing soak.

Safe usage *Use well diluted (less than 1 per cent). Avoid using during pregnancy and when breastfeeding.*

The plant

Parsley is native *to the Mediterranean region, but is now grown in gardens worldwide as a versatile culinary herb. The seeds contain most of the essential oil, although the entire plant can be used for making the oil.*

The essential oil

Parsley oil is *steam-distilled from the seeds of the plant. It is a colourless to pale yellow oil with a surprising sweet, warm, woody–spicy, herbaceous aroma.*

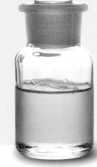

DIFFUSER OINTMENT

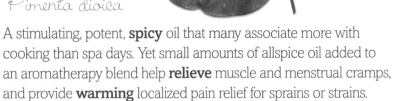

Allspice

Pimenta dioica

A stimulating, potent, **spicy** oil that many associate more with cooking than spa days. Yet small amounts of allspice oil added to an aromatherapy blend help **relieve** muscle and menstrual cramps, and provide **warming** localized pain relief for sprains or strains.

What is it **good for?**

Acts as a painkiller The oil has a local numbing effect that is useful for treating pain caused by neuralgia, muscular injuries, and joint strain, as well as pain from insect bites and stings.

Relieves muscle cramps Allspice has a warming, calming effect that soothes muscle cramps and spasms.

Acts as a mild sedative Its relaxing effect on the body and mind makes the oil useful for treating tension and anxiety. The oil's gently soothing action can help induce sleep.

Relieves indigestion Add to a massage oil blend to relieve indigestion, nausea, and trapped wind.

Eases cold symptoms Use in an inhalation to help relieve congestion.

Best **uses**

In a diffuser Diffuse 3–4 drops to ease anxiety.

As a rub A very small amount of the oil in a base oil or ointment can be used in a warming chest massage to help clear catarrh, congested coughs, and bronchitis.

Safe usage Non-irritant in dilution, sensitization possible. Potentially toxic with prolonged use. Dilute extremely well (less than 0.25 per cent). Avoid in pregnancy, when breastfeeding, and in children under 15 years old.

The plant

Native to the *Caribbean Islands and South America, the pimento tree produces small berry-like fruits, which are ground for use as a cooking spice. Both the leaves and berries are aromatic and are used to make the essential oil.*

The essential oil

Sometimes called pimento oil, *the light to pale brown oil is steam-distilled from the leaves and fruits. The oil's warm, spicy aroma is akin to that of clove and cinnamon essential oils.*

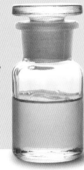

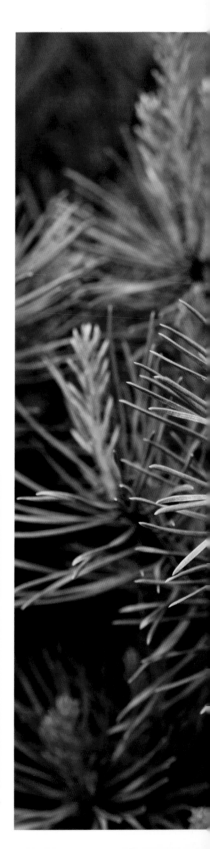

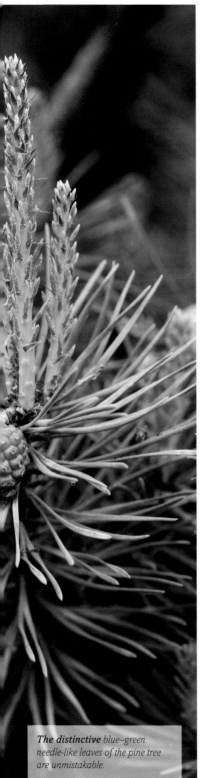

The distinctive blue–green needle-like leaves of the pine tree are unmistakable.

FRAGRANCE

Pine

Pinus sylvestris

Uplifting pine has a **warming** effect on sore joints and muscles, and its **clearing** action helps to unblock sinuses and **ease** breathing. The oil is valued by perfumers for the sweetness it adds to fragrance blends.

A PERFECT **BLEND**

Blends well with cedarwood, eucalyptus, lavender, lemon, rosemary, sage, and juniper.

What is it **good for?**

Eases breathing Decongesting and antiviral, pine oil protects against viruses, helps to clear catarrh, and eases hay fever symptoms.

Acts as a painkiller A warming oil, pine's analgesic and anti-inflammatory properties soothe muscular aches and painful joints. It can be applied locally to boost circulation to affected areas.

Acts as an antiseptic The oil can be used to treat infectious skin problems such as impetigo and boils.

Acts as an insect repellent Add a few drops to a strip of fabric or piece of wood and place with clothes to protect them from moths.

Supports urinary health The oil is effective for soothing cystitis, prostate problems, and urinary infections.

Enhances wellbeing A grounding oil, pine's aroma revitalizes mind and spirit, relieving exhaustion, tension, and other stress-related symptoms.

Freshens air Pine is ideal for clearing stale smells and eliminating odours.

Best **uses**

As an air freshener Add 20–30 drops to 60ml (2fl oz) each of vodka and water. Pour into a spray bottle and use to clear the air, avoiding furniture.

Safe usage Non-toxic, non-irritant in dilution. Ensure you use the variety Pinus sylvestris as other varieties may be toxic or irritant.

The plant

There are 90 species of pine tree. The essential oil comes from the Scots, or forest, pine, grown in Europe and Asia. Oil is distilled from the evergreen needles and twigs year round.

The essential oil

The pale yellow oil is steam-distilled from the twigs and buds of the tree. It has the distinctive fresh, sweet, resinous aroma of a pine forest.

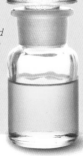

DIFFUSER

MASSAGE OIL

Black pepper

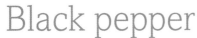
Piper nigrum

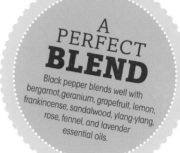

A warming, spicy oil, black pepper has strong **antiseptic** properties. Its **stimulating** aroma has a clearing effect on the **mind,** making this a useful oil for improving **focus,** while its ability to boost circulation can **revive** tired muscles and joints and speed the healing of bruises.

What is it **good for?**

Eases aches and pains Black pepper's main constituent, piperine, is an anti-inflammatory, which makes this essential oil a potent ingredient in ointments and salves for aching limbs and sore muscles. The oil also has a warming action that is effective for relieving sports injuries and improving muscle tone.

Stimulates circulation Black pepper essential oil helps to encourage circulation to the extremities, so use for cold hands and feet. Regular use may also help to improve the appearance of cellulite.

Aids detox The oil encourages perspiration and can be used in small doses to support the effective functioning of the lymphatic system. It also has a mild diuretic effect.

Boosts immunity If you are feeling run down, this essential oil is a good choice as it bolsters the body's defences against infections.

Eases breathing A penetrating oil, black pepper can help loosen and clear congestion in the lungs.

Helps to quit smoking Studies have shown that inhaling black pepper vapours can help reduce cravings for cigarettes.

Enhances alertness The oil imbues a general feeling of warmth that can enhance the senses, and it also helps to clear the mind and bring a sense of clarity that can aid focus, motivation, and stamina, while combating mental fatigue.

Best **uses**

In a diffuser If your "can do" attitude is feeling a little worn out, add 3–4 drops of black pepper essential oil to a diffuser, vaporizer, or oil burner to improve motivation and help your levels of concentration.

As a massage oil For a general massage, black pepper essential oil is best used as part of an oil blend. To make a quick oil blend to reduce bruising and relieve sore muscles and joints, add 15 drops of black pepper oil to 1 tablespoon of base oil, and apply locally.

Safe usage *Non-toxic, non-irritant in dilution.*

The plant

Black peppercorns *are actually the dried fruits of a climbing vine-like shrub native to Indonesia, where the spice is still mainly cultivated today. Best known as a cooking spice, black pepper also has a long established history of use as a medicinal spice in India and China. Black pepper essential oil is valued by perfumers for adding a warming spicy note to perfume blends.*

The essential oil

The essential oil *of the black peppercorn is steam-distilled from the dried, crushed unripe fruit. The thinly textured oil is an amber to yellow–green colour and has a distinctive pungent, spicy aroma that is both warming and fresh.*

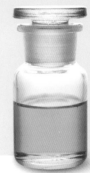

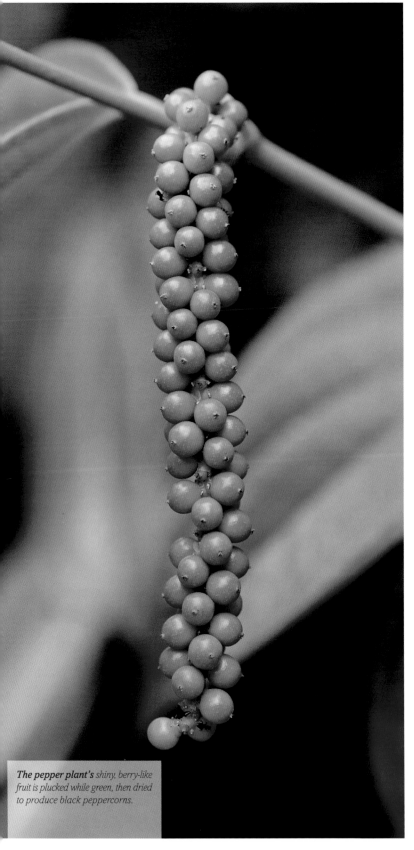

Soothing and warming, black pepper essential oil eases aches and pains and stimulates the circulation.

The pepper plant's shiny, berry-like fruit is plucked while green, then dried to produce black peppercorns.

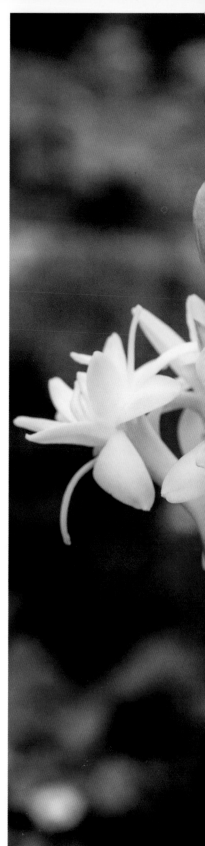

FRAGRANCE   MASSAGE OIL

Patchouli
Pogostemon cablin

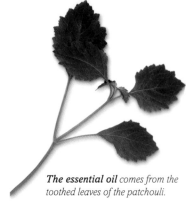

The essential oil comes from the toothed leaves of the patchouli.

A tried and tested aromatherapy favourite, patchouli oil **soothes** and **heals** the skin, improving the appearance of scar tissue and stretch marks. It also **revitalizes** ageing complexions, and its **antiseptic** properties help to treat pimple-prone skin.

What is it **good for?**

Repairs, tones, and cleanses skin Patchouli oil regenerates skin cells, helping scars and stretch marks to fade, and moisturizes dry skin. An astringent, the oil balances sebum secretions to normalize oily and acne-prone skin. It helps to control acne, and to treat sores and impetigo. Its antifungal action is useful for treating athlete's foot.

Repels insects The oil can ward off insects. Use neat on bites and stings.

Aids detox Patchouli oil has a diuretic effect, making it useful in anti-cellulite skincare products and massage oils.

Enhances wellbeing The oil acts as an anti-depressant, and is useful for treating exhaustion, stress, and anxiety. It's also used as an aphrodisiac.

Aids digestion Its balancing effect relieves diarrhoea and constipation.

Best **uses**

As a perfume Patchouli and rose makes a classic scent. Add 10 drops of patchouli and 20 drops of rose absolute to 2 tablespoons base oil or vodka.

As a massage oil Add patchouli oil to a base oil for an uplifting and relaxing massage that relieves tension and anxiety, and can also help to boost a sluggish digestion.

Safe usage *Non-toxic, non-irritant in dilution.*

The plant

***The patchouli bush**, native to India and Malaysia, is called "puchaput". To produce the oil the leaves are lightly fermented or scalded to break the cell walls and release the aroma.*

The essential oil

***The leaves are steam-distilled** to produce a pale yellow to pale green oil with a spicy, woody, musky scent prized by perfume makers. The smell is rather "love it or hate it", so it's best used in small amounts and in blends.*

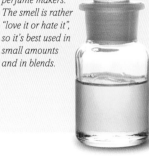

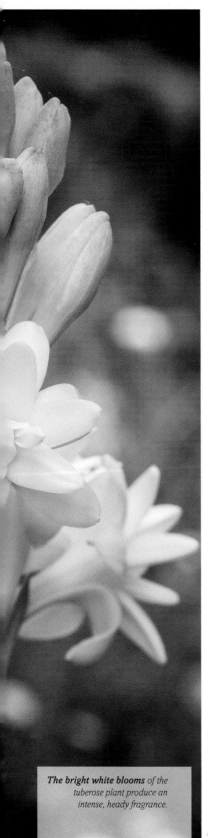

The bright white blooms of the tuberose plant produce an intense, heady fragrance.

MASSAGE OIL

DIFFUSER

Tuberose
Polianthes tuberosa

Tuberose helps to **calm** the nervous system and is widely used to provide **relief** from depression, anger, nervous exhaustion, stress, and tension. The same calming and uplifting properties make it a natural **aphrodisiac** for both men and women.

What is it **good for?**

Acts as a mild sedative Calming on the nervous system, the oil acts like a sedative to help promote restful sleep.

Boosts circulation This warming oil can help to improve circulation and chase away winter chills.

Balances emotions Tuberose is a grounding oil. It increases emotional stamina, relieving stress, tension, anxiety, depression, and anger, and also inspires creativity and calm.

Acts as an aphrodisiac A relaxing oil, the heady, sensual aroma helps to release inhibitions and lift a low libido, especially when due to stress.

Combats body odour A strong, long-lasting, floral aroma combined with antibacterial properties helps to eliminate body odour.

Best **uses**

As a massage oil Make a warming massage oil by adding 10–20 drops of tuberose to 2 tablespoons base oil. As it has a strong, heady aroma, a little goes far, so it's best to dilute well.

In a diffuser Spice up the atmosphere in a room by adding 3–4 drops of the oil to a diffuser, vaporizer, or oil burner.

***Safe usage** Use well diluted (less than 1 per cent). Avoid use on hypersensitive skin and on children under seven years old.*

The plant

***The night-blooming tuberose** is also known as the "Night Queen". It takes around 1550kg (3000lb) of handpicked flowers to extract 0.5kg (1lb) of the absolute oil. Tuberose is related to narcissus and jonquil and has distinctive tubular flowers.*

The essential oil

***The dark orange–brown viscous** absolute is solvent-extracted from the flowers. It has a strong, spicy–sweet, creamy aroma.*

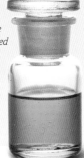

STEAM
INHALATION

OINTMENT

Ravensara, Ravintsara

Ravensara aromatica, Cinnamomum camphora

A warming, stimulating oil with **antiviral** and **antiseptic** properties, this oil is a natural choice during the cold and flu season. Confusion around the oil's source (see box, below), means the oil is now commonly called ravintsara, though the name ravensara is still seen.

What is it **good for?**

Provides cold and flu relief
The oil's decongestant and antiviral properties can ease cold and flu symptoms such as coughs and sinusitis, and cleanse air in sick rooms.

Combats viruses Its antiviral properties are useful for treating cold sores, shingles, and herpes.

Enhances wellbeing Stimulating and reviving, ravintsara eases nervous exhaustion and stress, and helps to lift depression and negative thoughts.

Boosts immunity Ravintsara has immunostimulant properties, which means it can help support immunity, especially when defences are low due to stress and overwork.

Aids digestion Gently massaged into the abdomen, the oil stimulates digestion, while its antiseptic properties make it a useful treatment for tummy upsets and gastric flu.

Relieves pain The oil has a relaxing and analgesic action on aching muscles and joints, and can be used in a compress to soothe and treat sprains and strains.

Best **uses**

In a steam inhalation To relieve sinus or respiratory tract infections, add 3–4 drops to a bowl of hot water, cover your head and the bowl with a towel, and breathe deeply for 15 minutes. Blend with oils that have similar decongestant properties, such as eucalyptus, thyme, or pine.

As a cold-sore treatment The oil can be used neat to treat cold sores. Dab on with a cotton swab as needed.

Safe usage Non-toxic, non-irritant in dilution.

The plant

There is confusion *around this oil. In the past, the name ravensara was used for oil from the Agatophyllum aromaticum tree. However, ravensara is used in perfumery; the aromatherapy oil ravintsara is from the leaf of a variety of camphor tree in Madagascar.*

The essential oil

The essential oil *is steam-distilled from the young, leafy twigs. It is a thin, clear to yellow oil with a camphor-like aroma that is somewhere between lavender and tea tree essential oils.*

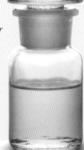

This immune-boosting oil offers protection in the winter months.

SKIN CARE

MASSAGE OIL

Rose

Rosa damascena, R. centifolia

Roses have been used as **medicinal** plants since antiquity, and are celebrated for their calming, **uplifting** aroma. The oil has a toning, **anti-inflammatory**, and **rejuvenating** effect, and its mild detoxifying and antiseptic properties can relieve pain and nausea.

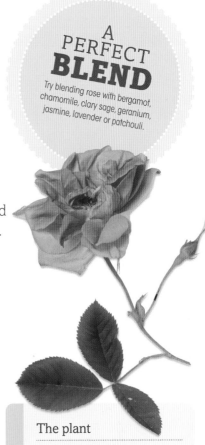

A PERFECT **BLEND**

Try blending rose with bergamot, chamomile, clary sage, geranium, jasmine, lavender or patchouli.

What is it **good for?**

Rejuvenates skin Rose oil supports cell and tissue regeneration, which helps to maintain the skin's elasticity and reduce the appearance of fine lines. It makes an excellent choice for minimizing the appearance of broken capillaries on the skin.

Heals skin The oil helps to repair sun-damaged skin and damage from burns and scalds, as well as reduce the appearance of stretch marks. Its skin-calming and anti-inflammatory properties can soothe dry, hot, itchy skin.

Fights bacteria Rose oil has been shown to have antimicrobial properties. In one study, Damask rose demonstrated antibacterial activity against 15 strains of bacteria.

Enhances wellbeing The oil creates a sense of relaxed wellbeing and can help to increase feelings of vitality. This calming property makes it useful for taking the edge off stress-related conditions.

Supports women's health Rose oil has a toning effect on the uterus, which can help to ease heavy, clotted or painful periods. It is also used to limit the effects of, and provide relief from, premenstrual tension.

Relieves digestive discomfort A mild detoxifying and antiseptic effect, combined with nerve-soothing properties, help relieve tummy upsets, nausea, and constipation. The oil has a fortifying effect on the gallbladder and liver, supporting efficient digestion and absorption of nutrients.

Best **uses**

As a skin toner Make a toner by combining 2 tablespoons witch-hazel and 4 tablespoons rose flower water with 4 drops of rose absolute oil. Put in a plain bottle or spray bottle and use as needed. Shake well before use.

As a massage oil Rose can relieve feelings of depression, anxiety, and grief. Blend 4 drops of rose, 4 drops of geranium and 4 drops of orange essential oils with 2 tablespoons base oil for an uplifting body massage.

Safe usage *Non-irritant. Absolute is non-toxic; use essential oil in dilutions of less than 1 per cent due to its methyl eugenol content.*

The plant

A popular garden shrub, roses are widely grown for their beauty and, with some species, for their fragrance.

The essential oil

When steam-distilled, the essential oil is known as rose otto, and is a clear or pale yellow oil with an intense floral aroma. Rose absolute is also available, which is somewhat less costly, and is an amber-coloured, more viscous, liquid.

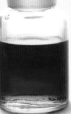

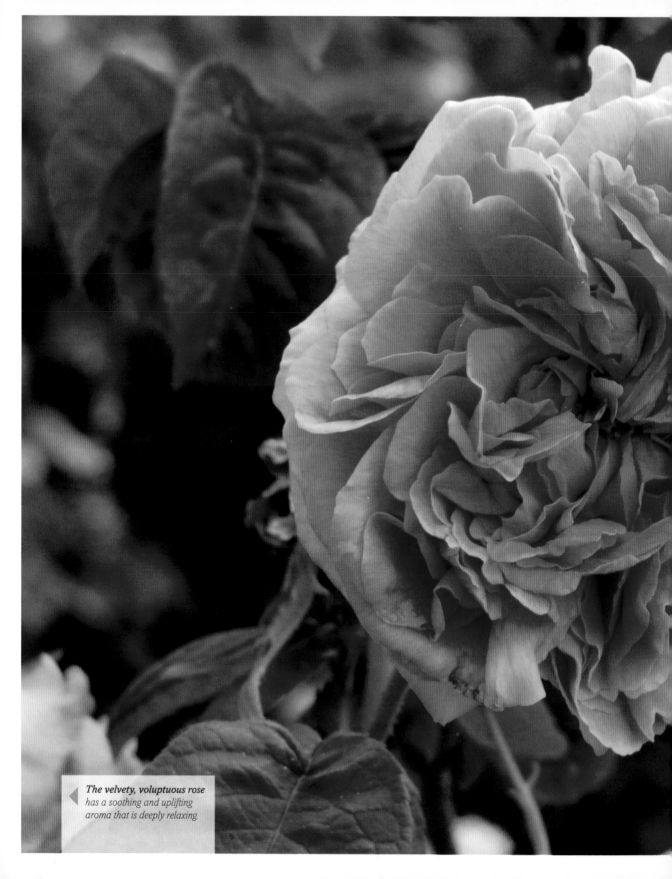

The velvety, voluptuous rose *has a soothing and uplifting aroma that is deeply relaxing.*

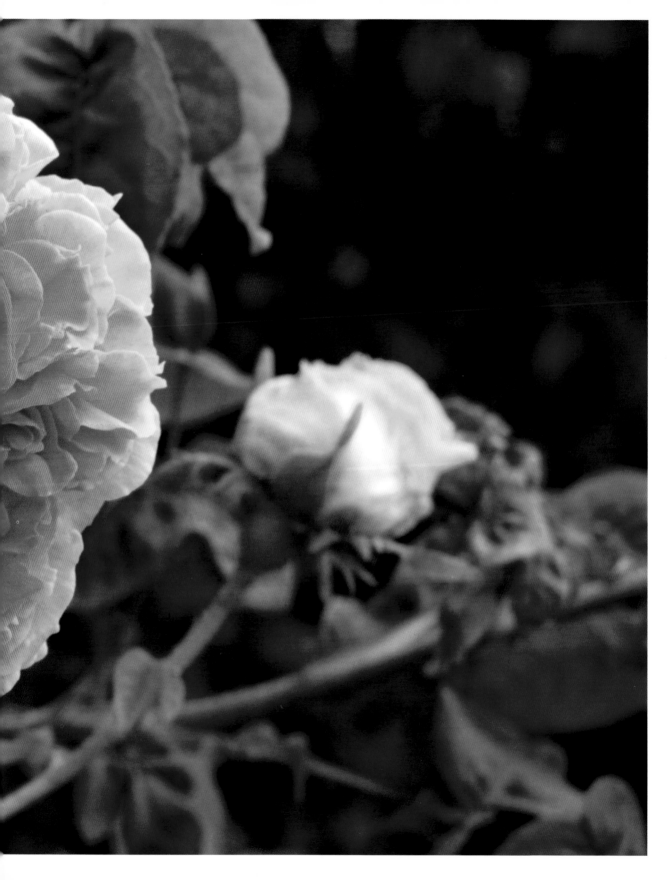

SHOWER

MASSAGE OIL

Rosemary
Rosmarinus officinalis

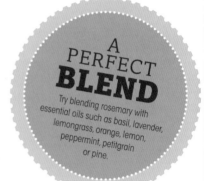
A PERFECT BLEND
Try blending rosemary with essential oils such as basil, lavender, lemongrass, orange, lemon, peppermint, petitgrain or pine.

Toning and **cleansing** rosemary oil helps to clear the mind. It contains potent **antibacterial** and antifungal substances that can fight infection, and has a warming **anti-inflammatory** action that helps relieve pain. Its **stimulating** effect on the lymphatic system aids detox and improves circulation.

What is it **good for?**

Helps fight germs Rosemary essential oil contains rosmarinic acid, which in addition to being anti-inflammatory, is also antiviral and antibacterial. This makes rosemary useful for fighting off respiratory infections and for using topically on skin infections. The oil can be dabbed neat on sores, bites, and scabies to reduce inflammation and aid healing.

Acts as a hair tonic The oil helps to stimulate the circulation, which in turn combats hair loss and dandruff.

Aids detox The oil stimulates both the circulation and lymphatic systems, aiding the removal of waste products and relieving water retention, which in turn helps to fight cellulite.

Boosts circulation Rosemary is useful for treating low blood pressure and warming cold hands and feet. Its boost to circulation also brings some relief to sprains and strains, and soothes sore muscles after exercising.

Improves focus Rosemary essential oil stimulates the nervous system and increases circulation to the brain, which in turn helps to improve memory, concentration, and mental alertness. The oil has a reviving effect when you are feeling tired, debilitated, or lethargic, which also makes it an especially useful remedy for jet lag.

Relieves menstrual cramps The oil's warming and anti-inflammatory properties help to relieve painful period cramping.

Best **uses**

As a shower gel To revive both body and mind, try this after-sport scented shower gel. Add 55 drops of rosemary, 30 drops of peppermint, and 40 drops of lemon essential oils to a 250-ml (9-fl oz) bottle of unfragranced shower gel, and enjoy a refreshing and stimulating shower.

As a massage oil Add 10 drops of the essential oil to 1 tablespoon base oil to create a simple, warming, pain-relieving, and detoxifying massage oil.

Safe usage Non-irritant in dilution. Avoid use near the nose in children under seven years old.

The plant

Rosemary is a popular aromatic herb with silvery green leaves and pale blue flowers. The plant is a Mediterranean native and today is still produced mainly in France, Spain, Croatia, Tunisia, and Morocco. This ubiquitous herb has been used widely in food, medicine, and during religious ceremonies for thousands of years.

The essential oil

The virtually colourless oil that is extracted from rosemary is steam-distilled from the fresh flowering tops of the herb. The essential oil has a pungent, fresh, and pleasant herbaceous aroma.

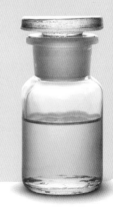

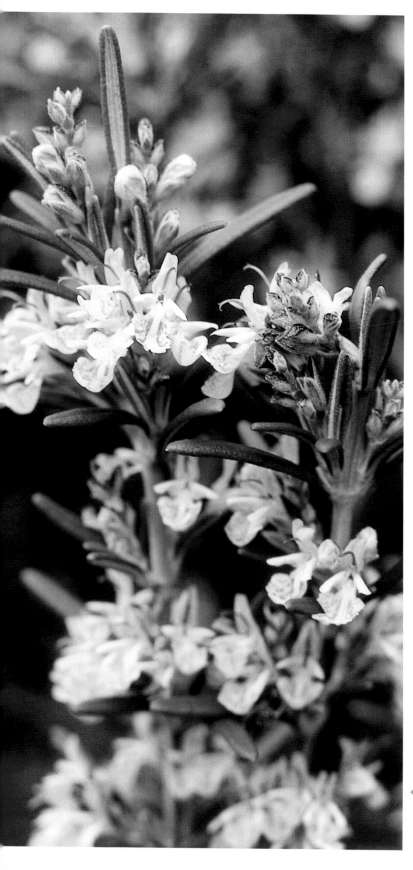

This refreshing and cleansing oil is a popular addition to hair treatments, adding shine to lacklustre hair.

◀ **Rosemary has** *highly fragrant needle-shaped leaves with delicate lavender blue to purple blooms.*

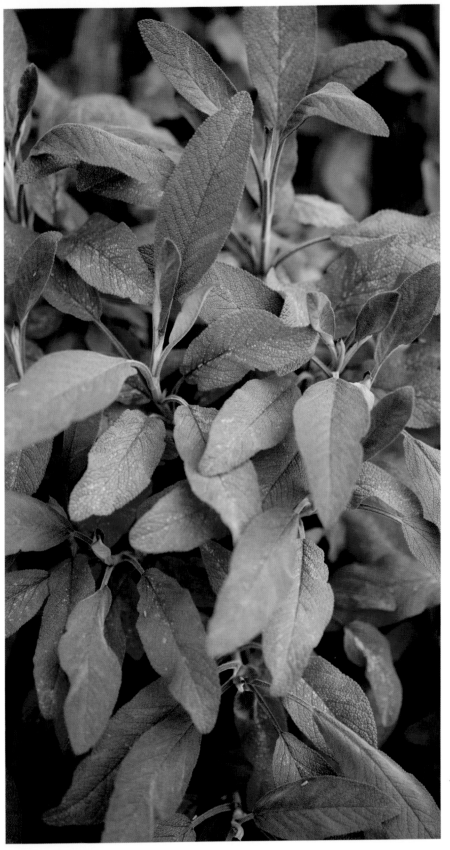

This warming, antibacterial oil has a potent effect and should be diluted well before use.

The finely veined, distinctive leaves of this evergreen shrub are highly aromatic.

MOUTHWASH

FOOT BATH

Sage (Dalmatian)
Salvia officinalis

An extremely stimulating oil, sage is primarily used as a warming oil that can help to relieve aching muscles. The oil also has an **astringent** quality that makes it a useful skin toner. Use it to **relieve** stress and improve mental **focus** when you are tired or under pressure.

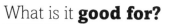

A
PERFECT
BLEND
Essential oil blending partners for sage include bergamot, lavender, lemon, and rosemary.

What is it **good for?**

Acts as an antiseptic Sage essential oil has a particular affinity to the gums, and its antibacterial properties can help to eliminate the bacteria that can harbour in the mouth and cause bad breath and gum disease.

Brightens the complexion Sage has circulation-boosting properties that help to improve skin tone and minimize the appearance of open pores. Its antioxidant action reduces the harmful effects of free radicals, which can make skin look dull, so can help to brighten tired-looking complexions.

Acts as a hair and scalp tonic Sage has an effective anti-fungal action and so is a useful oil to help control dandruff.

Calms nerves During periods of stress and exhaustion, sage can have a tonic effect on the nervous system. It revives and stimulates, bringing renewed vitality.

Acts as a deodorant Sage essential oil has a naturally deodorizing effect that can help to fight body and foot odour. It's useful for relieving excessive sweating, particularly during the menopause.

Best **uses**

As a mouthwash Make an antiseptic mouthwash to treat inflamed gums or combat bad breath by adding 1 drop of sage essential oil to 1 teaspoon glycerine or calendula tincture, then dilute the mixture in half a glass of water. Rinse the mouthwash around the mouth and gums and then spit it out.

In a foot bath To fight foot odour, add 4–5 drops of sage essential oil to a shallow basin of warm water. Soak the feet for 10–15 minutes, then dry them thoroughly.

Safe usage *Use very well diluted (less than 0.5 per cent). Avoid using during pregnancy and when breastfeeding, and avoid using on children under 15 years old. Toxic if ingested.*

The plant

Another popular culinary herb, with an established history of medicinal use, the name "sage" is derived from the Latin word "salvare", which means "heal" or "save". The plant, which has silver–grey leaves and blue to purplish flowers, is a native of the Mediterranean region, but now grows throughout much of the world.

Spanish sage (Salvia lavandulifolia) is often preferable to use rather than Dalmatian sage as it is considerably less harsh, although should still be avoided during pregnancy and when breastfeeding.

The essential oil

Steam-distillation of the dried leaves of the sage plant produces a thin, clear essential oil that has a sharp, slightly spicy, fresh, and herbaceous aroma.

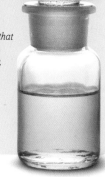

BATH OIL

MASSAGE OIL

Clary sage
Salvia sclarea

Renowned for **uplifting** the mind and emotions, clary sage also has a **tonic** effect on many body systems, including the digestive and circulatory systems. It can **revive** tired muscles, relieve menstrual and labour pains, and is considered an **aphrodisiac**.

What is it **good for?**

Lifts mood Clary sage lifts depression and calms nerves, creating a sense of peace and, in some, euphoria. It is used to return vitality after an illness.

Relieves aches and pains A powerful muscle relaxant, clary sage can ease muscular aches and pains.

Aids digestion Massaged over the abdomen, the oil can aid digestion and relieve tummy upsets and wind.

Boosts circulation Its tonic effect is partly due to it boosting the circulation. It can help lower high blood pressure.

Supports women's health The oil can be used to treat the symptoms of PMS, ease period cramps, and relieve anxiety and hot flushes in menopause.

Acts as an aphrodisiac Clary sage can help restore libido and vitality.

Best **uses**

As a bath oil For menstrual pain or stress, add 5–6 drops to 1 tablespoon base oil or full-fat milk and disperse in a bath. Soak for at least 10 minutes.

In a massage oil Add 1–2 drops of clary sage and 2 drops of lavender oils to 1 tablespoon base oil for a massage to aid digestion and boost circulation.

Safe usage Use well diluted to avoid potential skin irritation (less than 0.5 per cent). Avoid on hypersensitive skin and on children under seven years old.

The plant

Related to sage, but with tall, dramatic flower stems, clary sage is a native of southern Europe. The herb has long been prized as a medicinal plant and is also a popular ingredient in perfumes.

The essential oil

The oil is a colourless to pale green liquid with a herbaceous, sweet, slightly nutty aroma. It is steam-distilled from the flowering tops and leaves.

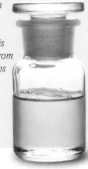

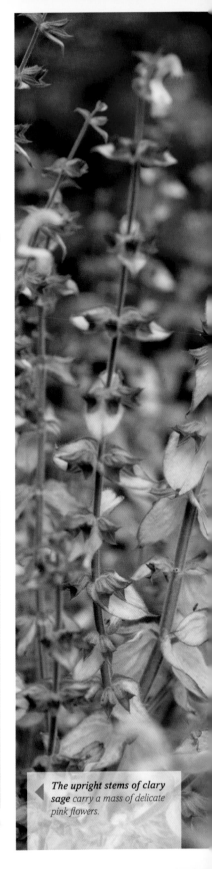

The upright stems of clary sage carry a mass of delicate pink flowers.

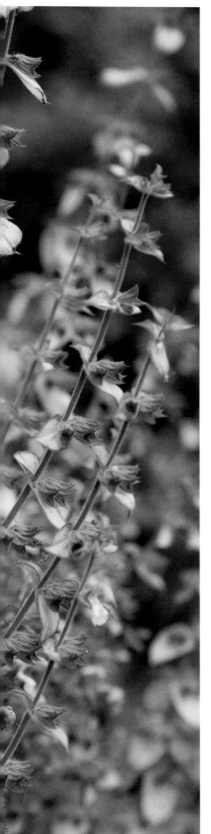

DIFFUSER

FRAGRANCE

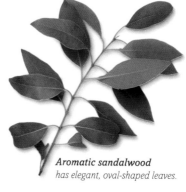

Aromatic sandalwood has elegant, oval-shaped leaves.

Sandalwood

Santalum album

Sandalwood has a long history in Ayurvedic and Chinese medicine. Its **anti-inflammatory** and antiseptic properties **revive** and **heal** dry and damaged skin. It has a **restorative** effect on mind and emotions, and calms respiratory conditions.

What is it **good for?**

Protects and balances skin The oil's anti-inflammatory and astringent effects help to balance skin. It treats oily skin effectively, while also soothing dry, itchy, or inflamed skin. It can reduce the appearance of scars and blemishes and soothe razor burn.

Restores vitality Sandalwood can dispel anxiety and lift depression, aiding sleep and helping to reignite a passion for life. The oil is considered an aphrodisiac, especially for men.

Acts as an antiseptic Its mild antiseptic action is used to ease the effects of genito-urinary tract infections.

Eases breathing Sandalwood has a cooling and anti-inflammatory effect on the mucous membranes and can help calm chronic coughs. A mild decongestant and antiseptic, it can help to treat bronchitis, laryngitis, and respiratory tract infections.

Best **uses**

In a diffuser Add 3–4 drops to a diffuser or to water in a room spray to perfume air and promote calm.

As an aftershave balm For a reviving and calming aftershave balm, add 1 drop of sandalwood essential oil to 1 teaspoon almond base oil. Warm the oil between the palms and then use to soothe skin after shaving.

Safe usage Non-toxic, non-irritant in dilutions of less than 2 per cent.

The plant

The sandalwood tree, a native of India, was for many years such a popular source of essential oil that it became seriously endangered. When buying the oil, it is important to check that it comes from a sustainable source.

The essential oil

The essential oil is steam-distilled from the heartwood of the tree. It is pale yellow to pale gold in colour and has a subtle, sweet, and soothing woody aroma.

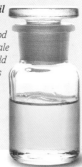

FIRST AID

MASSAGE OIL

STEAM
INHALATION

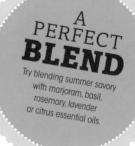

A
PERFECT
BLEND

Try blending summer savory
with marjoram, basil,
rosemary, lavender
or citrus essential oils.

Summer savory

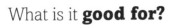

Satureja hortensis

Once believed to be a powerful **aphrodisiac,** monks of the Benedictine
order were banned from growing summer savory in their gardens. Today it is
recognized for its **calming** effect on the digestive system, helping to ease trapped
wind. It is helpful for **boosting strength and resolve** in times of stress.

What is it **good for?**

Helps fight infection Savory has
effective antiseptic properties that
help to combat the bacteria that
can cause skin infections. This makes
it a useful remedy to have on hand
for first-aid applications. Research
has shown that savory essential oil
can inhibit the growth of *Candida
albicans,* the fungus responsible for
athlete's foot and thrush.

Aids digestion The gentle aromatic,
carminative, and digestive properties
of savory essential oil make it a useful
treatment for digestive problems such
as flatulence, nausea, and diarrhoea.

Relieves stress Savory essential oil
has a bolstering effect when you are
feeling stressed to the point of giving
up. It is also helps to motivate when
you feel exhausted at the prospect
of a difficult task.

Soothes sore throats Using the oil
in a diffuser or steam inhalation helps
ease coughs, colds, and sore throats.

Treats bites and stings Dab the
diluted oil on to skin for instant relief
from insect bites and stings.

Promotes hair growth Summer
savory is a traditional remedy for
encouraging hair growth. The diluted
oil can be massaged into the scalp.

Best **uses**

For first aid Mix 3–4 drops of the
essential oil in 1 tablespoon St John's
wort macerated oil or 2 tablespoons
vodka and dab onto insect bites,
or patches of athlete's foot or other
fungal infections.

In a massage oil For a soothing
massage after you've over-indulged,
mix 2–3 drops of the essential oil in
1 tablespoon base oil. Massage
the abdominal area gently in a
clockwise motion.

In an inhalation Add a few drops
to a bowl of warm water and inhale to
relieve congestion and cold symptoms.

*Safe usage Use well diluted (less
than 1.5 per cent). Avoid using on
hypersensitive skin and on children
under seven years old.*

The plant

*The Saxons named savory after its
spicy, pungent taste. A member of the
mint family, summer savory is a
Mediterranean native, with small
leathery leaves and light purple
flowers. It is widely used in cooking.*

*Winter savory (Satureja montana)
is thought to have a stronger antiseptic
action and aroma that makes it less
popular in aromatherapy, but useful
in small quantities to boost the
medicinal properties of other oils.*

The essential oil

*Steam-distilled from the leaves
and stems, the essential oil is pale
yellow to pale orange with a spicy,
herbaceous aroma.*

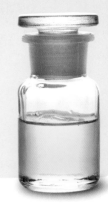

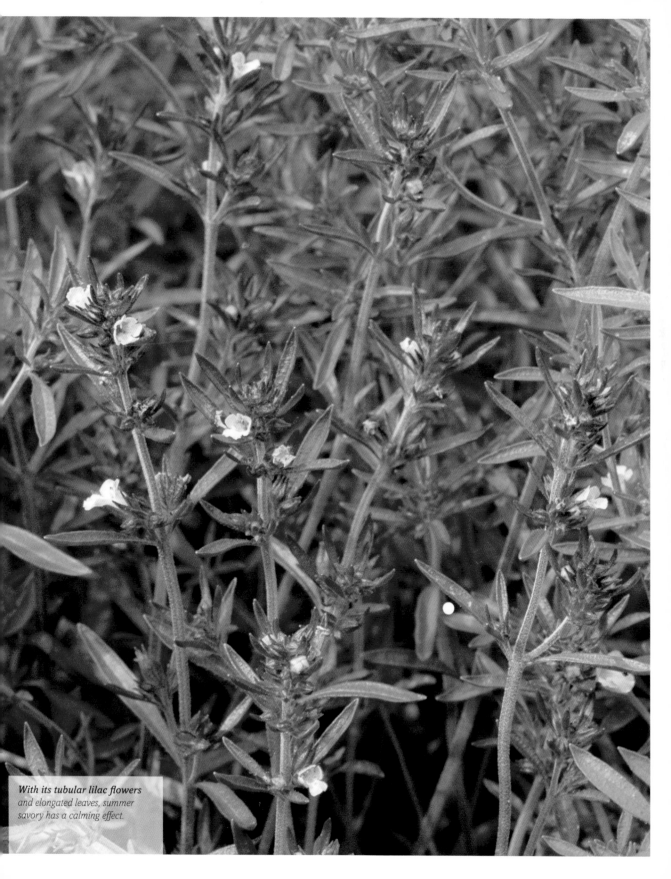

With its tubular lilac flowers and elongated leaves, summer savory has a calming effect.

HAIR CARE

DIFFUSER

STEAM
INHALATION

Benzoin

Styrax benzoin

Benzoin, also known as gum benzoin, is a traditional ingredient in **incense**. Today the oil is added to skin creams for its antiseptic, **healing**, and **calming** properties. In scents, it is a popular fixative, slowing the evaporation of the perfume to help it last longer.

What is it **good for?**

Calms itchy skin Benzoin is an effective remedy for a range of dry, irritable, and itchy skin conditions, including sun- and wind-damaged skin and conditions such as eczema and psoriasis. The oil gives mature skin a boost by increasing elasticity.

Heals wounds The oil has useful antibacterial properties that help heal cuts and wounds. It can be used to treat acne and other skin eruptions.

Eases aches and pains Benzoin essential oil has a local stimulating effect that improves circulation. Used in a massage blend, it can help to loosen stiff muscles and relieve the soreness of arthritis and rheumatism.

Enhances wellbeing Soothing and warming, benzoin is known to have a calming effect on the mind and to help ease depression.

Best **uses**

For hair For an itchy scalp, add 5 drops to a mild unscented shampoo.

In a diffuser Add to a diffuser, vaporizer, or oil burner, for a sweet scent.

In an inhalation A steam inhalation helps clear congestion.

Safe usage Use well diluted (less than 2 per cent). Avoid on hypersensitive skin and on children under two years old.

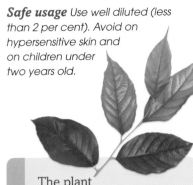

The plant

This large tropical tree is native to Thailand and its adjacent islands. Benzoin resin is collected by making an incision in the trunk that allows the sap to escape. As it flows, the fresh gum is yellowish, but becomes a darker red–brown colour as it dries.

The essential oil

Benzoin oil is golden brown with a sweet, vanilla-like scent. Too thick and sticky to be used undiluted, it is sold as an oleoresin or tincture to be used like an essential oil.

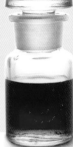

DIFFUSER

OINTMENT

Clove

Syzygium aromaticum, Eugenia caryophyllata

Clove yields a **warming** oil that can be used in small amounts to add **antiseptic** and **analgesic** properties. It is a useful mouthwash for oral infections, and its spicy aroma is comforting and relaxing.

What is it **good for?**

Cares for teeth and gums Widely used in both conventional and complementary dental health products, clove is both an antiseptic and anaesthetic, helping to fight the germs that cause bad breath and relieve swollen gums and toothache.

Calms and treats skin Added to acne treatments, clove oil helps to reduce red, painful inflammation and kill the bacteria that causes acne. It can also be used to treat warts.

Clears congestion Expectorant properties make the oil useful for respiratory infections, such as coughs, colds, sinusitis, and asthma. As a room scent, it clears and disinfects the air.

Relieves anxiety Clove oil has a relaxing, comforting aroma that can reduce anxiety and enhance focus on the task at hand.

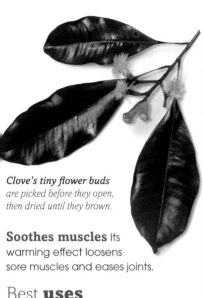

Clove's tiny flower buds are picked before they open, then dried until they brown.

Soothes muscles Its warming effect loosens sore muscles and eases joints.

Best **uses**

In a diffuser Diffuse 2–3 drops to clear or disinfect air.

As a muscle rub Add 3 drops to 1 tablespoon base oil for a warm rub.

Safe usage Use very well diluted (less than 0.5 per cent). Avoid on hypersensitive or damaged skin and on children under seven years old.

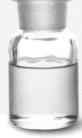

The plant

We tend to think of clove as a spice, but it is actually a herb derived from the dried flower buds of the tree.

The essential oil

The essential oil can be steam-distilled from the leaves, stems, and buds. This yields a clear to pale yellow liquid with a rich and appealing spicy aroma.

DIFFUSER

OINTMENT

Tagetes
Tagetes erecta

Tagetes is traditionally used to treat infections and wounds, **repel** insects, and to clear congestion. The oil also has a **mild sedative** effect that **calms** anxiety and nerves. With its **uplifting** aroma, it is a popular perfumery ingredient, especially in men's fragrances.

What is it **good for?**

Heals wounds The oil has an antiseptic action that can help to treat infection in wounds, cuts, and abscesses, as well as fungal infections.

Relieves cramping Tagetes calms digestive irritation and inflammation and its antispasmodic action relieves menstrual and muscle cramps.

Clears congestion The oil helps to open up the bronchial passages and encourage the removal of phlegm from the sinuses and lungs.

Calms nerves With its mild sedative effect, tagetes eases anxiety, panic, and stress, lifts depression, dispels anger, and can induce relaxation.

Acts as an insect repellent The oil's insecticidal properties can help to repel flies and mosquitoes. Pop some in your bag for holidays.

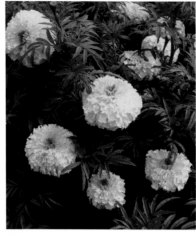

This popular shrub is festooned with bright yellow and orange blooms in summer and autumn.

Best **uses**

In a diffuser Add 3–4 drops to a diffuser, vaporizer, or oil burner to ease coughs, bronchitis, and chest infections, or to use as an insect repellent.

In an ointment To treat fungal infections, add 10–15 drops to an ointment base. Apply as needed.

Safe usage Use well diluted (less than 2 per cent). Highly photo-toxic even in low dilutions so avoid on the skin for 24 hours before exposure to the sun.

The plant

Also called Southern marigold, this member of the marigold family, a popular border shrub, has bright yellow–orange flowers.

The essential oil

The essential oil is steam-distilled from the flowers. It has a golden colour and an aromatic, earthy, floral aroma with hints of citrus.

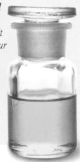

BATH OIL   SKIN CARE

Thyme

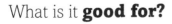
Thymus vulgaris

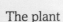

A popular oil for baths and ointments, thyme **boosts** circulation and **relieves** tired and sore muscles and joints. The oil is an effective **antiseptic**, helping to clear fungal infections, as well as fight colds and loosen stubborn phlegm. Its **stimulating** aroma can help clear and **refresh** the mind.

What is it **good for?**

Soothes coughs The antiseptic and antispasmodic properties of thyme essential oil make it a great remedy for easing the symptoms of colds, such as coughs and sore throats, and for soothing the symptoms of chronic bronchitis.

Fights fungal infections Try adding thyme essential oil to hair rinses, or massaging the diluted oil into the scalp, nails, or feet to help clear conditions such as dandruff and seborrheic dermatitis, athletes foot, and fungal nail infections.

Eases aches and pains The oil has a warming effect that helps to loosen tight muscles and ease aching joints.

Helps clear acne Studies show that constituents in thyme can be more effective than benzoyl peroxide, the active ingredient in most anti-acne creams or washes, at killing propionibacterium – the bacterium that causes acne.

Enhances wellbeing Thyme essential oil brings relief when you are feeling anxious, stressed or low.

Treats urinary infections Thyme essential oil's antiseptic and antifungal properties make this oil an ideal choice to help deal with uncomfortable urinary tract infections, such as cystitis.

Improves circulation Thyme essential oil has a stimulating and general toning effect on the circulatory system, which makes it a useful treatment for low blood pressure, weakness, and anaemia.

Best **uses**

As a bath oil Add 5–6 drops of thyme essential oil to 1 tablespoon base oil or eggcupful of milk and disperse in a warm bath to help treat urinary tract infections.

As a skin toner Try blending 2 drops each of thyme and mandarin essential oils in a base of 2 teaspoons aloe vera juice to 90ml (3fl oz) witch hazel. Shake the blend well and apply with a cotton wool ball, or pour the blend into a spray bottle and use as a refreshing facial spritzer.

Safe usage Use well diluted (less than 2 per cent).

The plant

This is a low, creeping aromatic herb that is a member of the mint family. Thyme is native to the Mediterranean region where it thrives in the hot, sunny locations and the well-drained soil. Thyme is widely used as both a culinary and medicinal herb.

The essential oil

The flowering tops and leaves of the popular herb, thyme, can be steam-distilled to create the essential oil. Several different chemotypes are used in the aromatherapy essential oil. Thyme linalol (Thymus vulgaris ct linalol) is more gentle and the most suitable essential oil for general aromatherapy use.

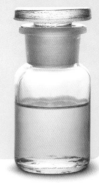

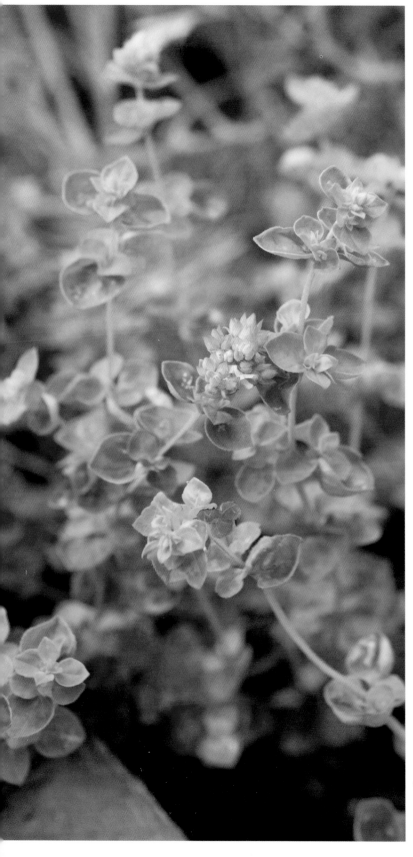

With its antiseptic properties, thyme essential oil is a useful oil for fighting winter colds.

This evergreen shrub has tiny oval-shaped leaves with white or pink flowers in early summer.

SKIN CARE

MASSAGE OIL

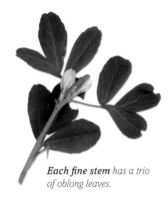

Each fine stem has a trio of oblong leaves.

Fenugreek

Trigonella foenumgraecum

A well-known **digestive aid** and laxative, fenugreek also has a **relaxing** effect on the nerves and an **antiseptic** and expectorant action on respiratory infections. It **stimulates** the circulation and can treat bruises and swelling when applied to the skin.

What is it **good for?**

Clears and soothes skin The oil's antibacterial and antifungal properties help treat skin infections such as boils. It also has an anti-inflammatory quality that relieves itchy, dry skin conditions.

Aids relaxation The oil has a relaxing effect on the nerves that can soothe anxiety and help lower blood pressure.

Eases congestion Fenugreek acts as an expectorant and soothes and relaxes inflamed respiratory tissues.

Aids detox Its tonic and antioxidant properties encourage perspiration and boost the metabolism. A mild laxative, it helps the body to remove waste.

Aids digestion Fenugreek soothes digestive upsets and aids digestion.

Supports women's health The oil can help to ease period pains, regulate cycles, and calm hot flushes.

Best **uses**

As a facial oil Add 4–6 drops of the oil to 1 tablespoon of a light base oil for use on inflamed or acne-prone skin.

In a massage oil Make a relaxing and skin-soothing massage blend by adding 15 drops of fenugreek essential oil to 1 tablespoon base oil. You can also use this to ease indigestion, gently massaging the oil into the abdomen in a clockwise motion.

Safe usage *Non-irritant in dilution.*

The plant

Native to the Middle and Near East, *the spice is also known as methi. Fenugreek produces distinctive, triangular, oil-rich seeds. Its round leaves can be dried and used as herbs.*

The essential oil

The essential oil *is actually an absolute extracted from the seeds. This produces a yellow–brown waxy liquid with a potent, sweet–spicy, earthy scent.*

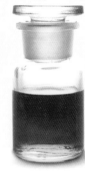

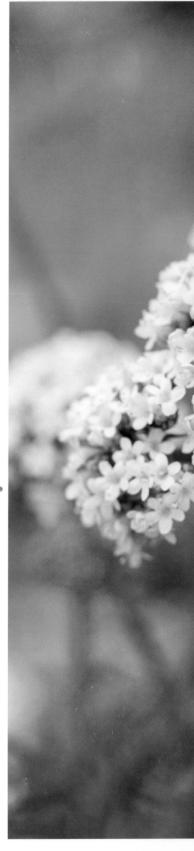

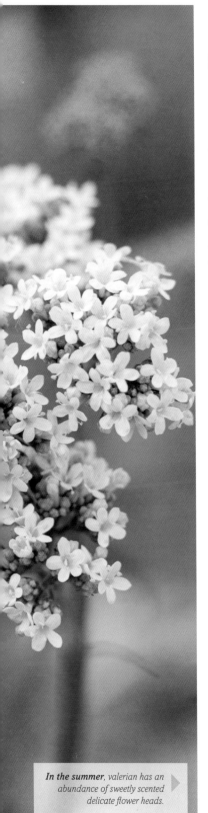

In the summer, valerian has an abundance of sweetly scented delicate flower heads.

BATH OIL

MASSAGE OIL

Valerian

Valeriana officinalis

The most widely used herbal **sedative**, valerian is a recognized treatment for **insomnia** and tension. Its other psychological benefits include **lifting depression** and anxiety. It can help regulate blood pressure, slow palpitations, and settle digestion.

What is it **good for?**

Promotes restful sleep A powerful sedative, valerian can treat insomnia and improve sleep quality.

Balances emotions The oil can help to soothe nerves, and calm anxiety, depression, and restlessness. A good treatment for stress and tension.

Lowers blood pressure Valerian can help to regulate blood pressure and calm a rapid heartbeat.

Aids detox The oil's mild laxative effect encourages healthy bowel movements, and its diuretic action promotes urination. It can also calm an upset stomach, especially when this is linked to stress, and aid the effective metabolism of nutrients.

Supports women's health Valerian soothes stomach cramps and can ease pre-menstrual tension.

Best **uses**

In a bath oil Add 2 drops each of rose, valerian, and sandalwood essential oils to 1 tablespoon base oil or full-fat milk and disperse in a bath.

In a massage oil Added to an oil blend, valerian essential oil can be used to help encourage a state of deep relaxation. Try blending 4 drops each of valerian, lavender, and cedarwood essential oils to 2 tablespoons base oil.

Safe usage Non-toxic, non-irritant in dilution.

The plant

Native to parts of Europe and Asia, the plant has distinctive leathery leaves and clusters of pink or white flowers. The name valerian is derived from the Latin "valere", which means "to be well" or "to feel good".

The essential oil

Steam-distilled from the root, the yellow to yellow–green oil has an earthy, musky, woody aroma that can be overpowering. For the best effect, blend with softer, sweeter oils.

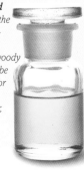

HAIR CARE

DIFFUSER

Vanilla

Vanilla planifolia

A relative newcomer to aromatherapy, vanilla is familiar to most as a flavouring for desserts and baked goods. Its **soothing** and softening properties can help **repair** rough or **damaged** skin. It is a mild **pain-reliever** and has antiseptic properties.

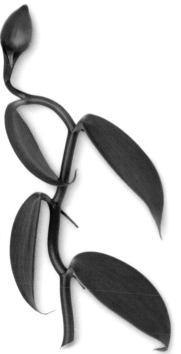

The green vanilla pods are dried prior to use.

What is it **good for?**

Soothes dry skin Vanilla essential oil has skin- and hair-softening and soothing properties. It is also rich in antioxidants that can help protect the skin from the damage caused by environmental pollutants and toxins.

Acts as a painkiller The main aromatic chemical in vanilla is vanillin, which has similar pain-relieving properties to the capsaicin found in chilli peppers. When vanilla oil is diluted, it can be used on the skin to provide temporary, localized relief from general aches and pains and from toothache.

Helps relieve stress Vanilla can be used to help dispel general feelings of negativity as well as feelings of anxiety. This uplifting property is also thought to contribute to its aphrodisiac effect.

Helps to treat acne A mild antibacterial action enables vanilla essential oil to help fight the bacteria that cause acne and to reduce the occurrence of more minor pimples, blackheads, and spots.

Best **uses**

As a hair conditioner Add 10 drops of vanilla essential oil to 1 tablespoon coconut oil to make a hair mask that will condition and add shine to hair. Coat hair thoroughly and wrap in a towel for 10–15 minutes before shampooing and rinsing.

In a diffuser To help relieve stress and ease anxiety, add 1–2 drops of vanilla absolute to a diffuser, vaporizer, or oil burner.

Safe usage Non-toxic and non-irritant.

The plant

The vanilla bean is actually the fruit pod from a type of orchid. The green pods are dried slowly until they turn black. Once they start to curl, the pods are ready to use either as a culinary flavouring or to produce an essential oil absolute.

The essential oil

A thick, dark brown oil, vanilla absolute is solvent-extracted from the cured seed pods. Its familiar, sometimes overwhelming, scent, should be used sparingly in any blend.

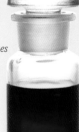

With its strong scent, just small amounts of vanilla are needed.

BATH OIL

DIFFUSER

Vetiver

Vetiveria zizanioides

Working mostly on an emotional level, vetiver has a profoundly **grounding** effect for those who are distressed or panicky. The essential oil can help to improve circulation and is a useful **antiseptic** and **astringent** in the treatment of oily and combination skin.

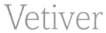
A PERFECT **BLEND**
Vetiver blends well with clary sage, cedarwood, jasmine, lavender, patchouli, rose, ginger, ylang ylang and citrus oils.

What is it **good for?**

Soothes sore muscles Vetiver oil makes a warming and pain-relieving remedy for muscular aches and pains, sprains, general stiffness, and for rheumatism and arthritis.

Helps heal wounds Its antiseptic and slightly astringent properties make this oil a good treatment for cuts, grazes, wounds, and sores.

Helps fade scars and marks By promoting skin-healing and the growth of new tissue, vetiver is ideal for reducing the appearance of stretch marks, scars, and burns.

Has a cooling action Add vetiver to a cold compress to cool fever, sunstroke, and soothe headaches.

Promotes emotional balance Vetiver is grounding and calming when you are feeling emotionally overwhelmed, weepy, under pressure, and uncertain which direction to take. It can help relieve distress, anger, and hysteria in both adults and children.

Acts as an aphrodisiac Vetiver is thought to enhance libido and is often used to awaken sexual desire in men and women, especially when libido has been dampened by overwork and mental fatigue.

Promotes restful sleep A natural sedative, the oil is often used to promote relaxation and restful sleep.

Best **uses**

As a bath oil Make a relaxing bath oil by mixing 4–6 drops in 1 tablespoon base oil or full-fat milk. Disperse in a warm bath and have a quiet soak for at least 15 minutes.

In a diffuser Promote a peaceful, grounding atmosphere in your home or office by adding 3–4 drops of the essential oil to a diffuser, vaporizer, or oil burner.

Safe usage *Non-toxic, non-irritant in dilution.*

The plant

A tall perennial grass *native to India, vetiver is a relative of other fragrant grasses such as citronella, lemongrass, and palmarosa. Roots over 24 months old have the highest oil content, but take longer to distil, making this an expensive oil.*

The essential oil

The oil is steam-distilled *from the chopped up rootlets, which are soaked in water prior to distillation. The resulting oil is a thick, dark amber liquid with a spicy, earthy fragrance that has a hint of lemon.*

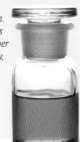

STEAM
INHALATION

SKIN CARE

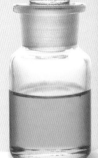

A
PERFECT
BLEND

Ideal blending partners for violet essential
oil include tuberose, clary sage, lavender,
benzoin, cumin, basil, sandalwood,
geranium, and citrus
essential oils.

Violet

Viola odorata

Violet is renowned for its **relaxing,** soothing, and inspiring properties.
It is a traditional remedy for calming irritations to the respiratory tract,
rejuvenating mature or weather-damaged skin, and **soothing** sensitive skin
conditions. Its elegant floral aroma is **calming** on the mind and emotions.

What is it **good for?**

Soothes dry skin Violet essential
oil has a gentle and reviving effect on
the skin and is well-known for its ability
to help hydrate and soothe dry and
sun- or wind-damaged skin. It is used
to help minimize the appearance of
spider veins and enlarged pores.

Acts as a painkiller The oil contains
anti-inflammatory compounds that
can relieve pain and inflammation in
muscles and joints; applied locally, it
can encourage circulation to an
affected area. It can also provide relief
for headaches and migraines.

Helps treat anxiety The oil is
comforting and calming when you are
feeling nervous, anxious, or exhausted.
This grounding effect can also help to
ease feelings of dizziness brought on
by anxiety and stress.

Eases congestion Violet has
expectorant properties that help to
shift phlegm and relieve the pressure
caused by blocked sinuses.

Best **uses**

As an inhalation Make a steam
inhalation by adding 5–6 drops of
violet essential oil to a bowl of hot
water. Place a towel over your head
and inhale deeply to loosen catarrh
or relieve anxiety. This is also an
effective way to condition and
cleanse the skin.

As a facial elixir Make a quick,
but luxurious, facial oil by adding
2 drops of violet absolute and carrot
seed oil to 1 tablespoon rosehip
seed oil.

Safe usage *Non-toxic, non-irritant
in dilution.*

The plant

*The essential oil of violet is an
absolute, concentrated in the downy
heart-shaped leaves rather than in
the purple flowers. It takes around
1000kg (2200lb) of violet leaves to
produce just 1kg (2¼lb) of the
absolute, which is why true violet
absolute is so expensive, and mostly
used in high-end perfume products.*

The essential oil

*The absolute essential oil of violet
is solvent-extracted from the crushed
leaves of the plant. This process
produces a thick oil that is a green
to brown colour. It has an earthy
aroma with intense, elegant
floral notes that
make it a
valuable
ingredient
in perfumes.*

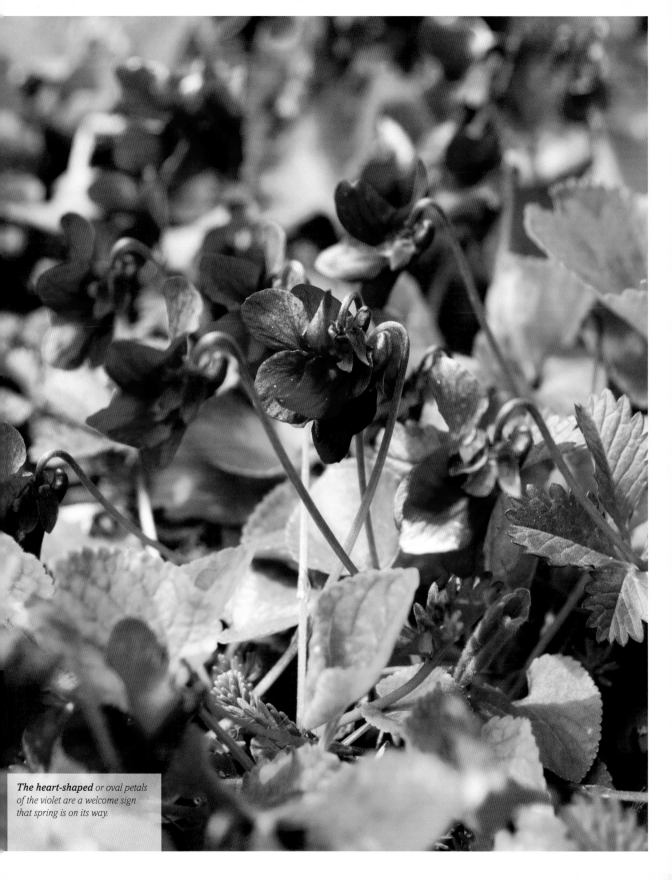

The heart-shaped or oval petals of the violet are a welcome sign that spring is on its way.

COMPRESS

DIFFUSER

Plai

Zingiber cassumunar, Z. montanum

Although plai is related to ginger, it is a **cooling,** rather than a warming, oil, making it ideal for feverish conditions and inflammation. It has a general **tonic** effect on the body and is highly valued for its ability to **relieve** the pain of arthritis and rheumatism and even post-operative pain. Plai is also a traditional Thai treatment for stretch marks.

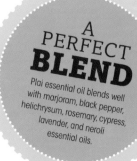

A
PERFECT
BLEND

Plai essential oil blends well with marjoram, black pepper, helichrysum, rosemary, cypress, lavender, and neroli essential oils.

What is it **good for?**

Acts as an antihistamine With its cooling, anti-inflammatory action, plai makes a natural antihistamine that can be helpful for managing conditions such as hay fever. Its soothing action has the potential to reduce the severity of asthma attacks in some individuals, where it can be used as a complementary treatment alongside prescribed medication.

Acts as a painkiller Plai essential oil is a popular analgesic that helps to ease many types of pain, including pain caused by injury, strained muscles, arthritis, and rheumatism. Some evidence suggests it may help relieve post-operative pain and inflammation.

Fades scars and stretch marks In Thailand, plai is a traditional remedy used to reduce the appearance of stretch marks and scars.

Relieves abdominal cramps Plai essential oil has antispasmodic and analgesic properties that can help to relieve menstrual cramping as well as the pain that is caused by irritable bowel syndrome.

Best **uses**

As a compress To help soothe and relieve sprains and strains, add 4–5 drops of plai essential oil to a shallow bowl of cool water, then soak a small, clean cloth in the mixture, wring it out well, and apply the cloth to the affected area.

In a diffuser To relieve the misery of hay fever and help reduce the severity of asthma attacks, try adding 3–4 drops of plai essential oil to a diffuser, vaporizer, or oil burner to disperse in a room.

Safe usage Non toxic, non-irritant in dilution.

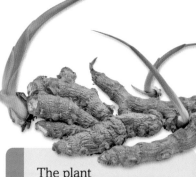

The plant

The therapeutic properties of the plai plant are concentrated in its distinctive root. It is also an ornamental plant with its distinctive blade-shaped leaves and brightly coloured "pseudo-stem" that resembles a pine cone.

The essential oil

Steam-distilled from the fresh roots of the plai plant, the colourless to pale yellow oil has an uplifting herbaceous, spicy aroma with hints of eucalyptus.

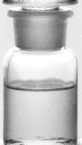

MOUTHWASH   MASSAGE OIL

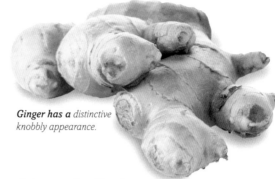

Ginger has a distinctive knobbly appearance.

Ginger
Zingiber officinale

Most of us know ginger as the remedy of choice for reviving and **relieving** the nausea that often accompanies pregnancy or travel sickness. In addition, it is also a useful **antiseptic** in cases of cold or flu, and it has an **analgesic** property that can help to ease tension headaches and muscular pain.

What is it **good for?**

Eases digestion Ginger has a wonderfully calming effect on the digestive system, helping to soothe unsettled digestion caused by stress or over-indulgence. It also relieves pregnancy-related nausea and nausea caused by motion sickness or the side effects of medication.

Revives a tired mind Comforting and warming, ginger essential oil helps to lift feelings of general fatigue and is also reviving when you are suffering from nervous fatigue or mental confusion.

Helps to combat colds Antiseptic and pain-relieving, ginger essential oil can help to ward off cold viruses, and once a cold has set in, it can soothe the pain and discomfort of sore throats, and ease congestion.

Relieves muscle pain Applied locally, ginger oil boosts circulation and provides warmth that revives and eases the pain of sore, tired muscles.

Relieves headaches Its anti-inflammatory and analgesic properties make ginger a natural choice for relieving headaches and migraines.

Best **uses**

For a gargle Add 2 drops of ginger essential oil to 1 teaspoon vodka and dilute in a small tumblerful of hot water. When sufficiently cooled, use as a gargle to treat sore throats.

In a massage oil For quick relief from headaches, migraines, and/or nausea, blend 2 drops of ginger essential oil with 1 teaspoon base oil. Massage gently into the temples and pulse points as needed.

Safe usage Non-toxic, non-irritant in dilution.

The plant

The ginger plant produces a distinctive, knobbly root that has been used as a culinary and medicinal ingredient for thousands of years, especially by the Chinese. Its enduring popularity is testament to the plant's therapeutic healing properties and its widespread culinary appeal.

The essential oil

Ginger essential oil is steam-distilled from the fleshy root of the ginger plant. The oil can vary in colour from pale yellow to dark amber and has a warm, spicy, woody scent with a hint of lemon and pepper.

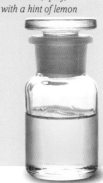

Naturally soothing, ginger is the go-to remedy for digestive upsets.

Base Oils

Base, or carrier, oils provide a medium for **diluting and dispersing** concentrated essential oils, which can otherwise irritate skin. Derived from **vegetable, nut, or seed sources**, or made by macerating a **herb in a plant** oil, base oils have their own benefits.

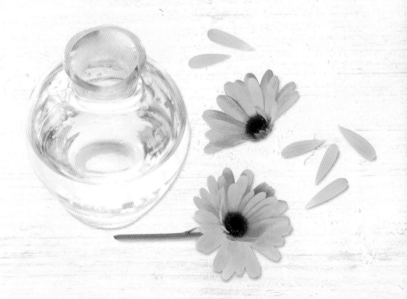

Argan

Argania spinosa

Argan oil comes from a tree found growing only in Morocco. With high levels of antioxidant **vitamin E** and essential fatty acids, it's a soothing oil for all skin types, and for hair and nails. It is **moisturizing** and protective against environmental factors, such as weather and pollutants.

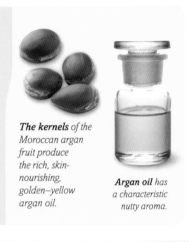

The kernels of the Moroccan argan fruit produce the rich, skin-nourishing, golden–yellow argan oil.

Argan oil has a characteristic nutty aroma.

What is it **good for?**

Makes an all-round moisturizer
A non-greasy, dry oil that can be used under make-up during the day and for skin repair at night, argan can minimize the appearance of scars and stretch marks and help to soften sun- or wind-damaged skin. Apply sparingly to lips before bedtime to aid healing and repair skin overnight.

Acts as a hand conditioner
Warm a few drops of the oil in the palms, then massage well into the hands, taking extra time to work into the nails and cuticles.

Conditions hair For damaged or dry hair, argan oil conditions and restores shine. Use as a pre-wash deep treatment, or for frizzy hair, rub a few drops into the hair just after washing for light control.

Tones skin With regular use, the oil helps to balance oily skin and reduce inflammation around spots and acne.

Borage

Borago officinalis

This oil is pressed from the seeds of the borage, or starflower, plant. Added to a base oil blend, it has a **beneficial effect** on mature, damaged, **sensitive skin**, or skin prone to breakouts due to hormonal fluctuations.

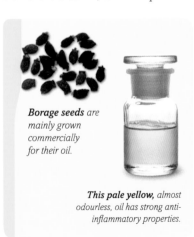

Borage seeds are mainly grown commercially for their oil.

This pale yellow, almost odourless, oil has strong anti-inflammatory properties.

What is it **good for?**

Rejuvenates skin Borage is a great choice for mature or damaged skin. It contains the fatty acid gamma linolenic acid (GLA), which helps to tone and rejuvenate skin. It has a hydrating effect and is regenerating, increasing skin-cell strength and improving elasticity.

Reduces inflammation Its anti-inflammatory properties make borage a good choice for skin prone to eczema, psoriasis, seborrheic

The borage herb is native to the Mediterranean region.

dermatitis, and breakouts due to hormonal fluctuations.

Keeps nails healthy Use the oil regularly on nails to maintain strength and keep cuticles healthy.

Enriches skin Just a small amount of this oil enriches a base oil blend. In blends and serums, borage is used at 2–10 per cent of the total base oil mix.

Canola

Brassica napus

Also known as rapeseed oil, canola has the benefits of being **widely available**, relatively **inexpensive**, and effective on dry, sensitive, or mature skin. However, it's often genetically modified and highly processed so choose organic brands.

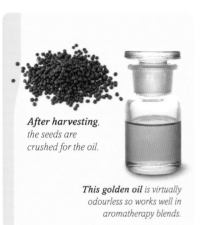

After harvesting, the seeds are crushed for the oil.

This golden oil is virtually odourless so works well in aromatherapy blends.

What is it **good for?**

Moisturizes skin Light and easily absorbed, canola helps to maintain the moisture balance of dry skin.

It is a widely available base oil You don't need to go to a specialist shop to find canola. Good, food-quality canola is available in the supermarket. Canola is also very stable so keeps for a long time.

Provides a neutral base The oil is almost odourless, so works well with

From the brassica family, canola has delicate yellow blooms.

most blends. Enrich it with avocado, borage or rosehip seed oil, or enhance its skin-soothing properties by adding a healing macerate such as calendula or St John's wort.

Safe usage *Ideally, choose organic oil to avoid possible pesticide residues that can be present in some genetically modified organisms (GMOs).*

Shea nut butter

Butyrospermum parkii

Extracted from the nuts of African karite trees, shea butter has a long history in cooking, but has more recently found its way into cosmetic formulations where its thick, **waxy texture** acts like an **emulsifier** and provides **skin-enriching** properties.

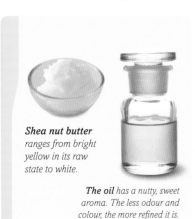

Shea nut butter ranges from bright yellow in its raw state to white.

The oil has a nutty, sweet aroma. The less odour and colour, the more refined it is.

What is it **good for?**

Repairs damaged skin Rich in fatty acids, antioxidant carotenoids, and vitamin E, shea nut butter helps to improve the condition of dry and mature skin and soothes eczema, psoriasis, skin allergies, and blemishes. It can also be used to treat dry, itchy scalp conditions.

Hydrates skin The fatty acids in shea nut butter are a good match for those in human skin. By helping to form a thin protective layer on the

skin, the oil helps prevent moisture loss and encourages healing of chapped lips. It also helps to soften cracked, dry skin on heels, elbows, and knees.

Can be used as a shaving balm Adding shea nut butter to shaving cream formulations helps to achieve a smoother shave.

Calendula macerated oil

Calendula officinalis

Calendula macerated oil is made by infusing marigold flowers into an oil such as sunflower. The result is a **rich** herbal oil with recognized **healing** properties. Calendula is especially popular for sensitive and dry skin due to its ability to **soothe** irritated skin quickly and **repair** skin tissue.

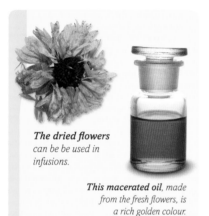

The dried flowers can be be used in infusions.

This macerated oil, made from the fresh flowers, is a rich golden colour.

What is it **good for?**

Repairs skin Calendula is mildly antiseptic so it can help ulcers, skin eruptions, cuts, and dermatitis to heal more quickly.

Can be used as after-sun skin care Calendula oil helps to condition and restore skin, and reduces inflammation after sun exposure.

Acts as a healing massage oil Calendula makes a good choice when a large area of skin requires attention as the oil spreads more easily over a large surface area than a cream-based product does.

Can be used for first aid Hypercal cream, which is a mainstay of most natural first-aid kits, is a mixture of hypericum (St John's wort) and calendula. If you are making a skin salve or ointment, add calendula macerate to help speed healing time.

Coconut

Cocos nucifera

This is a light, **moisturizing**, and **nourishing** semi-solid that quickly melts at body temperature. Coconut oil is suitable for all skin and hair types, but is especially beneficial for dry skin and hair. Raw, unrefined, unbleached organic coconut oil is best and adds a **pleasant aroma** to blends.

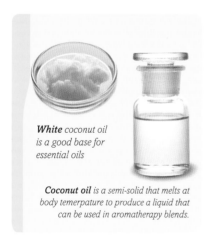

White coconut oil is a good base for essential oils

Coconut oil is a semi-solid that melts at body temerpature to produce a liquid that can be used in aromatherapy blends.

What is it **good for?**

Conditions hair Coconut oil helps combat dandruff and can restore lustre and shine to dry or damaged hair. Use the oil as a pre-shampoo conditioner or, for deeper conditioning, leave in overnight and wash the oil out in the morning.

Acts as a make-up remover Warm a little bit of coconut oil between the palms, then gently massage over the face and use a tissue or a damp facecloth to remove make up.

Heals rough, irritated skin The oil has an anti-inflammatory effect that can help to heal wounds, blisters, and rashes and to soothe razor burn after shaving. Use in place of mineral oil for chapped lips and for eczema and dermatitis.

Cares for teeth and gums The practice of "oil pulling" – swishing around 1 tablespoon coconut oil in the mouth for 20 minutes – helps to reduce bacteria, control plaque, and fight decay and infection. Don't swallow; there's also no need to rinse afterwards.

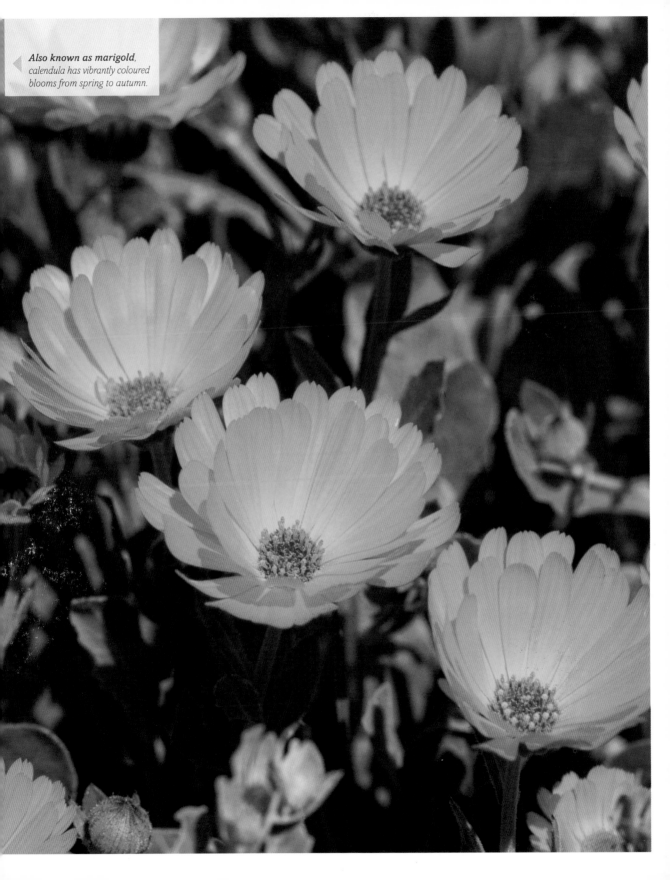

Also known as marigold, calendula has vibrantly coloured blooms from spring to autumn.

Hazelnut

Corylus avellana

A light oil with a fine texture and mild, nutty aroma, hazelnut is **rich in nutrients**, including vitamin E and linoleic acid, an essential fatty acid that protects the outer layer of skin. A **nourishing** oil, it is ideal for **reviving** dull, damaged, or dry skin. Its gentle **astringent** action improves skin tone.

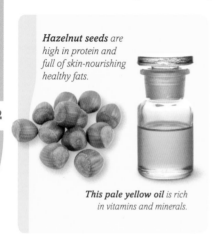

Hazelnut seeds are high in protein and full of skin-nourishing healthy fats.

This pale yellow oil is rich in vitamins and minerals.

What is it **good for?**

Balances skin Hazelnut oil is an excellent choice for a facial massage oil, especially for oily or acne-prone skin types. Its astringent action helps to tone and balance skin, while its emollient properties provide moisture and protection for skin. The oil can also be used to balance and condition oily hair.

Protects skin Its light texture makes this oil a good choice for wind- and sun-damaged skin. It can be added to skin creams to take advantage of its mild SPF factor, and to after-sun treatments to help repair and condition skin.

Works in a blend Hazelnut can be used on its own or as an enriching oil for a base-oil blend. For example, if skin is very dry but still needs toning, try blending this oil with a deeply moisturizing oil such as rosehip seed or avocado oil to create the combination that's right for your skin.

Sunflower

Helianthus annuus

A popular and affordable all-purpose oil, sunflower blends easily with other bases and essential oils. It is very high in **vitamin E**, which repairs and protects skin, and is easily absorbed into the skin.

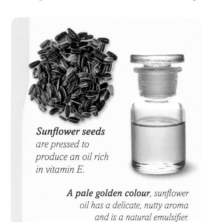

Sunflower seeds are pressed to produce an oil rich in vitamin E.

A pale golden colour, sunflower oil has a delicate, nutty aroma and is a natural emulsifier.

What is it **good for?**

The cheery sunflower produces edible seeds.

Hydrates skin There is evidence that sunflower oil can help to improve the barrier function of the skin, helping skin to retain moisture and fight off infection. This effect is due to the presence of light waxes, which help form a protective emollient barrier on the skin.

Heals skin The oil is protective and helps to repair sun-damaged skin. Healing vitamin E and carotenoids (a vegetable form of vitamin A) can reduce scarring and smooth the appearance of existing wrinkles and fine lines. In addition, the oil contains omega-6 linoleic acid, which helps decrease skin inflammation in acne, eczema, and sunburn, and helps to generate new skin cells.

Treats acne The carotenoids in the oil are excellent for cleansing and moisturizing acne-prone skin.

St. John's wort macerated oil

Hypericum perforatum

The well-known **sedative** effects of St John's wort herb also exist in the macerated oil, which is made by infusing a base oil with the fresh or dried herb. It has a **pain-relieving** effect, and its **anti-inflammatory** properties have a calming action on red, sore or inflamed skin conditions.

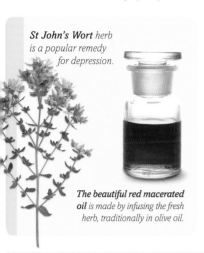

St John's Wort herb is a popular remedy for depression.

The beautiful red macerated oil is made by infusing the fresh herb, traditionally in olive oil.

What is it **good for?**

Calms inflammation Try using this oil to treat dry, painful inflamed skin conditions, such as eczema, psoriasis, and some types of lupus. It can also be used at the first sign of a tingle to treat cold sores and viral skin lesions.

Acts as a painkiller The oil can help calm nerve pain and soothe inflamed joints and tendonitis, as well as reduce inflammation in sunburn, minor scalds, cuts, and grazes. It can also relieve muscle and nerve pain.

Is a good massage base St John's wort adds a grounding, earthy aroma to a massage. It can be used on its own or added to massage oil blends to boost the effects of a relaxing massage. It also works well added to blends intended to treat nervousness, depression, and premenstrual or menopausal symptoms.

Safe usage *Do not apply before sun exposure as the oil may increase the photo-sensitivity of the skin.*

Flaxseed oil

Linum usitatissimum

Pressed from the tiny seeds of the plant, flaxseed oil is **rich in omega-3 fatty acids** and vitamin E, making it a **rejuvenating** oil for tired, dry or mature skin. Also known as linseed oil, it has **antioxidant** and **anti-inflammatory** qualities that can benefit acne-prone skin.

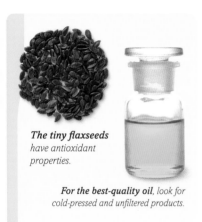

The tiny flaxseeds have antioxidant properties.

For the best-quality oil, look for cold-pressed and unfiltered products.

What is it **good for?**

Fades scars and stretch marks The high vitamin E content of flaxseed oil helps to reduce the appearance of scarring and stretch marks.

Hydrates skin Flaxseed oil seals in moisture, making a reviving remedy for dry skin conditions. Its anti-inflammatory action calms eczema and psoriasis.

Has anti-ageing effects The omega-3 fatty acids in flaxseed oil help protect and rejuvenate skin cells, brightening dull-looking skin and smoothing the appearance of lines.

Treats acne Use the oil to cleanse and condition oily or acne-prone skin and rosacea. It contains omega-3 alpha-linolenic acid (ALA), a powerful anti-inflammatory that reduces the soreness and redness around acne.

Enriches base oil blends Flax seed generally isn't used on its own, but is added to other base oils, creams, and lotions to add skin-strengthening properties.

Macadamia

Macadamia ternifolia

This **protective silky oil** is pressed from the native Australian nut. It has a sweet, nutty aroma and contains naturally high amounts of **palmitoleic acid**, also found in human sebum. This acid helps to protect skin from premature ageing and weather damage.

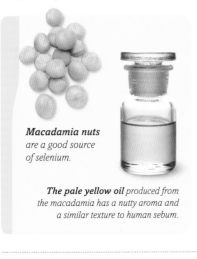

Macadamia nuts are a good source of selenium.

The pale yellow oil produced from the macadamia has a nutty aroma and a similar texture to human sebum.

What is it **good for?**

Protects skin Macadamia oil contains nourishing fatty acids and sterols, or plant hormones, that help to moisturize and repair skin. It is a great choice for healing skin after too much exposure to the sun, wind, or cold weather conditions. The oil is also great for conditioning hair.

Has anti-ageing effects Macadamia is rich in omega-7 palmitoleic acid, which has been shown to help delay skin ageing.

The oil has a particularly regenerating, moisturizing, and hydrating effect on mature skin. It is also non-irritating to the skin around the eyes – try patting the tiniest amount around the eyes to fight bags and sagging skin.

It is long-lasting Macadamia will keep longer than most nut and seed oils (up to 12 months), but it needs to be stored in a cool dark place to keep it at its best.

Neem

Melia azadirachta

Pressed from the fruit and seeds of the tree, neem oil is highly **antiseptic** – a little goes a long way. It has a strong, pungent odour so is best used to **enrich** other oils. It is particularly good at helping to **heal** infections and for dry skin conditions, and makes an effective **insect repellent**.

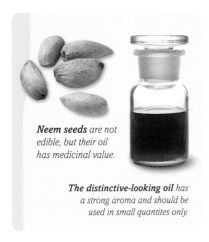

Neem seeds are not edible, but their oil has medicinal value.

The distinctive-looking oil has a strong aroma and should be used in small quantites only.

What is it **good for?**

Treats dandruff Neem is a useful dandruff remedy. Try blending with coconut oil for a pre-wash hair mask. Leave in for 10 minutes, then rinse off.

Works well in blends Neem is effective even in small amounts and blending it helps to counter its strong aroma. To find what works for you, start with just a few drops diluted in a neutral base oil, such as sunflower or almond, and gradually increase the amount to no more than 5 per cent of the blend.

Acts as an insect repellent Neem is a powerful insecticide that has become a staple of many natural head-lice treatments and mosquito repellents. For head lice, apply neat from root to tip and comb through with a nit comb, then wash out.

Heals skin The oil can be dabbed neat on to cold sores and contains anti-inflammatory compounds that help ease eczema and psoriasis. Its skin-softening properties can improve the appearance of scaly, dry skin.

Moringa

Moringa oleifera

Also known as ben oil, moringa is pressed from the seeds of the plant. It contains high levels of the fatty **oleic acid** and is a deeply penetrating oil with skin-softening properties. It is rich in **antioxidants**, which help to protect skin from premature ageing due to free radicals.

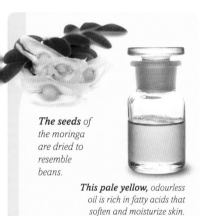

The seeds of the moringa are dried to resemble beans.

This pale yellow, odourless oil is rich in fatty acids that soften and moisturize skin.

What is it **good for?**

It makes a good massage base Highly lubricating and similar in composition to olive oil, but much lighter and odourless, moringa oil makes an ideal oil base for aromatherapy massage blends. Its light texture in particular helps to make a pleasant facial massage or elixir.

Conditions skin Moringa can help to reduce the appearance of large pores, as well as fine lines, wrinkles, stretch marks, and scars.

Moisturizes skin Its high fatty-acid content nourishes skin and helps prevent moisture loss. The oil provides instant hydration for dry, damaged, or mature skin. Blend with coconut oil to make a hair and scalp treatment that restores shine and fights dandruff.

Helps controls acne With antibacterial and anti-inflammatory properties, the oil is useful for acne-prone skin. Studies show that moringa can help to kill off the germs that can cause skin infections.

Evening primrose

Oenothera biennis

Cold-pressed from the oil-rich seeds, evening primrose is an **enriching** oil that contains **skin-loving fatty acids**, such as omega-6 linoleic acid, which strengthens membranes around the skin, and **anti-ageing** gamma linolenic acid (GLA).

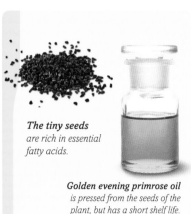

The tiny seeds are rich in essential fatty acids.

Golden evening primrose oil is pressed from the seeds of the plant, but has a short shelf life.

The fragrant flowers of the evening primrose are edible.

What is it **good for?**

Has anti-ageing effects Light and easily absorbed, the oil has anti-inflammatory and skin-rejuvenating properties that can improve tone and elasticity in mature skin.

Conditions skin Evening primrose helps skin retain moisture and increases skin cells' ability to absorb oxygen and fight off infection. The oil penetrates deep into the skin, helping to heal conditions such as eczema and acne. To help soften brittle and easily breakable nails, rub in 1–2 drops daily.

Can be added to cosmetics If you are adding evening primrose oil to home-made cosmetics, it should make up 5–10 per cent of the blend. The oil has a short shelf life, so once opened, it should be stored in the fridge and used within 6–9 months. If you need just a small amount for a massage blend or cream, add from capsules, rather than open a bottle.

Olive

Olea europea

Rich in skin-nourishing **fatty acids**, **antioxidants**, and **vitamin E**, over the years olive oil has earned its reputation as an affordable, but also superior, **moisturizing** and healing treatment. Use it neat or in a multitude of cosmetic formulations for skin and hair.

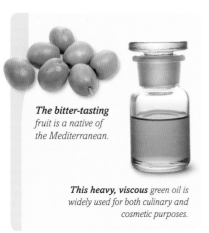

The bitter-tasting fruit is a native of the Mediterranean.

This heavy, viscous green oil is widely used for both culinary and cosmetic purposes.

What is it **good for?**

Conditions skin This deeply penetrating oil helps to keep skin soft and well-conditioned. A naturally occurring compound, squalene, provides a barrier against water loss. Rub a few drops into the nails and cuticles to protect and condition them.

Has anti-ageing effects Its antioxidant properties help maintain the integrity of skin cells and fight off the effects of free radicals, which cause premature skin ageing.

Can be used as a hair tonic
Olive oil can be used as a pre-treatment before shampooing, or as an overnight hair mask to treat dry and damaged hair and irritated, sensitive scalps.

Acts as a make-up remover
Olive oil makes an effective and simple make-up remover, helping to lift all traces of grime and dirt and leave skin well moisturized and conditioned.

Avocado

Persea gratissima

Avocado is one of the best oils for **soothing** dry skin and softening rough skin patches, such as those on the elbows and heels. Naturally high in vitamins, minerals, and **antioxidants**, the rich oil is cold-pressed from the fruit and used in small amounts to **enrich** lighter oil bases.

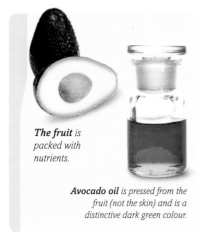

The fruit is packed with nutrients.

Avocado oil is pressed from the fruit (not the skin) and is a distinctive dark green colour.

What is it **good for?**

Conditions and soothes skin
Avocado helps to hydrate parched skin and aid the regeneration of skin cells. A high fatty acid content means this is a great oil for conditioning rough skin on the feet, knees, or elbows, and also for reviving hair damaged by styling or the sun.

Repairs and protects skin
If used regularly, the oil can help to prevent or minimize the appearance of stretch marks.

Acts as an anti-ageing oil
Avocado oil gives lustre and shine to tired or dull complexions. It contains fatty acids and phytosterols (plant hormones) that help to replenish and revitalize mature skin.

Acts as a natural SPF While it can't be used as a sunscreen on its own, avocado oil does contain a natural SPF factor at a low level that can help to protect skin and hair from sun exposure. The oil also relieves the pain of sunburn.

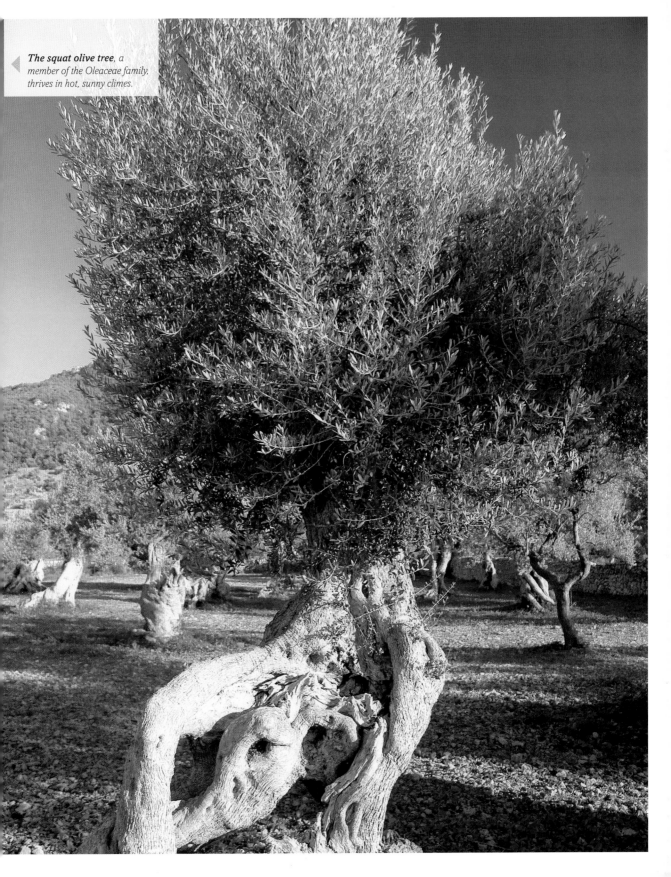

The squat olive tree, a member of the Oleaceae family, thrives in hot, sunny climes.

Almond

Prunus amygdalus dulcis

This light general-purpose oil is cold-pressed from the seeds of the sweet almond tree. Vitamin rich, the oil is suitable for **all skin types**, but especially for **sensitive skins**, and it is gentle enough to be used on children. It helps **soothe** dry, irritated skin and prevent moisture loss.

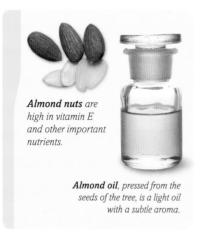

Almond nuts are high in vitamin E and other important nutrients.

Almond oil, pressed from the seeds of the tree, is a light oil with a subtle aroma.

What is it **good for?**

Acts as a natural moisturizer
Almond oil provides a long-lasting barrier against the elements that helps prevent moisture loss, soothes and encourages the healing of dry, irritated skin, and relieves inflamed skin conditions, such as eczema.

It is suitable for babies and young children Almond oil is gentle enough to use on babies and young children, for example to treat nappy rash or cradle cap. Other gentle oils, such as olive and sunflower are also recommended for babies.

Helps lubricate massage blends The oil is absorbed slowly, which makes it a popular choice as a massage oil base. It also has a delicate aroma that will not compete with the essential oils in a blend.

Acts as a make-up remover
Almond oil removes dirt and make-up effectively, leaving the skin feeling soft and supple.

Apricot kernel

Prunus armeniaca

Apricot kernel oil is a **light cold-pressed oil**, rich in the fatty acid known as gamma linoleic acid, or GLA, which helps skin to maintain its moisture balance. Light enough to leave no greasy residue, the oil is particularly suitable as a base for facial serums and light **moisturizing** lotions.

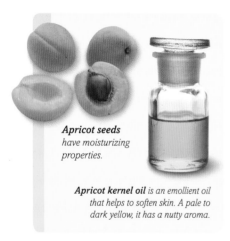

Apricot seeds have moisturizing properties.

Apricot kernel oil is an emollient oil that helps to soften skin. A pale to dark yellow, it has a nutty aroma.

What is it **good for?**

Helps restore moisture If skin feels dry, itchy, or tight after bathing or cleansing, this is the perfect oil to apply lightly to damp skin before towelling off. For mature skin, it is softening and improves skin elasticity, helping to smooth out fine lines.

It is suitable for sensitive skin
Apricot oil soothes sensitive skin and provides a thin barrier against irritants. It makes an ideal substitute for petroleum-based baby oils.

Acts as a massage base Apricot kernel absorbs more slowly than some oils, which makes it a great base for massage blends and night-time skin treatments. A little goes a long way, so buy the best you can afford.

Conditions hair The oil makes an effective treatment for flyaway hair and also minimizes the appearance of split ends. Work a few drops into damp hair and allow it to dry naturally to seal in moisture all day long.

Rosehip seed

Rosa canina

The oil from the seeds of the rose plant is a luxurious source of **skin-nourishing** fatty acids. Renowned for its **soothing** anti-inflammatory effect, it is suited to dry, mature, and weather-damaged skin.

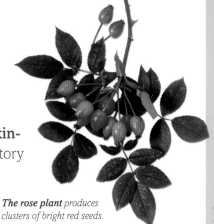

The rose plant produces clusters of bright red seeds.

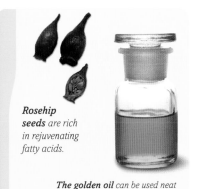

Rosehip seeds are rich in rejuvenating fatty acids.

The golden oil can be used neat on small areas of skin, or added to blends to enrich other oils.

What is it **good for?**

Has anti-ageing effects Rosehip contains the essential fatty acids omegas 3 and 6 that support cell and tissue regeneration, helping to keep skin supple and reduce the appearance of fine lines around the eyes. It is great for treating spider veins.

Prevents scarring The oil can be added to body lotions and creams to minimize the appearance of stretch marks. It can also help reduce scarring from wounds, burns, and after surgery.

Treats acne The oil is a source of trans-retinoic acid, a form of vitamin A, which is a recognized treatment for acne-prone skin. Rosehip helps balance the skin's oils and its toning action minimizes pores. It is also good for calming pimples and boils.

Eases itching Soothing and easily absorbed, when the skin is dry and itchy rosehip seed's cooling, anti-inflammatory action brings quick relief.

Sesame

Sesamum Indicum

Pressed from the familiar sesame seed, this oil is **packed with nutrients**, including vitamin E and potassium, both of which help to **rejuvenate** and **protect** the skin. The oil also has inherent **anti-inflammatory** properties, making it especially suited to healing dry skin conditions.

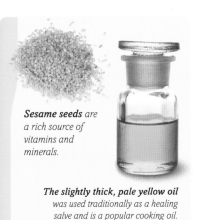

Sesame seeds are a rich source of vitamins and minerals.

The slightly thick, pale yellow oil was used traditionally as a healing salve and is a popular cooking oil.

What is it **good for?**

Tones skin This deeply penetrating oil helps to repair damaged cells and improve circulation, which in turn gives tired or weather-damaged skin a healthy glow.

Useful for head and face massage Ayurvedic practitioners believe that even without the addition of essential oils, sesame oil produces a calming and warming effect that boosts circulation and aids detox, while relieving stress and promoting sleep.

Moisturizes skin Sesame helps to keep skin hydrated, and is particularly well suited to those with dry to normal skin. The oil also relieves itchy, burning, and inflamed skin conditions.

Acts as a sunscreen While sesame oil can't be used on its own to protect the skin against the sun's damaging rays, adding some of the oil to facial and body preparations will boost their SPF factor, while also helping to protect skin from the harmful effects of free radicals that are generated by the sun's rays.

Jojoba

Simmondsia chinensis

Jojoba is actually a **liquid wax** rather than an oil, and because it is so similar to human sebum, it is considered one of the main treatments for dry and mature skin. Its waxy nature adds a **protective** layer that helps skin retain moisture. Readily absorbed, it can be used on all skin types.

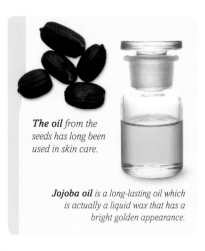

The oil from the seeds has long been used in skin care.

Jojoba oil *is a long-lasting oil which is actually a liquid wax that has a bright golden appearance.*

What is it **good for?**

Conditions skin and hair Jojoba can be used to soften hard, dry or rough skin and to relieve the symptoms of skin conditions such as eczema and psoriasis. Just a little added to hair gives instant shine and it can also be used to treat dry scalp conditions and dandruff.

Has anti-ageing effects Jojoba is a good oil for dry, chapped, weather-worn, and mature skins. It helps to reduce water loss and improves suppleness and elasticity, helping to reduce the appearance of fine lines, wrinkles, and scars.

Acts as a make-up remover Jojoba oil is suitable for all skin types, and can be used to lift and dissolve the dirt and oil that clogs pores, leaving skin instantly moisturized. Its thick texture makes it a great substitute for soap when shaving. A little applied to the legs or face helps to lubricate the skin, enabling an extra close shave that also helps to prevent razor irritation.

Cocoa butter

Theobroma cacao

A natural and effective **emollient** with a distinctive chocolate–vanilla aroma, cocoa butter can be added to body and face creams and balms to **provide a barrier** against moisture loss and environmental damage. It is good for dry and damaged skin, and helps to fade stretch marks.

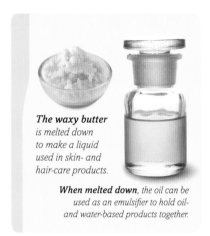

The waxy butter is melted down to make a liquid used in skin- and hair-care products.

When melted down, *the oil can be used as an emulsifier to hold oil- and water-based products together.*

What is it **good for?**

Prevents moisture loss Cocoa butter acts as a barrier to prevent water loss and keep skin hydrated. The oil aids skin elasticity and tone by supporting collagen production, helping to prevent premature wrinkles and reduce stretch marks. It also helps soften and hydrate the hair.

Thickens creams and acts as an emulsifier Solid and pale yellow at room temperature, cocoa butter can be gently melted into face and bodycare formulations to thicken them and add benefits. Cocoa butter is a natural emulsifier, helping oil- and water-based lotions to hold together.

Best for clear skin and dry complexions Cocoa butter can be occlusive, which means it can clog pores. For this reason it may not be suitable for skin that is prone to acne or pimples.

Wheatgerm

Triticum vulgare

A **nurturing** and **skin-protecting** oil, wheatgerm oil has the highest vitamin E content of any vegetable oil and is also rich in betacarotene. While too sticky and thick to use on its own, the oil adds multiple **skin-conditioning** benefits to base oil blends and lotions and creams.

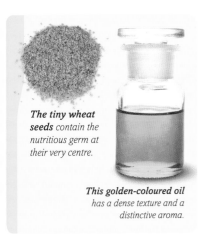

The tiny wheat seeds contain the nutritious germ at their very centre.

This golden-coloured oil has a dense texture and a distinctive aroma.

What is it **good for?**

Repairs skin Wheatgerm oil moisturizes and heals dry or cracked skin, and also helps to fade scarring and stretch marks. It is an especially rich source of vitamin E, which helps to protect skin from the effects of the weather, to moisturize and heal dry or cracked skin, and to maintain an even skin tone.

Has anti-ageing effects Vitamin E helps fight the effects on the skin of damaging free radicals and supports cellular regeneration and collagen formation. Vitamin E-rich wheatgerm has a revitalizing effect on mature or weather-worn skin, helping to rejuvenate and prevent the development of premature fine lines around the eyes and mouth.

Works well in a blend With its thick, sticky consistency and distinctive grassy–nutty aroma, wheatgerm oil is best used to enrich the powers of other lighter base oils. It should make up 5–10 per cent of the final base oil blend.

Grapeseed

Vitis vinifera

This light, odourless, and inexpensive all-purpose oil can be used in a wide array of applications from massage to skin care. High in **antioxidants**, it is mild, but very nourishing. It has good **emollient** properties and a gentle **toning** effect that benefits both mature and acne-prone skin.

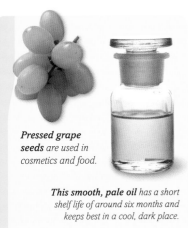

Pressed grape seeds are used in cosmetics and food.

This smooth, pale oil has a short shelf life of around six months and keeps best in a cool, dark place.

What is it **good for?**

Has anti-ageing effects Rich in the emollient linoleic acid (omega-6), grapeseed oil leaves the skin with a satiny finish. The oil is easily absorbed and has a mildly astringent effect that helps to tone and condition tired or dull-looking skin.

Is suitable for allergenic and sensitive skin This non-allergenic oil is suitable for those who cannot use nut oils. It is mild enough to use on infants and on sensitive skin.

Treats acne Grapeseed's astringent properties help to balance oily and acne-prone skin, refreshing the complexion and reducing redness and irritation.

Is a good massage base Grapeseed oil makes a great non-greasy base oil for massage blends. It also has the added benefit of dispersing in water, making it an ideal choice for bath-oil blends.

Essential Oil Recipes

Create your very own **home spa.**
With these simple recipes and all-
natural ingredients you can make a
range of gorgeous products to revive
body and mind, from aromatic blends
to fragranced candles and **pampering**
bath and beauty products.

Blending essential oils

The **art of blending** oils successfully to create **pleasing** and uplifting scents comes with practice. The fragrance families on pages 166–67 will help you understand which scents work especially well together. Below are a few practical **guidelines** to help you get started. Enjoy **experimenting** with scent combinations and discovering which aromas appeal to you. Over time, your confidence will grow and you will develop an **instinct** for blending.

How oils work **together**

Each essential oil is made up of multiple components, all of which are responsible for the different attributes and properties of the oil. The beauty of essential oils is that a fragrance is not just one individual note, but is composed of a complex harmony of notes (see box, right). You can work with these different notes to create favourite blends, adding citrus notes by blending with lemon, grapefruit, or lime, for example; or enhancing a blend with spicy notes by adding cardamom or black pepper.

The art of creating a beautiful blend of oils often comes down to practice, but there are some tips you can use to make life easier. And while you won't want to waste oils, a little trial and error can help you to understand how they work together and to gain confidence blending, so don't be afraid to make a few mistakes.

Blending guidelines Start off by creating very simple blends. As you work with the essential oils and become more familiar with them, you will notice that some are stronger smelling and more pervasive than others. These oils will dominate the ones that have a more subtle smell, so do bear this in mind and blend carefully, drop by drop, while you are practising and gaining confidence.

● **Always dilute essential oils** before applying to the skin (see the blending table on page 37 for guidelines of quantities of essential oil to base oil).

Aromatherapists use the following guidelines: 1 per cent dilution in a base oil for a product for sensitive skin, for a facial oil, for children, the elderly or for those with a weak immune system; 2.5 per cent dilution in a base oil for a product for the body of a healthy adult; and 5 per cent dilution for a local or topical application, for example for a compress.

● **Aim to use four to seven oils** per blend and avoid adding more than seven oils. When you start blending, you might prefer to blend just two or three oils at once, and these simple blends can be effective. As you gain confidence and discover scent combinations you like, you can begin to add a few more oils.

● **If you make a mistake** while blending oils, perhaps adding an oil whose smell you aren't keen on, it is hard to rectify the mistake. In this case, it's best to abandon the blend and start again.

● **Blend oils** in a small beaker or cup. If you need to store a blend, transfer it to a sterilized dark glass bottle and label the bottle with the date and the ingredients of the blend.

Top, middle, and base notes

Fragrances are built using "accords", which means that individual scents, or notes, are blended to create a new, unified aroma. Each fragrance is made up of top, middle, and base notes, which are combined to give structure to the blend and to create appealing, balanced, long-lasting fragrances.

● *Top notes* are light and refreshing and give the first impression.

● *Middle notes* are the heart of the fragrance and include most of the herbaceous scents, such as geranium.

● *Base notes* are rich aromas, such as sandalwood and ylang ylang, which give a scent body and longevity.

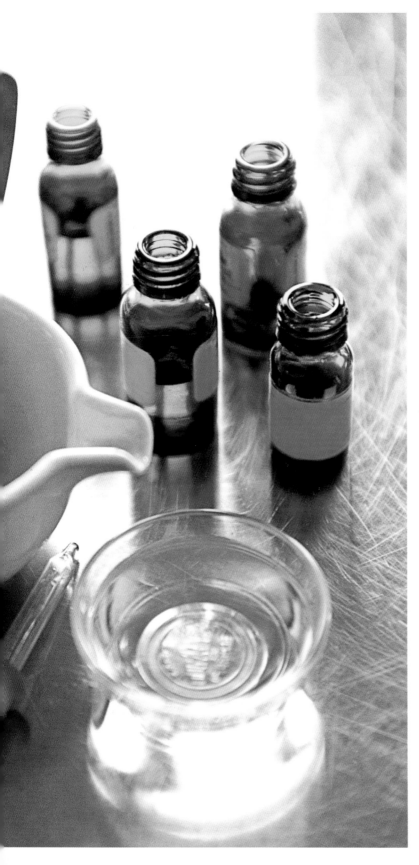

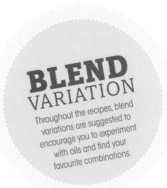

BLEND
VARIATION

Throughout the recipes, blend
variations are suggested to
encourage you to experiment
with oils and find your
favourite combinations.

Mix small
quantities of
oil to start with
as you learn the
art of blending.

Perfect blends

Essential oils can be categorized into **fragrance "families"**, which can guide your blending choices. Typically, the **aromas** each of us most enjoy belong to just one or two families. Here, families are arranged in a circle. While there are no rules, scents tend to marry well with those in their own family, and also with **neighbouring families**.

Floral oils

Florals are full-bodied scents such as rose that form the heart of an aroma. They can be used alone, or blended for more complex scents. Add citrus oils to lighten heady florals; spicy oils for a warm scent; or herbaceous oils for a cool aroma.

Essential oils
- Rosewood • Violet • Geranium
- Neroli • Rose • Ylang ylang
- Jasmine • Lavender
- Tagetes • Helichrysum
- Palmarosa • Mimosa

Floral lavender

Herbaceous oils

Herbaceous oils, such as basil, parsley, and chamomile, have a natural, elegant "green" scent and often form the "middle" note (see p164) of an aroma. Their clear scent can temper sweeter floral oils, and they can soften sharper citrus ones.

Essential oils
- Basil • Clarysage • Oregano • Parsley
- Tarragon • Thyme • Yarrow • Dill
- Mugwort • Caraway • Carrot seed
- Chamomile • Fennel • Marjoram
- Myrtle • Summer savory • Manuka

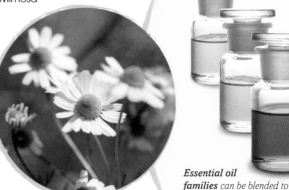

Herbaceous chamomile

Essential oil families can be blended to create more complex aromas.

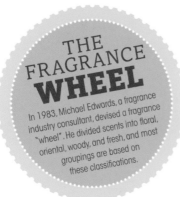

THE FRAGRANCE **WHEEL**
In 1983, Michael Edwards, a fragrance industry consultant, devised a fragrance "wheel". He divided scents into floral, oriental, woody, and fresh, and most groupings are based on these classifications.

Citrus oils

Zingy and vibrant, the citrus family includes citrus oils, as well as oils such as fragonia that have scents reminiscent of citrus. These oils add tartness to floral and herbaceous oils, and make a crisp scent when blended with medicinal oils.

Essential oils
- Bergamot • Lemon • Grapefruit
- Mandarin • Orange • Lemon verbena • Lemongrass • Lemon balm • Lime • Buchu • Fragonia
- Petitgrain • Citronella • Litsea

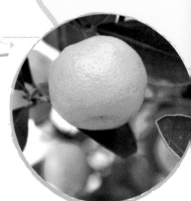

Citrus orange

Spicy oils

This exotic family of scents is made up of warm, sensual, spicy, and velvety aromas. Oils such as cinnamon can form the central note in a scent, and rich oils such as vanilla create a "base" note (see p164), giving longevity to a scent. Try marrying spicy oriental oils with woody ones, such as sandalwood, to create blends that are earthy and deep. Oriental oils also blend naturally with many floral scents, such as ylang ylang, jasmine, and lavender, where the floral note tempers the oriental one to prevent it overpowering.

Essential oils
- Vanilla ● Cinnamon ● Nutmeg ● Cardamom ● Clove ● Juniper
- Coriander ● Black pepper ● Cumin ● Galangal ● Litsea ● Fenugreek
- Ginger ● Star anise ● Tuberose ● Allspice ● Cistus

Spicy cinnamon

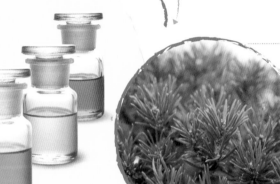

Woody pine

Woody oils

Earthy, mossy, musky, and dense, these complex scents contain many dominant aromas. Woody scents tend to be deeply grounding and are often sensual, as with sandalwood; and oils such as cedarwood and myrrh accentuate oriental aromas. Adding zesty citrus notes to woody oils creates a lively, fresher scent, while mixing woody oils with medicinal ones, such as eucalyptus, creates cool, resinous, minty aromas that offset the deep woody tones.

Essential oils
- Frankincense ● Cypress ● Pine ● Myrrh
- Patchouli ● Sandalwood ● Cedarwood
- Angelica ● Elemi ● Benzoin ● Valerian ● Vetiver

Medicinal oils

Crisp and clean, these, often lighter, scents produce a refreshing "top" note (see p164) to complement heavier woody aromas. Try also blending with woody or herbaceous oils to create a layered scent.

Essential oils
- Camphor ● Sage ● Wintergreen ● Birch ● Tea tree ● Cajuput ● Niaouli
- Ravintsara ● Rosemary ● Bay laurel ● Peppermint ● Eucalyptus ● Plai

Medicinal sage

Additional ingredients

Essential oils can be combined with various ingredients to make a **range** of bath and body products and treatments. For **basic blends**, the oils on pages 148–61 make the ideal base for essential oils. In the following recipes, additional ingredients are used, such as **waxes**, floral waters, mineral salts, and citric acid to create **creams**, lotions, balms, scents, and infusions.

Castor oil is an excellent skin emollient as it creates a barrier. It's also an effective cleanser.

Aloe vera juice provides a hydrating base for essential oils. Calming and cooling, it has healing properties and can repair damaged skin, making it a useful ingredient in skincare products.

Beeswax is used in skincare products to form a protective film on the skin that helps reduce water loss. A rich moisturizer, this is a good base for creams and ointments. You can buy beeswax in a block or in pellets that are easier to melt down.

Emulsifying waxes help essential oils and water to combine in creams and lotions and remain stable over a period of time.

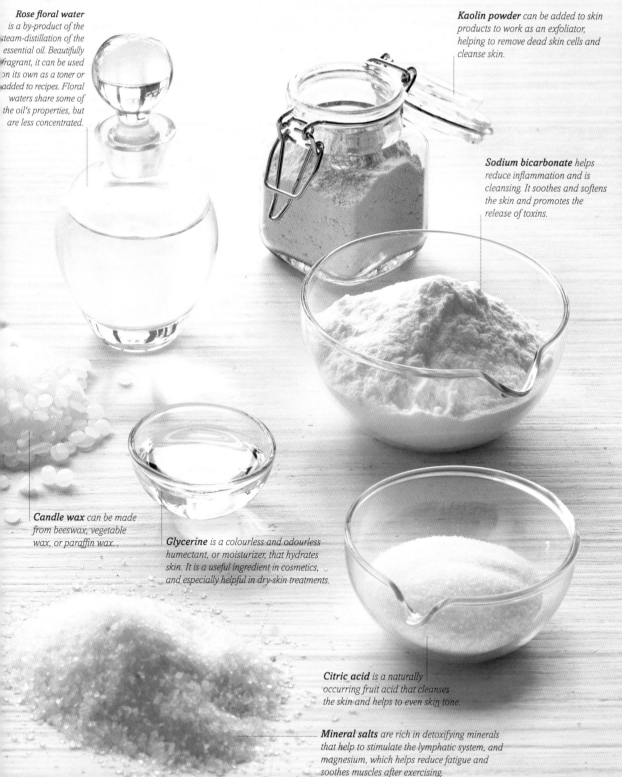

Rose floral water is a by-product of the steam-distillation of the essential oil. Beautifully fragrant, it can be used on its own as a toner or added to recipes. Floral waters share some of the oil's properties, but are less concentrated.

Kaolin powder can be added to skin products to work as an exfoliator, helping to remove dead skin cells and cleanse skin.

Sodium bicarbonate helps reduce inflammation and is cleansing. It soothes and softens the skin and promotes the release of toxins.

Candle wax can be made from beeswax, vegetable wax, or paraffin wax.

Glycerine is a colourless and odourless humectant, or moisturizer, that hydrates skin. It is a useful ingredient in cosmetics, and especially helpful in dry-skin treatments.

Citric acid is a naturally occurring fruit acid that cleanses the skin and helps to even skin tone.

Mineral salts are rich in detoxifying minerals that help to stimulate the lymphatic system, and magnesium, which helps reduce fatigue and soothes muscles after exercising.

Aromatherapy blends

Using fragrant blends of essential oils in the way that best suits your lifestyle is a great way to enhance general wellbeing and health. Essential oils have wonderful properties that are calming, balancing, anxiety-reducing, uplifting, cleansing, and stimulating, all of which will help you to relax, unwind, and release stress, as well as provide an overall boost to your body.

MASSAGE OIL   BATH OIL   DIFFUSER

Blend for relaxation

Allowing ourselves time to relax is key to wellbeing. Lavender essential oil is well known for **aiding relaxation** and blends well with **calming** rose oil. Vetiver oil has a woody, earthy, slightly bitter fragrance with relaxing and **sedative properties**, making it ideal for use before bedtime.

Ingredients

Makes 30ml (1fl oz)
Almond oil 2 tbsp
Lavender essential oil 5 drops
Rose essential oil 3 drops
Vetiver essential oil 2 drops

How to **make**

For a massage oil, combine all the ingredients in a bowl, then transfer the blend to a sterilized dark glass bottle and seal with a cap or dropper, ready for use. Store the blend in a cool, dark place. It will keep for up to 3 months.

How to **use**

As a massage oil Massage into the skin on the body (avoiding your face). Allow the oil to absorb into the skin before you get dressed.

In the bath For a relaxing bedtime wind-down soak, mix the essential oils with just 1 tablespoon of the almond oil, or alternatively mix the essential oils with 1 tablespoon full-fat milk, then add to a warm bath.

In a diffuser Add the essential oils on their own to a diffuser, vaporizer or oil burner and gently fragrance your chosen environment as you relax and unwind.

Safe usage Take care not to slip when getting into and out of the bath.

Unwind and relax with a soothing aromatic blend.

BLEND VARIATION

For other relaxing blends with an almond base oil try chamomile, mandarin, and bergamot, or marjoram, lavender, and orange.

Once your blend is made up, you can add it to a bath or use for a massage as you wish.

SHOWER

Uplifting blend

This trio of **reviving** oils can lift spirits and boost flagging energy. Zesty, **energizing** grapefruit stimulates body and mind and geranium helps to balance emotions by being both **calming** and **uplifting**. Jasmine completes the blend perfectly, its heady aroma increasing feelings of wellbeing.

Ingredients

Makes 30ml (1fl oz)

Unscented shower gel 2 tbsp

Grapefruit essential oil 4 drops

Jasmine absolute or essential oil 4 drops

Geranium essential oil 1 drop

How to **make**

Mix the essential oil drops with the unscented shower gel.

How to **use**

In the shower Use this uplifting blend first thing in the morning for an energizing shower that will help you start the day on a positive note.

MASSAGE OIL   DIFFUSER

Soothing blend

Calming aromatherapy provides a natural and easy way to deal with the symptoms of stress and feelings of anxiety. **Uplifting** floral essential oils, such as neroli, can be blended with other mood-boosting oils, such as frankincense, to create a wonderfully **soothing** massage or diffusion.

Ingredients

Makes 30ml (1fl oz)

Almond oil 2 tbsp

Frankincense essential oil 3 drops

Neroli essential oil 3 drops

Orange essential oil 2 drops

How to **make**

For a massage oil, combine all the ingredients in a bowl, then transfer the blend to a sterilized dark glass bottle and seal with a cap or dropper, ready for use. Store in a cool, dark place. It will keep for up to 3 months.

How to **use**

As a massage oil Massage into the skin on the body (avoiding your face). Allow the oil to absorb into the skin before you get dressed.

In a diffuser Add the essential oils on their own to a diffuser, vaporizer or oil burner to create a calming and tranquil environment.

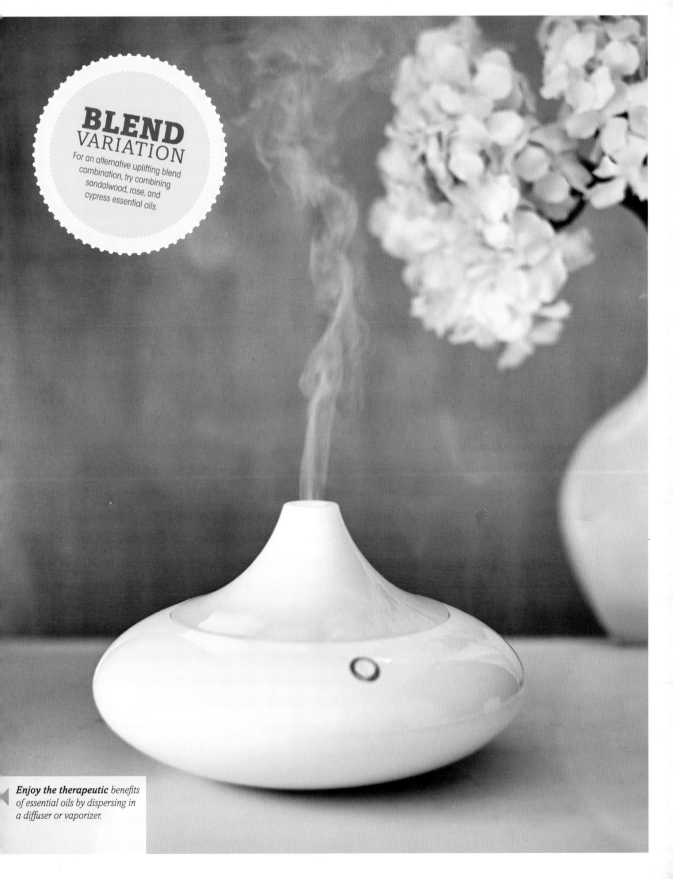

BLEND
VARIATION

For an alternative uplifting blend combination, try combining sandalwood, rose, and cypress essential oils.

Enjoy the therapeutic *benefits of essential oils by dispersing in a diffuser or vaporizer.*

MASSAGE OIL DIFFUSER BATH OIL

Calming blend

The aromatherapeutic properties of certain oils work on both mind and body, helping to **calm** and **balance** the emotions and soothe skin. Rose essential oil helps to calm skin, reducing redness and inflammation, while geranium oil can balance oily skin and calm unsettled **emotions**. Light, versatile, and gentle on the skin, almond base oil makes an ideal carrier for this blend.

Ingredients

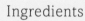

Makes 30ml (1fl oz)
Almond oil 2 tbsp
Rose absolute or essential oil 7 drops
Geranium essential oil 7 drops

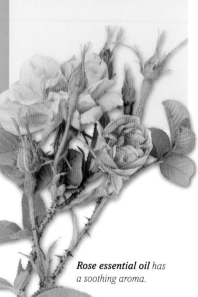

Rose essential oil has a soothing aroma.

How to **make**

For a massage oil, combine all the ingredients in a bowl, then transfer the blend to a sterilized dark glass bottle and seal with a cap or dropper, ready for use. Store in a cool, dark place. It will keep for up to 3 months.

How to **use**

As a massage oil Massage into the skin on the body (avoiding your face). Allow the oil to absorb into the skin before you get dressed. For a calming facial oil, blend 2 tablespoons almond or calendula oil with 1 drop each of rose and lavender essential oils.

In a diffuser Add the essentials oils on their own to a diffuser, vaporizer or oil burner and gently fragrance your environment with this soothing blend.

In the bath Mix the essential oils with just 1 tablespoon of the almond oil, or alternatively mix the oils with 1 tablespoon full-fat milk or a bath oil base, then add to a warm bath.

Safe usage *If using the oils in a bath, take care not to slip when getting into and out of the bath.*

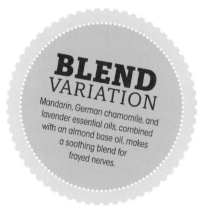

BLEND
VARIATION
Mandarin, German chamomile, and lavender essential oils, combined with an almond base oil, makes a soothing blend for frayed nerves.

Blend for focus

Essential oils have long been used to facilitate meditation as they help to deepen and slow breathing, as well as **balance** and **centre energy**. Rosemary essential oil has a **stimulating** effect on the central nervous system so is useful for improving poor concentration. Clove and peppermint essential oils help to keep sleepiness at bay, so they are an ideal combination for maintaining focus.

Ingredients

Makes 30ml (1fl oz)
Sunflower oil 2 tbsp
Rosemary essential oil 6 drops
Clove essential oil 2 drops
Peppermint essential oil 2 drops

How to **make**

Combine the ingredients in a bowl, then transfer to a sterilized dark glass bottle and seal with a cap or dropper, ready for use. Store in a cool, dark place. It will keep for up to 3 months.

How to **use**

On the skin Dab the fragranced blend onto the pulse points on the wrists and temples. Use a bottle with a roller ball for easy application.

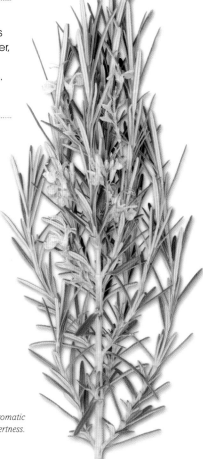

This centring group of oils helps to enhance concentration.

Reviving and stimulating, aromatic rosemary promotes mental alertness.

MASSAGE OIL

STEAM
INHALATION

DIFFUSER

Purifying and cleansing blend

Enjoy a **detox** massage or **cleanse** your environment by using essential oils with key **purifying** properties. You can also deep-cleanse skin by adding the oils to an unscented facial wash or oil blend, or to a steam inhalation to open pores. Juniper has stimulating and astringent properties, frankincense tones skin and helps to close pores, and lemon's citrussy scent refreshes, eliminating unwelcome odours.

Ingredients

Makes 30ml (1fl oz)

Jojoba oil 2 tbsp

Juniper essential oil 8 drops

Frankincense essential oil 4 drops

Lemon essential oil 2 drops

How to **make**

For a massage oil, combine all the ingredients in a bowl, then transfer the blend to a sterilized dark glass bottle and seal with a cap or dropper, ready for use. Store the blend in a cool, dark place. It will keep for up to 3 months.

How to **use**

As a massage oil Massage into the skin on the body (avoiding your face). Allow to the oil to absorb into the skin before you get dressed.

In an inhalation Add the essential oils on their own to hot water, cover your head with a towel, and allow the steam to act on your skin for 5 minutes. Wash skin with cool water and pat it dry with a clean towel.

In a diffuser Add the essential oils on their own to a diffuser, vaporizer or oil burner and diffuse in a sick room or your chosen room to cleanse and freshen the air.

Gently astringent and toning, this blend of essential oils has a potent cleansing action.

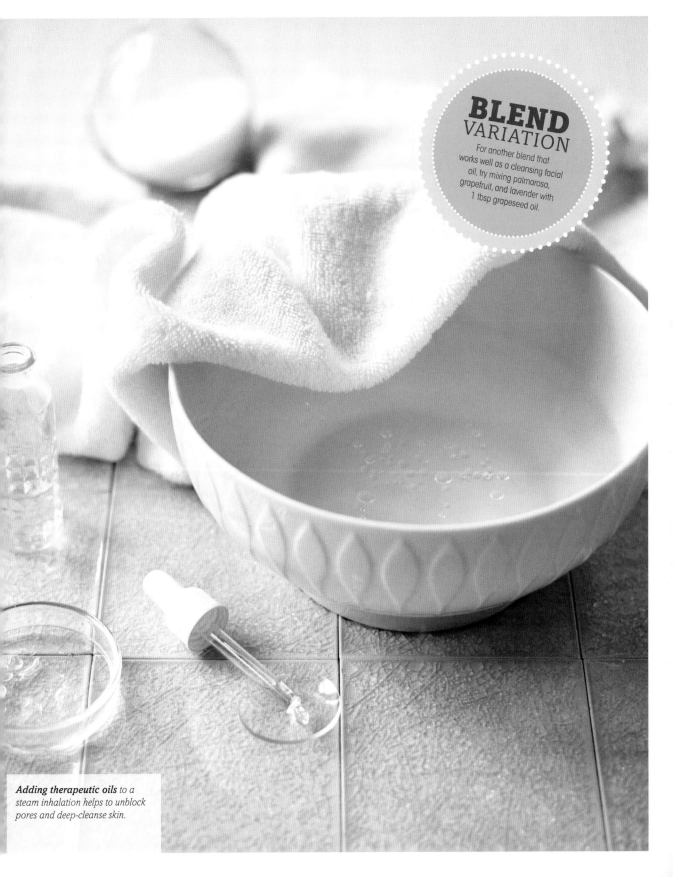

BLEND
VARIATION
For another blend that works well as a cleansing facial oil, try mixing palmarosa, grapefruit, and lavender with 1 tbsp grapeseed oil.

Adding therapeutic oils to a steam inhalation helps to unblock pores and deep-cleanse skin.

MASSAGE OIL

Sensual massage blend for him

Ylang ylang essential oil is exotically fragrant and intensely **uplifting** with calming properties. It blends well with **relaxing** and emotionally **grounding** sandalwood. Mix the oils with a nourishing base oil, light a candle or two, and treat your loved one to a massage.

Ingredients

Makes 30ml (1fl oz)

Jojoba oil 2 tbsp

Ylang ylang essential oil 6 drops

Sandalwood essential oil 6 drops

Nutmeg essential oil 2 drops

How to **make**

Combine all the ingredients in a bowl, then transfer the blend to a sterilized dark glass bottle and seal with a cap or dropper, ready for use. Store the blend in a cool, dark place. It will keep for up to 3 months.

How to **use**

As a massage oil Massage into the skin on the body (avoiding the face). Allow the oil to absorb into the skin before getting dressed.

MASSAGE OIL

Sensual massage blend for her

For a more feminine blend, mix rose absolute or essential oil with patchouli essential oil. Beautifully floral rose opens the heart and **soothes** nerves and feelings of anxiety, while patchouli has a sweet, earthy scent that is **grounding** and **calming.**

Ingredients

Makes 30ml (1fl oz)

Jojoba oil 2 tbsp

Rose absolute or rose essential oil 8 drops

Patchouli essential oil 4 drops

Vetiver essential oil 2 drops

Geranium essential oil 2 drops

How to **make**

Combine all the ingredients in a bowl. Transfer to a sterilized dark glass bottle and seal with a cap or dropper, ready for use. Store the blend in a cool, dark place. It will keep for up to 3 months.

How to **use**

As a massage oil Massage into the skin on the body (avoiding the face). Allow the oil to absorb into the skin before getting dressed.

Enjoy a sensual massage with this sweetly scented blend of oils.

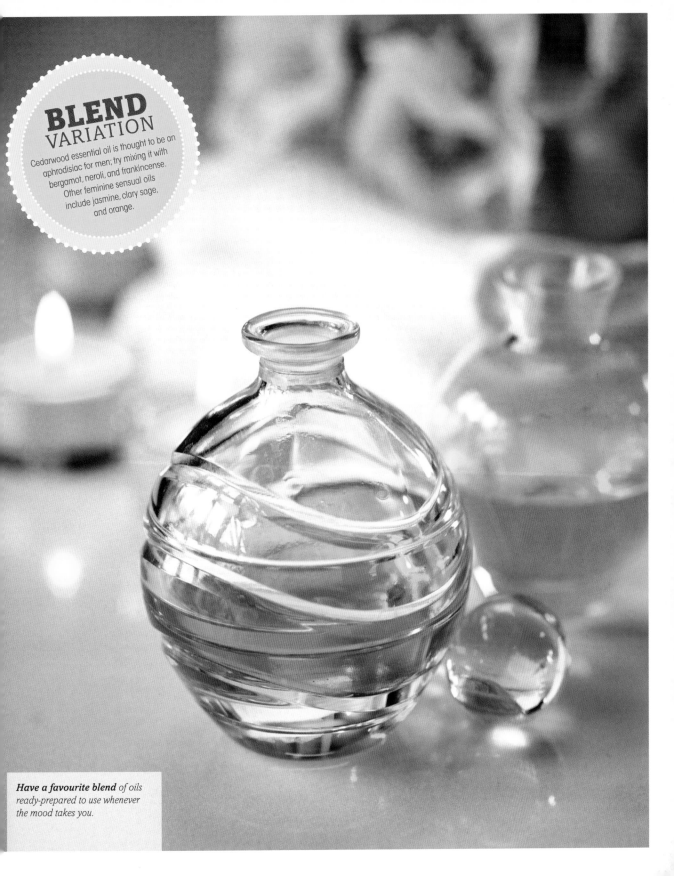

Have a favourite blend of oils *ready-prepared to use whenever the mood takes you.*

MASSAGE OIL

BLEND
VARIATION
For an alternative immune-strengthening blend, add lemon, thyme, and tea tree essential oils to a diffuser to refresh a room and protect against infection.

Immune-boosting blend

Immunity is the final line of **defence** against disease. Poor nutrition, lack of exercise, stress, and other lifestyle issues all place extra strain on the body's ability to function well, which can lead to an accumulation of toxins that can cause disease. Niaouli, lavender, and rosemary essential oils help **support** a compromised immune system and are strongly **antimicrobial**, helping the body to fight off infection.

Ingredients

Makes 30ml (1 fl oz)

Grapeseed oil 2 tbsp

Lavender essential oil 2 drops

Niaouli essential oil 2 drops

Rosemary essential oil 2 drops

How to **make**

Combine all the ingredients in a bowl, then transfer the blend to a sterilized dark glass bottle and seal with a cap or dropper, ready for use. Store the blend in a cool, dark place. It will keep for up to 3 months.

How to **use**

As a massage oil Massage into the skin on the body (avoiding the face). Allow to the oil to absorb into the skin before you get dressed.

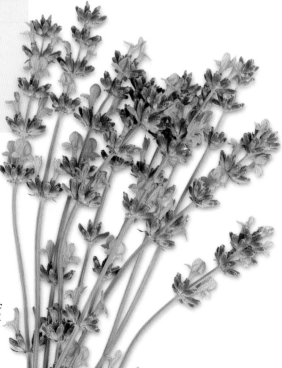

Harness the antiseptic properties of lavender essential oil.

MASSAGE OIL

BATH OIL

Regenerating blend

Essential oils can be used to encourage **skin-cell regeneration**, which is useful in the case of cuts, burns, scars, and stretch marks. Myrrh essential oil is ideal for slow-to-heal wounds and weepy eczema, while **anti-inflammatory** helichrysum can help speed up the **wound-healing** process, and frankincense encourages the growth of new cells – all of which help with skin healing and regeneration.

Ingredients

Makes 30ml (1fl oz)
Rosehip seed oil 1 tbsp
Calendula macerated oil 1 tbsp
Frankincense essential oil 6 drops
Helichrysum essential oil 4 drops
Myrrh essential oil 2 drops

How to **make**

For a massage oil, combine all the ingredients in a bowl. Transfer to a sterilized dark glass bottle and seal with a cap or dropper. Store in a cool, dark place. Keeps for up to 3 months.

How to **use**

As a massage oil Massage into the skin on the body (avoiding the face). Allow the oil to absorb into the skin before you get dressed.

In the bath Mix the essential oils with 1 tablespoon combined rosehip and calendula oil or 1 tablespoon full-fat milk. Disperse in a warm bath.

Safe usage Do not use the blend on broken skin. Take care not to slip when getting in and out of the bath.

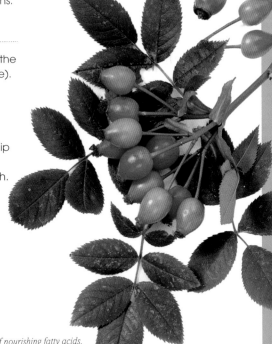

This healing blend of essential oils has a generally rejuvenating effect on the skin.

A rich source of nourishing fatty acids, rosehip is ideal for skin healing.

MASSAGE OIL

BATH OIL

Stimulating blend

Essential oils can be used to **stimulate** the appetite, digestive system, circulation, and lungs. This dynamic blend is ideal if you're feeling generally below par: ginger **calms** the digestive system and restores appetite; black pepper stimulates circulation; and tea tree helps **boost immunity**.

Ingredients

Makes 30ml (1fl oz)
Almond oil 2 tbsp
Ginger essential oil 6 drops
Black pepper essential oil 4 drops
Tea tree essential oil 4 drops

How to **make**

For a massage oil, combine all the ingredients in a bowl, then transfer the blend to a sterilized dark glass bottle and seal with a cap or dropper, ready for use. Store the blend in a cool, dark place. It will keep for up to 3 months.

How to **use**

As a massage oil Massage into the skin (avoiding the face). Allow the blend to absorb into the skin before you get dressed.

In the bath Mix the essential oils with just 1 tablespoon almond oil or, if you wish, 1 tablespoon full-fat milk. You can also enjoy a stimulating shower by mixing the essential oils with a fragrance-free shower gel.

Safe usage Take care not to slip when getting in and out of the bath.

DIFFUSER

Refreshing blend

If you feel sluggish and overcome by nervous exhaustion, this **energizing** blend could be the perfect pick-me-up. Pine oil has a **refreshing** effect, stimulating the nervous system and, along with eucalyptus, **enhancing concentration**, and peppermint is **reviving** and uplifting.

Ingredients

Makes 1 diffusion
Pine essential oil 2 drops
Peppermint essential oil 2 drops
Eucalyptus essential oil 1 drop

How to **make**

Add the essential oils to a diffuser, vaporizer or oil burner, according to the manufacturer's instructions.

How to **use**

In a diffuser Allow the oil blend to disperse and gently fragrance your chosen environment.

Safe usage Peppermint oil may be irritating to the skin. Don't use in concentrations above 2 per cent, and avoid near babies and young children.

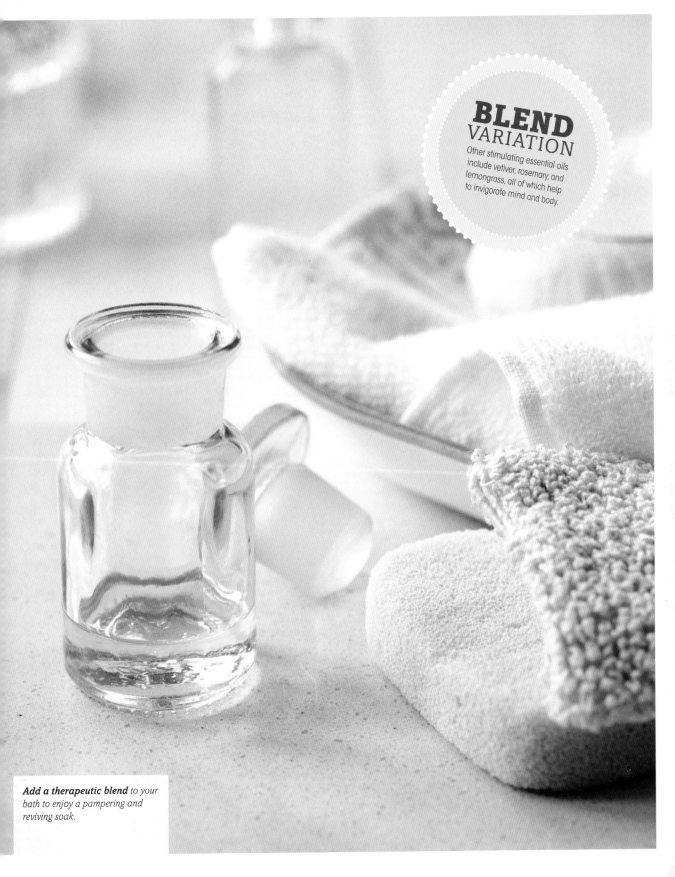

BLEND VARIATION

Other stimulating essential oils include vetiver, rosemary, and lemongrass, all of which help to invigorate mind and body.

Add a therapeutic blend to your bath to enjoy a pampering and reviving soak.

Home and body fragrances

Filling your home with aromatic essential oils, or using oils as favourite scents, allows you to enhance your environment and enjoy their therapeutic benefits throughout the day. Whether creating a personalized scent, dispersing a delicious aroma in a simple atomizer or making a perfumed candle, the following recipes will help you to create natural, uplifting fragrances for yourself and your home.

FRAGRANCE

Floral body mist

Body mists create a light alternative to more concentrated perfumes. Here, a **hydrating** base of aloe vera juice and rose floral water is blended with **exotically sweet** and **floral** ylang ylang, the deep undertones of vetiver, and the fresh **herbal** notes of clary sage.

Ingredients

Makes 120ml (4fl oz)

Rose floral water 75ml (2½fl oz)

Aloe vera juice or gel 2 tbsp

Glycerine 1 tbsp

Ylang ylang essential oil 10 drops

Bergamot essential oil 5 drops

Vetiver essential oil 5 drops

Clary sage essential oil 5 drops

How to **make**

1 Place the rose floral water, aloe vera juice or gel, and glycerine in a bowl. Add the essential oils and combine.

2 Transfer into a sterilized bottle with an atomizer and store in a cool, dark place. It keeps for up to 6 months.

How to **use**

As a fragrance Shake well before use then apply a burst of fragrance. As body mists are lighter than perfumes, reapply as required. Avoid spraying on clothes, fabrics or bed linen as the oils may stain.

Try out different blends to find your perfect signature scent.

Light and fresh, *body mist scents can be worn confidently throughout the day.*

FRAGRANCE

DIFFUSER

Lemon and lime room scent

Refresh and deodorize your living space with a **zesty** and **uplifting** blend of citrus oils. Use in an atomizer as a room spray or simply vaporize the oil blend in a diffuser to freshen and **scent** the air. The citrus oil combination in this blend has fresh, **sharp**, and **fruity** notes, as well as being uplifting and deodorizing, making this room fragrance an everyday must-have for the home and office.

Ingredients

Makes 60ml (2fl oz)

Vodka 2 tbsp

Lime essential oil 10 drops

Lemon essential oil 7 drops

Bergamot essential oil 6 drops

Mandarin essential oil 5 drops

Mineral water 2 tbsp

How to **make**

1 For a room spray, mix the vodka and the essential oils in a bowl. Add the mineral water and combine.

2 Transfer into a sterilized bottle with an atomizer. Store in a cool, dark place. It will keep for up to 6 months.

How to **use**

As a room scent Shake well, then atomize into the room.

In a diffuser Add the essential oils on their own to a diffuser, vaporizer, or oil burner.

This zesty citrus blend instantly freshens a room.

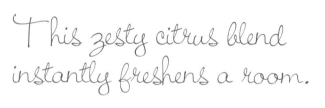

The refreshing aroma of lime helps to clear the mind.

FRAGRANCE   DIFFUSER

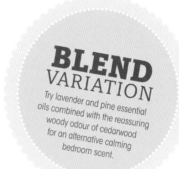
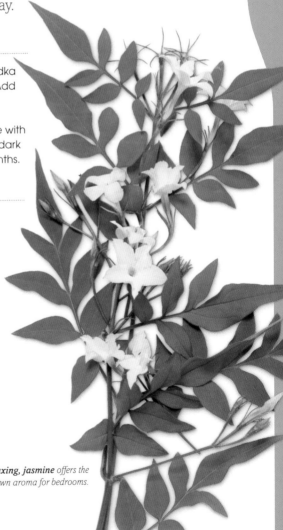

BLEND
VARIATION

Try lavender and pine essential oils combined with the reassuring woody odour of cedarwood for an alternative calming bedroom scent.

Relaxing bedroom blend

At the end of a long day we often need help to relax. This blend of oils can transport you to a place of **tranquillity**. The strongly **floral**, seductive fragrance of **jasmine** combines with frankincense, which deepens breathing and lifts feelings of anxiety. Use as a room spray, or simply vaporize in a diffuser to create a calm ambience. Light a candle or two and chill out after a long day.

Ingredients

Makes 60ml (2fl oz)

Vodka 2 tbsp

Jasmine absolute essential oil 8 drops

Frankincense essential oil 7 drops

Cardamom essential oil 6 drops

Mineral water 2 tbsp

How to **make**

1 For a room spray, mix the vodka and essential oils in a bowl. Add the mineral water and combine.

2 Transfer into a sterilized bottle with an atomizer. Store in a cool, dark place. It will keep for up to 6 months.

How to **use**

As a room scent Shake well before use, then atomize into your living space.

In a diffuser Add the essential oils on their own to a diffuser, vaporizer or oil burner.

Deeply relaxing, jasmine offers the perfect wind-down aroma for bedrooms.

FRAGRANCE

Uplifting candle

Candles can be made from different types of wax, such as paraffin wax, soy wax or, the most **traditional**, beeswax. Not all oils work well in a candle; **experiment** using cheaper oils. Some highly coloured oils will change the colour of paler waxes.

How to **make**

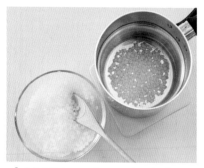

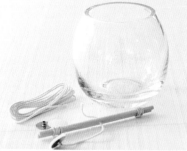

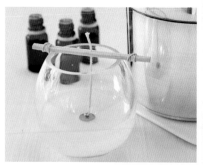

1 Melt the candle wax in a bain marie saucepan. Alternatively, place the candle wax in a heat-proof glass bowl. Half-fill a saucepan with boiling water and place the bowl on top of the saucepan to make a bain marie. Melt the candle wax gently.

2 For the candle wick, insert the end of a pre-waxed wick between two small wooden sticks held together with elastic bands. Using a wax button or a drop of wax, place the wick in the centre of a clean, dry votive mould or glass and stick the wick onto the base. Add the oils to the wax, mix thoroughly, then transfer half of the wax into a jug or vessel that is easy to pour from.

3 Pour the wax into the mould in three stages. First, half-fill the mould by slowly pouring the melted wax, taking care not to disturb the wick. Leave to set and cool. Reheat and stir the wax, then continue to part-fill the mould, allowing the wax to set and cool before filling it to the top level. By pouring in stages before the wax sets, the surface should be smooth.

Ingredients

Makes 1 x 90g (3oz) candle
Candle wax 90g (3oz)
Lemongrass essential oil 60 drops
Basil essential oil 40 drops
Lime essential oil 40 drops

How to **use**

As a room fragrance Place the candle in a safe place away from fabrics and with sufficient ventilation, and fragrance your chosen room with this uplifting blend.

BLEND
VARIATION

Add favourite floral scents, such as jasmine and rose, for a summery candle; or warming spicy oils, such as cinnamon and clove, for a cosy winter scent.

Creating your very own scented candles is a cost-effective and fun way to fragrance your home.

Pampering and beauty

Bring the spa experience into your own home with revitalizing and rejuvenating essential oil products and treatments. Simple recipes for moisturizing and refreshing bath products, nourishing and hydrating oils and scrubs for the face and body, and pampering hand and feet treatments will enable you relax, unwind, and enjoy the therapeutic benefits of essential oils in your own home.

BATH OIL

Soothing muscle soak

The essential oils in this blend work together to **improve circulation**, helping to repair muscle fibres and **relieve pain**. Mineral salts reduce fatigue and **soothe** aches and pains, and the arnica and comfrey herbs help muscles to recover from over-exertion.

Ingredients

Makes 530ml (17½fl oz)

Comfrey herb 1 tbsp

Arnica montana herb 1 tbsp

Water for the infusion 500ml (16fl oz)

Lavender essential oil 2 drops

Rosemary essential oil 2 drops

Black pepper essential oil 1 drop

Mineral salts 1 tbsp

How to **make**

1 Make the comfrey and arnica infusion by brewing the herbs for 10 minutes in a teapot with 500ml (16fl oz) boiled water. Strain the liquid.

2 Add the essential oils to the mineral salts and combine.

3 Add the salt and essential oil mixture to the strained herbal infusion and stir until dissolved.

Mineral-rich sea salt soothes skin and eases aching muscles.

How to **use**

As a bath infusion Add the infusion mixture to the bath immediately and bathe as usual.

Safe usage *Do not use on broken or newly shaved skin.*

Energizing mineral bath

Has your get-up-and-go disappeared? Use this combination of herbs, salts, and essential oils to give you renewed vigour. The **stimulating** and **invigorating** benefits of tea tree and black pepper essential oils will **energize** you for the hours ahead, and a rosemary and peppermint herbal infusion mixed with mineral salts helps to reduce tiredness and give you some added oomph!

Ingredients

Makes 530ml (17½fl oz)

Peppermint dried herb 1 tbsp

Rosemary dried herb 1 tbsp

Water for the infusion 500ml (16fl oz)

Peppermint essential oil 2 drops

Tea Tree essential oil 2 drops

Black pepper essential oil 1 drop

Mineral salts 1 tbsp

How to **make**

1 Make the rosemary and peppermint infusion by brewing the herbs for 10 minutes in a teapot with 500ml (16fl oz) boiled water. Strain the liquid.

2 Add the essential oils to the mineral salts and combine.

3 Add the salt and essential oil mixture to the strained herbal infusion and stir until dissolved.

How to **use**

As a bath infusion Add the infusion mixture to the bath immediately and bathe as usual.

Safe usage Do not use on broken or newly shaved skin.

Stimulating and cooling, the essential oil of peppermint is instantly invigorating.

Lie back and enjoy this invigorating mineral bath soak.

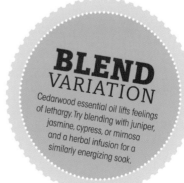

BLEND VARIATION

Cedarwood essential oil lifts feelings of lethargy. Try blending with juniper, jasmine, cypress, or mimosa and a herbal infusion for a similarly energizing soak.

BATH OIL

Rose bath bombs

Create bath bombs to suit your mood or the time of day. Here, **calming** rose and **balancing** geranium provide a perfect relaxing evening soak. Experiment with different dried flowers, such as lavender, and your favourite essential oils.

Ingredients

Makes 20
Sodium bicarbonate 400g (14oz)
Citric acid 200g (7oz)
Dried rose petals 2–3 tsp
Cocoa butter or vegetable oil 1 tsp
Geranium essential oil 10 drops
Rose absolute essential oil 5 drops
Water 1 tsp

How to **use**

In the bath Add the fragrant bath bomb to a warm bath and let it dissolve while you recline and relax.

How to **make**

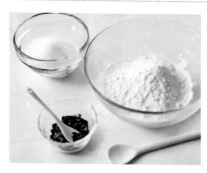

1 Lightly grease ice-cube moulds (a spray oil is ideal for this). Measure out the dry ingredients, then mix all of them together.

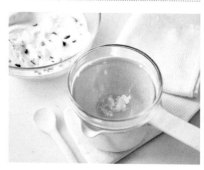

2 Melt the cocoa butter in a bain marie (see p188), and add the essential oils. Add the melted cocoa butter to the dry ingredients and mix.

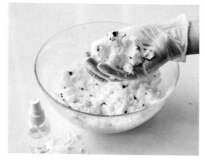

3 Add water with an atomizer and bind the mixture with your hands until it resembles damp sand and sticks together without fizzing. If it is crumbly, add a bit more water.

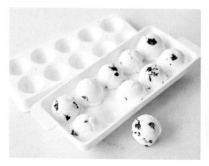

4 Firmly press into the moulds and allow to set for at least 1 hour. Turn from the moulds and use as required. The bombs keep for up to 3 months.

BLEND
VARIATION
Try adding citrussy essential oils such as orange and grapefruit for zesty bath bombs, or chamomile essential oil for a relaxing and soothing bedtime soak.

Make a batch of bath bombs, ready to pop in the bath whenever you like.

BATH OIL

Moisturizing bath melts

Quick and simple to make, these skin-softening bath melts contain a combination of **nourishing** shea nut butter, **moisturizing** cocoa butter, and coconut oil, blended with **balancing** geranium essential oil. The melts also work well in a warm shower as the heat from the water softens the butters, allowing you to massage the melt gently into the skin for a deeply moisturizing dry-skin treatment.

Ingredients

Makes 10

Shea nut butter 50g (2oz)
Cocoa butter 50g (2oz)
Coconut solid oil 2 tbsp
Geranium essential oil 20 drops

How to **make**

1 Place the shea nut butter and cocoa butter in a glass bowl and melt in a bain marie (see p188).

2 Add the coconut oil to the warm melted butters, then add the essential oil and mix. Pour into soap moulds or miniature cup cake cases.

3 Leave to cool and set. You can decorate the melts by pressing dried flowers into the surface as they cool. Keep them cool and dry in their cases and store in the fridge until needed. They keep for up to 3 months.

How to **use**

In the bath Add the bath melt to a warm bath. Alternatively, use it in a warm shower, allowing it to soften in the heat of the water then rubbing it into your skin for a moisturizing treat.

Safe usage Take care not to slip when getting into and out of the bath.

Enjoy an indulgent bath and feel silky smooth with these skin-replenishing bath melts.

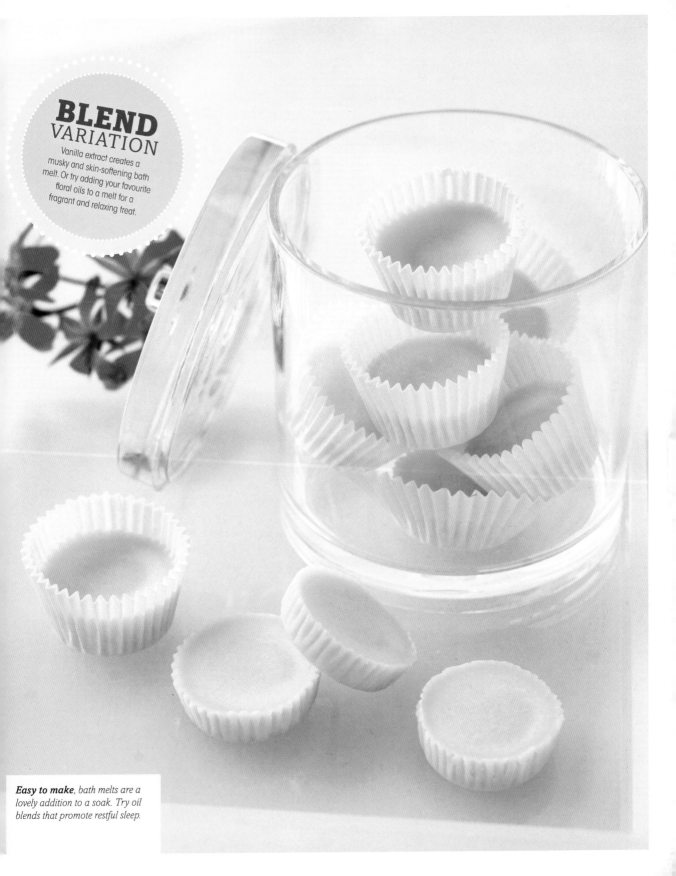

BLEND
VARIATION

Vanilla extract creates a musky and skin-softening bath melt. Or try adding your favourite floral oils to a melt for a fragrant and relaxing treat.

Easy to make, bath melts are a lovely addition to a soak. Try oil blends that promote restful sleep.

BATH OIL FOOT BATH

Lemon balm and lavender bath infusion

Try this mixture of herbs, petals, and fragrant oil to **soothe** body and mind. With its sweet, herbal scent, lavender oil is widely used for **relaxing**, while rose is **uplifting** and soothing. Lemon balm, a common garden plant, is wonderfully **calming**.

Ingredients

Makes 530ml (17½fl oz)

Dried lemon balm 1 tbsp

Dried rose petals 1 tbsp

Water for the infusion 500ml (16fl oz)

Lavender essential oil 10 drops

Mineral salts 1 tbsp

How to **make**

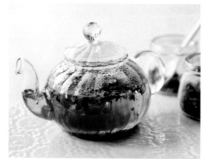

1 Make the infusion by brewing the lemon balm and rose petals for 10 minutes in a teapot with 500ml (16fl oz) boiled water.

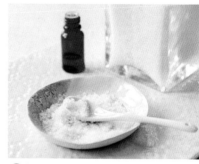

2 In a bowl, add the lavender essential oil to the mineral salts and combine to make a paste.

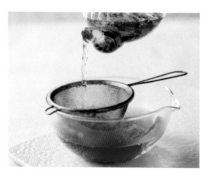

3 Strain the infused liquid into a bowl. Add the oil and salt paste to the strained infusion and stir until the salt is dissolved.

How to **use**

In the bath Add the infusion mixture to the bath immediately and unwind and relax.

As a foot bath Add the infusion mixture to a warm foot bath to soothe tired and aching feet.

Combining a herbal infusion
with therapeutic essential oils
relaxes the mind and body.

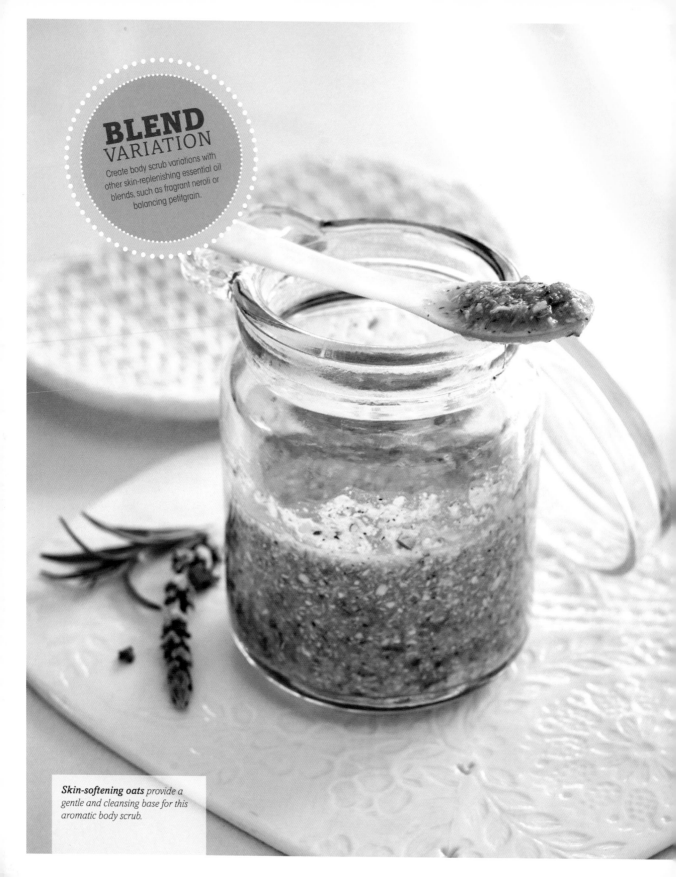

BLEND
VARIATION
Create body scrub variations with
other skin-replenishing essential oil
blends, such as fragrant neroli or
balancing petitgrain.

Skin-softening oats provide a
gentle and cleansing base for this
aromatic body scrub.

SKIN CARE

Exfoliating body scrub

Using a body scrub is a great way to boost the **circulation** and remove dead skin cells, leaving the skin soft, smooth, and invigorated. Almond oil is richly nourishing and great for **moisturizing** dry skin. Combined with **skin-softening** oats and calming Roman chamomile and lavender essential oils, this soothing scrub conditions and softens skin, giving a silky feel.

Ingredients

Makes 45ml (1½fl oz)

Jumbo oats 1 tbsp

Dried lavender flowers 1 tsp

Almond oil 2 tbsp

Lavender essential oil 4 drops

Roman chamomile essential oil 4 drops

How to **make**

1 Grind the oats and lavender flowers into a powder in a pestle and mortar or blender.

2 Mix the almond oil and essential oils together.

3 Mix the ground oats and flowers with the pre-mixed oils until they form a paste (add more almond oil if dry and more ground oats if too wet). Store in a sterilized jar with a tight-fitting lid. It will keep for up to 3 months.

How to **use**

As a scrub Gently massage the scrub into clean skin, and rinse off with warm water. Pat your skin dry with a clean towel.

Safe usage Do not use on broken or newly shaved skin.

Natural and nourishing, this fragrant scrub leaves skin feeling soft and invigorated.

MASSAGE OIL

Body toning oil

This **detoxifying** blend of essential oils promotes a healthy lymphatic system and tones and firms skin. Rosemary and peppermint combine a **diuretic** effect with **stimulating** and **decongesting** properties, while lemon stimulates the lymphatic system. Mandarin essential oil also has a diuretic action, and when massaged into the skin can help to reduce the appearance of stretch marks.

Ingredients

Makes 45ml (1½fl oz)

Wheatgerm oil 2 tbsp

Rosehip seed oil 1 tbsp

Peppermint essential oil 8 drops

Rosemary essential oil 5 drops

Lemon essential oil 4 drops

Mandarin essential oil 3 drops

How to **make**

Combine all the ingredients in a bowl, then transfer the blend to a sterilized dark glass bottle and seal with a cap or dropper, ready for use. Store the blend in a cool, dark place. It will keep for up to 3 months.

How to **use**

As a massage oil Massage into the skin with upwards circular movements, paying particular attention to any areas of dry skin. For maximum effect, dry-brush skin with a soft-bristled body brush to remove dead skin cells before using the oil.

This dynamic, toning group of essential oils can help tackle areas of stubborn cellulite.

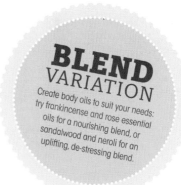

BLEND VARIATION
Create body oils to suit your needs: try frankincense and rose essential oils for a nourishing blend, or sandalwood and neroli for an uplifting, de-stressing blend.

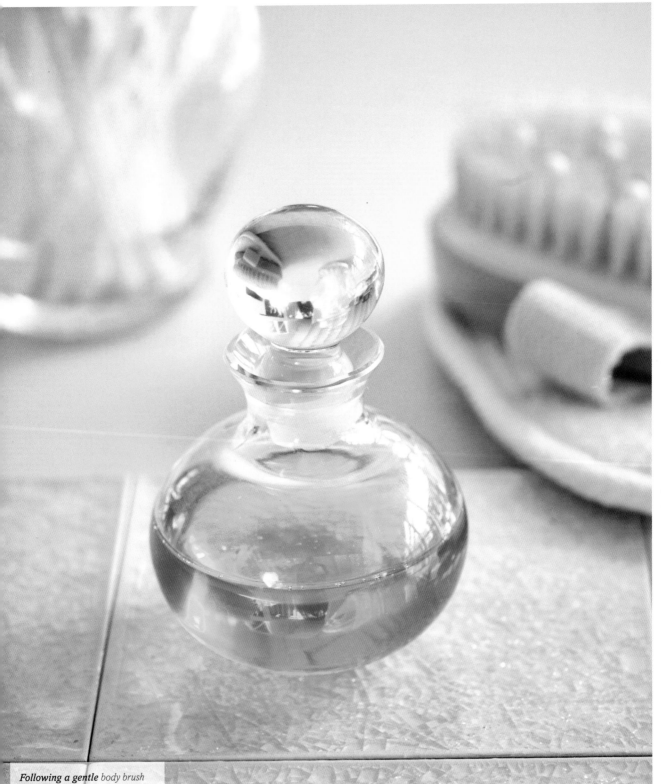

Following a gentle body brush with a stimulating massage blend maximizes the benefits to your skin.

HAIR CARE

Hair and scalp tonic

Stimulating and **cleansing** rosemary is excellent for hair and scalp conditions, including hair loss and dandruff, while cider vinegar helps to smooth the hair shaft and give added shine for healthy-looking hair. Combined with a herbal infusion, this **invigorating** hair tonic provides a fragrant rinse that not only leaves hair feeling **soft** and looking **glossy,** but can also help relieve a dry, flaking scalp.

Ingredients

Makes 220ml (7½fl oz)

Dried nettle leaves 1 tbsp

Water for infusion 200ml (7fl oz)

Cider vinegar 1 tsp

Sage essential oil 1 drop

Lemon essential oil 1 drop

Rosemary essential oil 1 drop

Cedarwood essential oil
1 drop

How to **make**

1 Make an infusion by brewing the nettles for 10 minutes in a teapot with 200ml (7fl oz) boiling water. Strain off the nettles.

2 Add the cider vinegar and the essential oils. Pour the mixture into a sterilized glass bottle. It will keep for up to 3 months.

Despite their sting, nettles have a host of benefits, and can help to cleanse and strengthen hair.

How to **use**

As a hair tonic Shake the bottle before use. Before shampooing, pour a cupful of the tonic over wet hair in the shower or bath. Massage into the hair or comb through, then follow with your usual shampoo. Continue to dry and style as usual.

Safe usage Avoid sage oil in pregnancy and when breastfeeding.

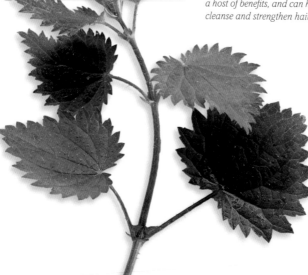

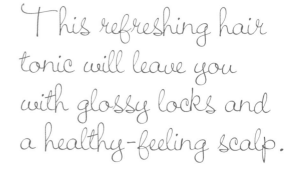

This refreshing hair tonic will leave you with glossy locks and a healthy-feeling scalp.

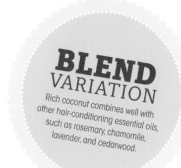

Conditioning hair oil

Coconut oil and shea nut butter are widely used in hair care thanks to their **nourishing** properties and their ability to add body, **lustre**, and **shine** to lank hair. Cypress essential oil helps to **revive** dull-looking and dry hair, lavender is soothing and **healing**, and lemon **moisturizes** the scalp. Apply the oil with a de-stressing scalp massage, working gently into any areas of tension.

Ingredients

Makes 45ml (1½fl oz)

Coconut oil solid 2 tbsp

Shea nut butter 1 tbsp

Cypress essential oil 3 drops

Lavender essential oil 2 drops

Lemon essential oil 1 drop

How to **make**

1 Melt the coconut oil and shea nut butter together in a bain maire (see p188). Remove from the heat and add the essential oils.

2 Pour into a sterilized glass jar. Leave to cool and then seal with a lid. It will keep for up to 3 months.

How to **use**

As a hair conditioner Depending on the length of your hair, a coin-sized amount of oil should be enough for one application. Massage into the hair, paying particular attention to the scalp, then wrap hair in a warm towel and leave for 30–60 minutes, or overnight. To remove the oil, rub shampoo through the hair before it comes into contact with any water, then rinse out the shampoo with warm water. Repeat to ensure the last traces of oil have been removed. Leave hair to dry naturally.

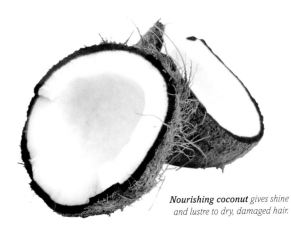

Nourishing coconut gives shine and lustre to dry, damaged hair.

SKIN CARE

Argan and avocado facial scrub

Frankincense oil has been used for centuries to **tone** and **firm** the skin, and is combined here with ground rice, a lovely natural exfoliator with a gentle scrubbing action. Mixed with **regenerative** argan oil and fatty acid-rich avocado oil, this facial scrub not only polishes, but also **replenishes** the skin. Aim to use twice a week to achieve smooth, glowing skin.

Ingredients

Makes 30ml (1fl oz)

Ground rice 1 tsp

Kaolin clay 1tsp

Argan oil 1 tbsp

Avocado oil 1 tbsp

Rose essential oil 1 drop

Frankincense essential oil 1 drop

How to **make**

1 Mix the ground rice, kaolin clay, and the argan and avocado oils together to form a paste (add more of the oils if too dry and more kaolin if the mixture seems too wet).

2 Add the essential oils. Use immediately.

How to **use**

As a facial scrub Gently massage the scrub into clean skin, avoiding the delicate area around the eyes, then remove with warm water. Pat your skin dry with a clean towel.

Using a facial scrub as part of your beauty regime keeps your skin supple and smooth.

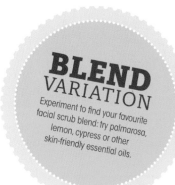

BLEND
VARIATION
Experiment to find your favourite facial scrub blend: try palmarosa, lemon, cypress or other skin-friendly essential oils.

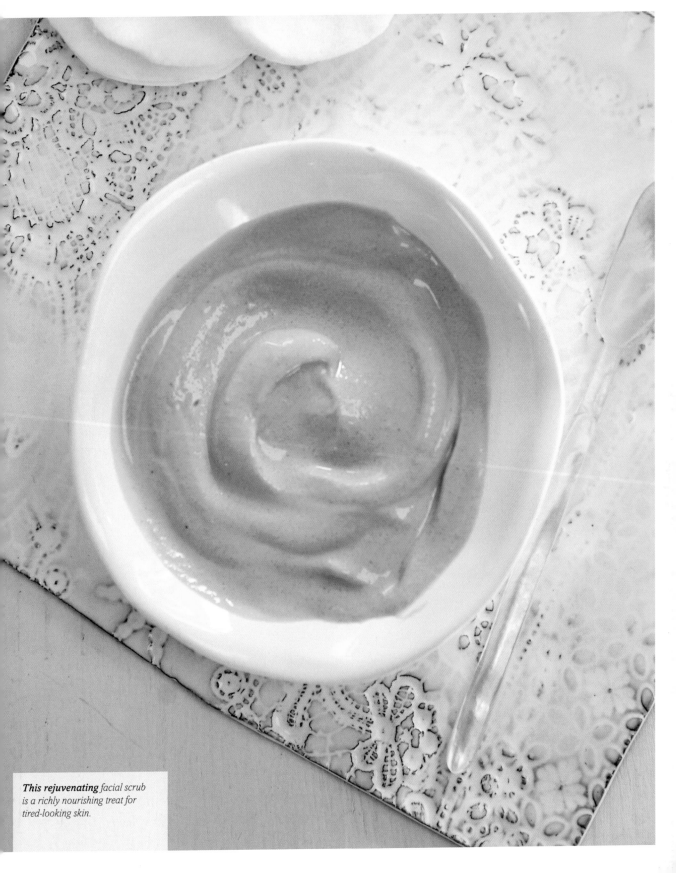

This rejuvenating *facial scrub is a richly nourishing treat for tired-looking skin.*

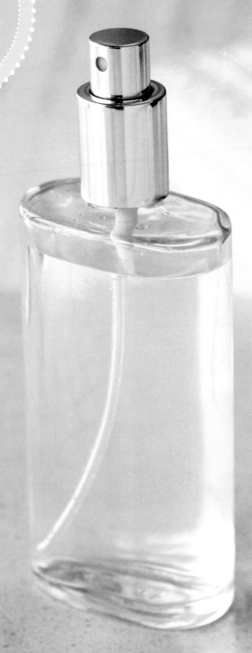

BLEND
VARIATION

Try other hydrating and refreshing essential oils for different "flavoured" spritzes, such as palmarosa, bergamot, and lemon.

Carry this facial spray with you on long journeys and revive and hydrate skin with a quick spritz.

STEAM INHALATION

Cleansing facial steam

One of the best ways to treat blocked facial pores is by giving them a **warm** steam facial. This sweats your skin, which opens pores and helps push any dirt out. Here, **antiseptic** tea tree, **skin-balancing** palmarosa, and **healing** lavender will help to give your skin a deep cleanse.

Ingredients

Makes Enough for 1 facial steam

Palmarosa essential oil 2 drops

Tea tree essential oil 1 drop

Lavender essential oil 1 drop

How to **make**

Half-fill a bowl with hot water, making sure that the bowl is set securely on a table. Add the essential oils.

How to **use**

As an inhalation Wash your face with a mild cleanser and rinse well. Keeping hair away from the face, drape a towel over your head and place your face over the bowl of steaming hot water. If at any point you feel the steam is too hot on your skin, move your face further away. Remain over the steam for about 10 to 15 minutes, or until the steam cools. Rinse your skin with lukewarm water and then pat it dry.

SKIN CARE

Facial spritz

Rose floral water can be used as a simple, beautifully **fragrant** skin remedy. The water contains some of the essential oil, which **calms** skin and reduces redness. Also useful for a **hydrating** boost, this mix is suitable for all skin types. Keep in the fridge for an ultra-refreshing spritz.

Ingredients

Makes 90ml (3fl oz)

Mineral water 75ml (2½fl oz)

Rose floral water 1 tbsp

Aloe vera juice 1tsp

Glycerine 1tsp

Rose absolute or essential oil
   5 drops

How to **make**

1 Combine the mineral water and rose floral water together.

2 Add the aloe vera juice and glycerine. Add the drops of essential oil.

3 Transfer to a sterilized bottle with an atomizer. Store in the fridge between uses. It will keep for up to 3 months.

How to **use**

As a skin spray Spritz the face or body after cleansing, or whenever you need a refreshing, hydrating boost. Perfect for travelling.

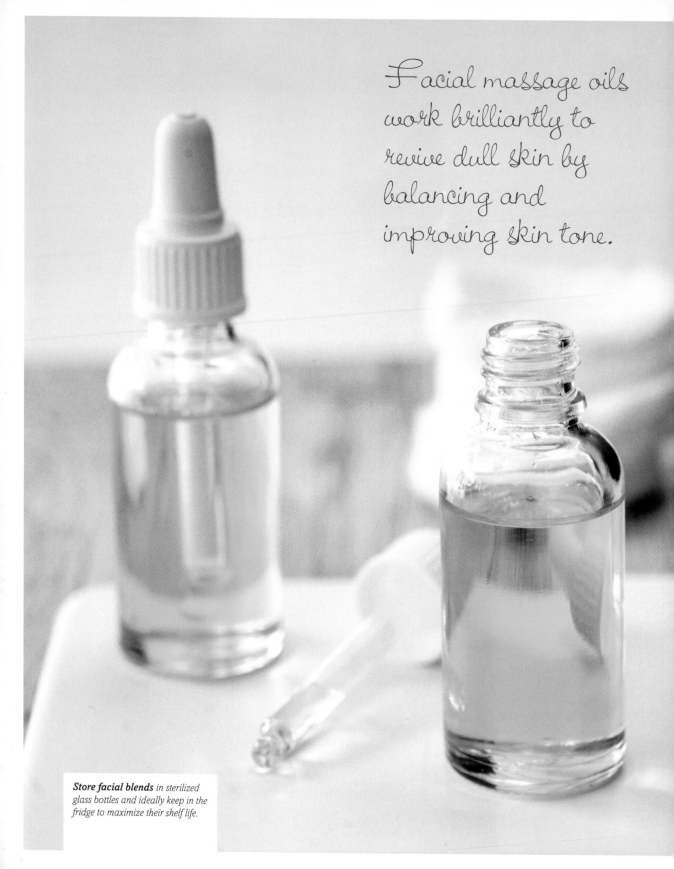

Facial massage oils work brilliantly to revive dull skin by balancing and improving skin tone.

Store facial blends in sterilized glass bottles and ideally keep in the fridge to maximize their shelf life.

MASSAGE OIL

Apricot and rose facial oil

Facial oils are simple to make and effective **moisturizers**. Here, beautifully **light** apricot oil makes an ideal facial massage oil for normal skin types, blending well with rosehip seed base oil, which helps tissue **regeneration** for facial lines and scars.

Ingredients

Makes 45ml (1½fl oz)

Apricot kernel oil 2tbsp

Rosehip seed oil 1 tbsp

Rose absolute or essential oil 2 drops

Cypress essential oil 2 drops

Clary sage essential oil 2 drops

Patchouli essential oil 1 drop

How to **make**

1 Combine the apricot and rosehip oils in a bowl. Add the essential oils to the mixture.

2 Transfer into a sterilized dark glass bottle and seal with a cap or dropper, ready for use. Store in a cool, dark place. It keeps for up to 3 months.

How to **use**

As a facial massage oil Apply a few drops to the fingertips and massage into the face and neck, using upward sweeping motions and avoiding the delicate eye area. Use at night, or under your everyday moisturizer if your skin is in need of additional hydration.

MASSAGE OIL

Tea tree and lemon facial oil

Suitable for combination and oily skin types, grapeseed and jojoba carrier oils help to restore normal oil production. **Astringent** lemon and **balancing** cedarwood essential oils tone and **balance** problem skin, and tea tree is strongly **antiseptic**, working on pimples and blackheads.

Ingredients

Makes 45ml (1½fl oz)

Grapeseed oil 2 tbsp

Jojoba oil 1 tbsp

Tea tree essential oil 4 drops

Lemon essential oil 2 drops

Cedarwood essential oil 1 drop

Rosemary essential oil 1 drop

How to **make**

1 Combine the grapeseed and jojoba oils in a bowl. Add the essential oils to the mixture.

2 Transfer into sterilized dark glass bottles and seal with a cap or dropper. Store in a cool, dark place. Keeps for up to 3 months.

How to **use**

As a facial massage oil Apply a few drops to the fingertips and massage into the face and neck, using upward sweeping motions and avoiding the delicate eye area. Use at night after washing the skin.

Safe usage Avoid exposure to the sun for 12 hours after using lemon essential oil.

HAND
CREAM

BLEND
VARIATION
For a different blend and aroma, substitute lemon and lime with other skin-nourishing essential oils, such as carrot, neroli, sandalwood, jasmine, or geranium.

Moisturizing nail balm

A daily hand and nail massage with this **refreshing** balm, concentrating on the cuticles, will **brighten** dull nails and help to stop them flaking and breaking. A combination of **nourishing** shea nut butter, cocoa butter, and coconut oil, along with **protective** beeswax, helps to improve cuticles and moisturize and strengthen nails, while lemon and lime essential oils **tone** and **revitalize**.

Ingredients

Makes 25ml (1fl oz)

Jojoba oil 1 tsp

Shea nut butter 1 tsp

Cocoa butter 1 tsp

Coconut oil solid 1 tsp

Beeswax ½ tsp

Lemon essential oil 5 drops

Lime essential oil 4 drops

How to **make**

1 Place the jojoba oil, shea nut butter, cocoa butter, coconut oil, and beeswax in a glass bowl. Heat in a bain marie until melted (see p188).

2 Remove from the heat. Add the essential oils and combine.

3 Pour into a sterilized glass jar, leave to cool, then seal with a lid. It will keep for up to 3 months.

How to **use**

As a nail balm Gently massage into the nails and cuticles as part of a daily hand-care regime. If your nails feel dry or brittle during the day, apply more frequently as required.

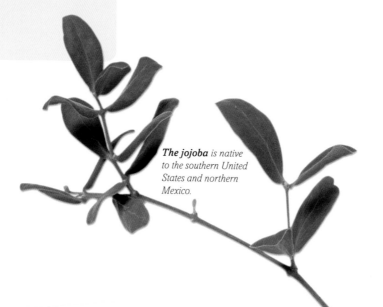

The jojoba is native to the southern United States and northern Mexico.

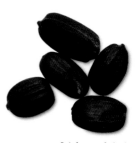

Jojoba seeds look similar to coffee beans, but are larger and less uniform.

HAND
CREAM

Rejuvenating hand cream

Revive the skin on your hands, which is over-exposed to the elements and often neglected, with this rich, protective cream that nourishes the hands and nails. The **soothing** and softening olive oil, **regenerative** hemp oil, nourishing cocoa butter, and **protective** beeswax moisturize and repair dry hands, while the **healing** and restorative essential oils are **uplifting** for the mind and increase wellbeing.

Ingredients

Makes 120ml (4fl oz)

Olive oil 1 tbsp

Hemp oil 1 tbsp

Cocoa butter 1 tsp

Beeswax 1 tsp

Emulsifying wax 1 tbsp

Mineral water 60ml (2fl oz)

Glycerine 1 tsp

Petitgrain essential oil 8 drops

Lemon essential oil 4 drops

Bergamot essential oil 4 drops

Myrrh essential oil 2 drops

How to **make**

1 Place the olive oil, hemp oil, cocoa butter, beeswax, and emulsifying wax in a glass bowl. Heat in a bain marie until melted (see p188).

2 Heat the water to 80°C (176°F). Add the glycerine. Add the hot oil mixture to the hot water and mix with a hand-held electric blender. Add the essential oils and continue to mix.

3 Pour into a sterilized glass jar, leave to cool, and seal with a lid. It will keep for up to 3 months.

How to **use**

As a hand cream Gently massage the cream onto dry hands, rubbing it into your nails and cuticles. Apply as often as required.

Treat your hands with this nourishing, rejuvenating, and beautifully scented hand cream.

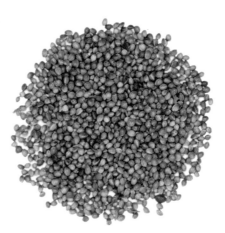

Rich in vitamin E and fatty acids, *hemp seeds produce a naturally skin-nourishing oil.*

FOOT BATH

Foot bath

Refresh and **soothe** aching feet with this foot bath, which contains a **cooling** peppermint infusion as well as the essential oil with its painkilling and **anti-inflammatory** properties. Honey **softens** skin, while cider vinegar relaxes muscles and fights foot bacteria. Use before the foot balm, below.

Ingredients

Makes 530ml (17½fl oz)

Peppermint dried herb 1 tbsp

Water for infusion 500ml (16fl oz)

Peppermint essential oil 2 drops

Lemon essential oil 2 drops

Mineral salts 1 tbsp

Honey 1 tbsp

Apple cider vinegar 1 tbsp

How to **make**

1 Make a peppermint infusion by brewing the herbs for 10 minutes in a teapot with 500ml (16fl oz) freshly boiled water. Strain the liquid.

2 Add the essential oils to the mineral salts and combine.

3 Add the honey and cider vinegar to the strained peppermint infusion and mix until dissolved.

4 Add the mineral salt and essential oil mixture to 1–2 cups of the infusion and stir until dissolved.

How to **use**

As a foot bath Add the infusion mixture to a warm foot bath and soak your feet immediately.

Safe usage Do not use on broken or newly shaved skin.

FOOT BATH

Foot balm

A combination of **restorative** essential oils, such as myrrh, **nourishing** vegetable oils, and **protective** and **moisturizing** beeswax, helps to soften hard skin to remedy dry or cracked heels. **Deodorizing** lemon essential oil helps lift odours, making this an all-round foot treatment.

Ingredients

Makes 90ml (3fl oz)

Beeswax 2 tbsp

Castor oil 1 tbsp

Hemp seed oil 1 tbsp

Sunflower oil 2 tbsp

Myrrh essential oil 2 drops

Lavender essential oil 2 drops

Lemon essential oil 2 drops

How to **make**

1 Place the beeswax and vegetable oils in a glass bowl. Heat in a bain marie (see p188) until melted.

2 Add the essential oils. Pour into a sterilized jar while warm then leave to set in the jar.

3 Seal the jar with a lid. It will keep for up to 3 months.

How to **use**

As a foot balm First exfoliate areas of dry skin on your feet with a pumice stone, then wash your feet thoroughly and pat dry. Massage the balm into the skin, paying particular attention to dry or cracked areas.

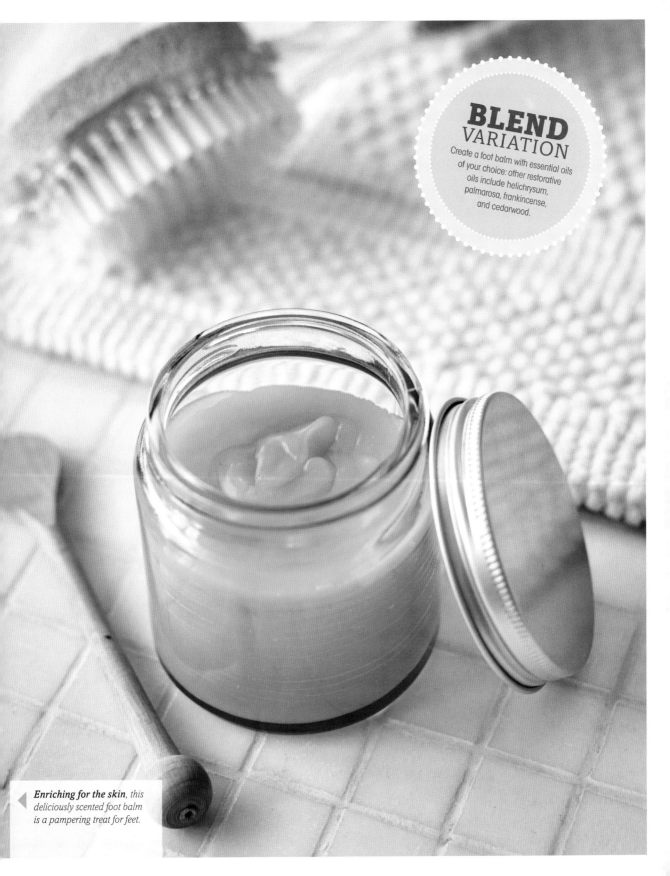

BLEND
VARIATION
Create a foot balm with essential oils of your choice: other restorative oils include helichrysum, palmarosa, frankincense, and cedarwood.

Enriching for the skin, this deliciously scented foot balm is a pampering treat for feet.

Healing
Remedies

Harness the healing powers of essential oils to provide relief from a range of common complaints. Learn how to use oils in therapeutic massages and baths, clearing inhalations, soothing compresses, and skin-healing ointments and creams.

Digestive problems

Lifestyle factors such as diet, as well as **stress** and emotional upset, can all impact on the **healthy functioning** of the digestive system, leading to blockages and other problems. Essential oils treat digestive upsets **holistically**, addressing both the root causes, such as anxiety, and providing relief for symptoms. If a condition persists or is acute, consult your doctor.

Bloating and constipation

The unpleasant feeling of being bloated occurs when your abdomen is stretched, puffy, and uncomfortable. It's common to feel this way during a festive period or celebrations. You can avoid feeling overfull by cutting down on fizzy drinks, monitoring portion sizes, sitting down to eat, and taking regular exercise. Constipation can be caused by poor diet and stress, and symptoms can be relieved by making dietary and lifestyle changes. Try increasing your daily intake of fibre to at least 18–30g (¾–1oz) a day. Fresh fruit, vegetables, and cereals are all high in fibre. You can also try including some bulking agents in your diet, such as oat bran, which helps to make stools softer and easier to pass. Drink plenty of water, too, exercise regularly, and keep active. The following remedies can help to ease digestive complaints.

Settling carrot and orange compress

The combination of carrot seed, orange, and fennel in this warming compress has a tonifying and soothing effect on the digestive system. Orange essential oil calms unsettled digestion and helps food move through the digestive tract, in turn relieving constipation, trapped wind, and easing indigestion. Carrot seed is mildly diuretic so helps to reduce fluid retention, and soothing fennel eases nervous indigestion caused by emotional upset, or indigestion after a rushed meal. This remedy is not suitable in pregnancy.

Ingredients

Makes 1 compress
Almond oil 1 tsp
Orange essential oil 3 drops
Fennel essential oil 2 drops
Carrot seed essential oil 2 drops

How to **make**

1 Fill a bowl with hot water. Add the essential oils to the base oil, then add to the water.

2 Soak a flannel in the bowl, then remove the flannel and squeeze out the excess water.

3 Wrap the flannel in a towel or cling film to insulate it. Place the compress on the abdomen. Leave the flannel in place while it cools to body temperature, then repeat 3 times.

Stimulating spearmint massage

Abdominal massage is an effective way to treat constipation and is easily self-administered. Cooling spearmint essential oil is extremely soothing for digestion as it helps to calm nausea and indigestion and can also improve a sluggish system.

Ingredients

Makes 30ml (1fl oz)
Grapeseed oil 2 tbsp
Spearmint essential oil 5 drops
Pine essential oil 5 drops
Rosemary essential oil 5 drops

How to **make**

1 Combine all the ingredients together in a bowl. Transfer to a sterilized dark glass bottle and seal with a cap or dropper.

2 Massage clockwise into the abdomen. Allow the oil to absorb into the skin before you get dressed. Store the remaining oil in a cool, dark place. Keeps for up to 3 months.

Soothing dill bath soak

This tummy-settling bath blend makes use of the antispasmodic properties of marjoram, together with the stimulating effect of black pepper and soothing dill to relieve trapped wind and pep up a sluggish digestion. It helps food to move along the digestive tract.

Ingredients

Makes 15ml (½fl oz)
Base oil or full-fat milk 1 tbsp
Black pepper essential oil 3 drops
Dill essential oil 3 drops
Marjoram essential oil 3 drops

How to **make**

1 Combine all the ingredients together in a bowl.

2 Disperse the blend immediately in a warm bath and enjoy a relaxing and soothing soak.

Indigestion

Indigestion can be felt as pain or discomfort in the upper abdomen, or as a burning sensation behind the breastbone. The symptoms of indigestion often appear shortly after eating or drinking, and may be caused by stomach acid coming into contact with the sensitive stomach lining. The stomach acid breaks down the lining, leading to irritation and inflammation. In most cases, indigestion is related to eating and is often followed by heartburn, or reflux (see below), although it can be triggered by other factors such as smoking, drinking alcohol, pregnancy, stress or taking certain medications. Try the massage below to ease symptoms.

Cardamom massage

Essential oils that are antispasmodic, calming, and warming, such as coriander, mandarin, and cardamom, can help to relieve indigestion.

Ingredients

Makes 30ml (1fl oz)
Almond oil 2 tbsp
Mandarin essential oil 5 drops
Coriander essential oil 3 drops
Cardamom essential oil 2 drops

How to **make**

1 Combine all the ingredients together in a bowl. Transfer to a sterilized dark glass bottle and seal with a cap or dropper.

2 Gently massage into the chest and abdomen. Allow the oil to absorb into the skin before you get dressed. Store the remaining oil in a cool, dark place. Keeps for up to 3 months.

Reflux

Acid reflux is a condition where stomach acid comes back up into the mouth and causes an unpleasant, sour taste. It can also be accompanied by symptoms such as wind and bloating, and indigestion and heartburn. Reflux can be caused by a number of things, such as eating big portions and high-fat meals, eating too many acidic foods, and chronic stress. Try this soothing massage to help calm the symptoms.

Peppermint and ginger massage

Essential oils can help relieve the symptoms of reflux when massaged onto the chest and abdomen. You may also find that a slice of lemon or fresh ginger, or a sprig of fresh peppermint infused in a glass of hot water is helpful.

Ingredients

Makes 30ml (1fl oz)
Sunflower oil 2 tbsp
Peppermint essential oil 7 drops
Ginger essential oil 5 drops
Dill essential oil 3 drops

How to **make**

1 Combine all the ingredients together in a bowl. Transfer to a sterilized dark glass bottle and seal with a cap or dropper.

2 Gently massage into the abdomen, chest, and upper back. Allow the oil to absorb into the skin before you get dressed. Store the remaining oil in a cool, dark place. Keeps for up to 3 months.

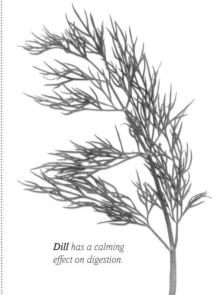

Dill has a calming effect on digestion.

Nausea and sickness

Nausea is the unpleasant sensation that can precede vomiting, or the feeling can be there without vomiting. Vomiting occurs when the stomach contents are forcefully expelled through the mouth. Nausea and vomiting may be due to a variety of causes, such as eating or drinking too much, hormonal changes in the first trimester of pregnancy, or an infection. These causes may need little or no treatment. However, if there is no obvious cause for prolonged bouts of sickness, talk to your doctor as it is important to identify the underlying cause. Try the remedies here to ease nausea.

Warming cardamom compress

If the abdomen is tender and painful to touch, gently applying a warm compress can be soothing and just as effective as an abdominal massage.

Ingredients

Makes 1 compress
Almond oil 1 tsp
Cardamom essential oil 2 drops
Black pepper essential oil 2 drops

How to **make**

1 Fill a bowl with warm water. Add the essential oils to the base oil and then to the water.

2 Soak a flannel in the bowl, then remove the flannel and squeeze out the excess water.

3 Wrap the flannel in a towel or piece of cling film to insulate it. Place the compress on the abdomen. Leave the flannel in place while it cools to body temperature, then repeat the process 3 times.

Ginger diffusion

Ginger is a classic remedy for overcoming nausea and tummy upsets, whether caused by over-indulgence, pregnancy hormones, or travel sickness. Here, ginger essential oil is partnered with Roman chamomile. A slightly gentler oil than German chamomile, Roman chamomile is suitable for young children and for those who have a delicate constitution.

Ingredients

Makes enough for 1 diffusion
Ginger essential oil 6 drops
Roman chamomile essential oil 3 drops
Peppermint essential oil 3 drops

How to **make**

1 Add the essential oil blend to a diffuser, vaporizer or oil burner.

2 Gently fragrance your chosen environment.

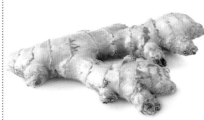

Ginger *can quell feelings of nausea.*

Diarrhoea

Diarrhoea is frequent, watery bowel movements. It can be caused by eating foods that irritate the gut, by a bowel infection, or by nerves and stress. Keep well hydrated if you have diarrhoea. These remedies can soothe intestinal lining.

Tummy-calming massage blend

Blend antispasmodic essential oils, such as cypress and ginger, with pain-relieving lavender for this therapeutic blend.

Ingredients

Makes 30ml (1fl oz)
Sunflower oil 2 tbsp
Cypress essential oil 6 drops
Ginger essential oil 5 drops
Lavender essential oil 3 drops

How to **make**

1 Combine all the ingredients together in a bowl. Transfer to a sterilized dark glass bottle and seal with a cap or dropper.

2 Massage clockwise into the abdomen. Allow the oil to absorb into the skin before you get dressed. Store the remaining oil in a cool, dark place. Keeps for up to 3 months.

Mandarin and geranium compress

Mandarin can settle digestion and is effective for overcoming feelings of nausea. Here it's combined with geranium and black pepper, which help to stimulate and support the digestive system. This compress will help to soothe an unsettled stomach and restore normal bowel movements. The heat also relaxes the abdominal muscles.

Ingredients

Makes 1 compress
Almond oil 1 tsp
Mandarin essential oil 3 drops
Geranium essential oil 2 drops
Black pepper essential oil 2 drops

How to **make**

1 Fill a bowl with hot water. Add the essential oils to the base oil, then to the water.

2 Soak a flannel in the bowl, then remove the flannel and squeeze out the excess water.

3 Wrap the flannel in a towel or piece of cling film to insulate it. Place the compress on the abdomen. Leave the flannel in place while it cools to body temperature, then repeat the process 3 times.

Appetite loss

There are a number of reasons why you might lose your appetite. Some conditions are temporary, or sometimes, appetite loss can indicate a serious condition such as anorexia nervosa, which is an eating disorder where a person keeps their body weight as low as possible. A condition such as anorexia requires specialist treatment. Always consult your doctor if you experience an unexplained loss of appetite. The bath soak below can help to stimulate appetite.

Peppermint soak

Ginger and peppermint stimulate the appetite. Added to a warm bath, they are absorbed into the skin and their scent inhaled. Peppermint and ginger herbal teas also help to stimulate appetite.

Ingredients

Makes 15ml (½fl oz)
Base oil or full-fat milk 1 tbsp
Peppermint essential oil 5 drops
Ginger essential oil 2 drops

How to **make**

1 Combine all the ingredients together in a bowl.

2 Disperse the blend immediately in a warm bath and enjoy a relaxing soak.

Mouth, gum, and tooth problems

Most oral disease is caused by bacterial infection. When bacteria forms in the mouth it produces a sticky, colourless film on the teeth called plaque, which hardens into tartar. Plaque and tartar irritate and inflame gums, which can destroy the gums and tissues. Research has linked gum disease to cardiovascular health and diabetes so a healthy mouth is thought to promote good health.

Bad breath (halitosis) has many causes, but is usually down to poor oral hygiene. If bacteria builds up in the mouth, it breaks down pieces of food lodged in the teeth and creates an bad odour. The following remedies help to improve oral hygiene.

Soothing gum oil

Myrrh essential oil, helps to reduce gum inflammation, while clove has a numbing effect to help relieve pain and soreness.

Ingredients

Makes 15ml (½fl oz)
Olive oil 1tbsp
Clove essential oil 1 drop
Myrrh essential oil 1 drop
Peppermint essential oil 1 drop

How to **make**

1 Combine all the ingredients together in a bowl. Transfer to a sterilized small glass jar.

2 Gently rub the oil blend into the gums, then rinse out with water.

Oregano gargle

To combat halitosis, try a gargle with antibacterial oils.

Ingredients

Makes 15ml (½fl oz)
Sunflower oil 1 tbsp
Peppermint essential oil 1 drop
Oregano essential oil 1 drop

How to **make**

1 Mix the oil blend with cold water.

2 Wash the solution around the mouth for 3–5 minutes, then spit it out. Rinse with water. Use 3 times daily.

Safe usage *Do not swallow. Not suitable in pregnancy.*

Respiratory complaints

While it is hard to avoid all cold viruses, there are steps you can take to **boost** immunity. Once a cold has set in, early treatment can also help to minimize its severity. Chronic conditions, such as asthma, require careful medical management, but there are ways to help control them. Essential oil's **decongesting**, **antiviral**, and **calming** properties can ease respiratory complaints.

Colds and sinusitis

A cold is a mild viral infection of the nose, throat, sinuses, and upper airways. This viral infection is very common and usually clears up on its own within a week or two. The main symptoms of a cold include an initial sore throat, blocked or runny nose, sneezing, and coughing.

Sinusitis is another common condition in which the lining of the sinuses becomes inflamed, and this usually follows a viral infection such as a cold. Symptoms of sinusitis include a green or yellow nasal discharge, blocked nose, pain and tenderness around the cheeks, eyes or forehead, a sinus headache and a temperature. The symptoms often improve within two to three weeks. While you can't "cure" a cold virus, there are several ways in which you can use essential oils to bring relief to colds and blocked sinuses.

Frankincense throat and chest rub

Frankincense essential oil helps to soothe the mucous membranes, calm breathing, and can also ease coughs, sore throats, and bronchitis. It is blended here with other soothing oils to create a warming upper-body rub to help combat colds and congestion.

Ingredients

Makes 30ml (1 fl oz)
Sunflower oil 2 tbsp
Frankincense essential oil 7 drops
Sandalwood essential oil 5 drops
Lavender essential oil 3 drops

How to **make**

1 Mix all the ingredients together in a bowl. Pour into a sterilized dark glass bottle. Seal with a cap or dropper.

2 Gently massage into the chest, throat, and upper back. Allow the oil to absorb before you get dressed.

Clearing eucalyptus diffusion

Eucalyptus has wonderful clearing properties that help to relieve blocked sinuses. Using a diffuser to disperse this essential oil in the air is an effective way to ease congested sinuses. Sit near the diffuser for the most direct effect.

Ingredients

Makes enough for 1 diffusion
Cedarwood essential oil 4 drops
Eucalyptus essential oil 4 drops
Ravensara essential oil 4 drops

How to **make**

1 Add the essential oil blend to a diffuser, vaporizer or oil burner.

2 Gently fragrance your chosen environment.

Cajuput and tea tree inhalation

Steam inhalations are very effective at treating sore throats and relieving congestion.

Ingredients

Makes enough for 1 inhalation
Cajuput essential oil 6 drops
Tea tree essential oil 4 drops
Lavender essential oil 4 drops

How to **make**

1 Add the essential oils to a bowl of hot water. Cover your head with a towel, making a tent over the bowl, lean over the bowl, and inhale deeply.

2 Allow the steam to soothe the throat for 5–10 minutes, taking a break from the steam if needed.

Asthma

Asthma is a common long-term condition that can cause coughing, wheezing, breathlessness, and tightness in the chest. The severity of the symptoms varies from person to person. In most people, the condition can be controlled well for most of the time, although some experience more persistent problems.

Occasionally, asthma gets gradually or suddenly much worse. This is known as an asthma attack, and these more severe attacks may require urgent hospital treatment and can even be life-threatening, although this is unusual.

No single cause for asthma has been identified, however there are several factors that may trigger an asthma attack. Inhaled or ingested allergens, such as dust mites and certain foods, can trigger an attack. Exercise and emotional stress can also produce asthmatic symptoms. Learning to manage the condition and avoid potential allergens is key to preventing attacks. The following remedies use oils to help calm mild symptoms so can be used alongside usual medical treatments. Consult your doctor before using these remedies, and always seek urgent medical help if you experience a severe asthma attack.

Eucalyptus and lemon inhalation

Sometimes asthma symptoms can be triggered by the presence of an infection such as a cold or flu virus. An inhalation using clearing essential oils can be useful to help ease asthma symptoms in these circumstances.

Ingredients

Makes enough for 1 inhalation
Lemon essential oil 4 drops
Eucalyptus essential oil 4 drops
Peppermint essential oil 4 drops

How to **make**

1 Place the oil drops directly on a tissue or handkerchief.

2 Keep the tissue with you and inhale by wafting the tissue under the nose. Do not cover the nose with the tissue.

Frankincense diffusion

Asthma symptoms can sometimes worsen if a person has had an emotional upset or specific trauma. In these circumstances, a diffusion with calming

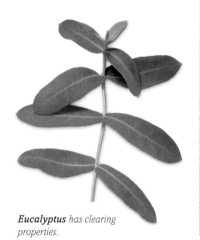

Eucalyptus *has clearing properties.*

essential oils such as frankincense, sandalwood, and lavender can be effective in easing the symptoms.

Ingredients

Frankincense essential oil 7 drops
Sandalwood essential oil 5 drops
Lavender essential oil 3 drops

How to **make**

1 Add the essential oil blend to a diffuser, vaporizer or oil burner.

2 Gently fragrance your chosen environment.

Calming chamomile massage

If asthma symptoms are typically brought on by exposure to allergens, such as dust mites or certain foods, have a ready-prepared massage blend to hand, made up of soothing essential oils such as chamomile, and an oil such as helichrysum, which has an antispasmodic action.

Ingredients

Makes 30ml (1fl oz)
Sunflower oil 2 tbsp
Helichrysum essential oil 4 drops
Lavender essential oil 4 drops
Roman chamomile essential oil 4 drops

How to **make**

1 Combine all the ingredients together in a bowl. Transfer to a sterilized dark glass bottle and seal with a cap or dropper.

2 Gently massage into the chest, throat, and upper back. Allow the oil to absorb into the skin before you get dressed. Store the remaining oil in a cool, dark place. Keeps for up to 3 months.

Circulatory problems

Circulatory problems can be caused by poor diet, smoking, having a sedentary lifestyle, and stress. Improving **lifestyle factors** such as diet and building a regular **exercise regime** can help to address problems. Essential oils can **stimulate** sluggish circulation and may help to provide the **motivation** to change your lifestyle.

Varicose veins and haemorrhoids

Varicose veins develop when the small valves inside the veins stop working properly. In a healthy vein, blood flows smoothly to the heart and the blood is prevented from flowing backwards by a series of tiny valves that open and close to enable it to pass through. If these valves weaken or are damaged, the blood can start to flow backwards and then collect in the vein, eventually causing the vein to become swollen and enlarged (known as varicose). Pregnancy, being overweight, and old age are all factors that can increase the chances of developing varicose veins.

Haemorrhoids, also known as piles, are related to varicose veins. These are swellings containing enlarged blood vessels that are found inside or around the rectum and anus. In many cases, haemorrhoids don't cause symptoms, and some people don't even realise that they have them. The compress below can help to ease and relieve symptoms such as pain or itching.

Soothing cypress compress

Cypress essential oil has a toning effect on the veins and is a useful oil for circulatory problems as it helps to regulate the flow of blood, making it particularly useful for conditions such as varicose veins. Here it is combined with detoxifying lemon and geranium essential oils, and juniper essential oil, which has an astringent action that is helpful for shrinking varicose veins and haemorrhoids.

Ingredients

Makes 1 compress
Sunflower oil 2 tsp
Cypress essential oil 3 drops
Lemon essential oil 3 drops
Juniper essential oil 3 drops
Geranium essential oil 1 drop

How to **make**

1 Fill a bowl with cold water. Add the essential oils to the sunflower oil, then add to the water.

2 Soak a flannel in the bowl, then remove the flannel and squeeze out the excess water.

3 Place the compress over the varicose veins, or for haemorrhoids, sit on the compress with a towel underneath. Leave in place for 10 minutes.

High blood pressure

Hypertension is another term for high blood pressure. Blood pressure is measured in millimetres of mercury (mmHg) and it is recorded as two figures: systolic pressure – the pressure of the

Essential oils can be used to stimulate or calm circulation.

blood when your heart pushes blood out, and diastolic pressure – the pressure of the blood when your heart rests in between beats, which reflects how strongly your arteries are resisting blood flow.

It is perfectly normal for the systolic blood pressure to increase on exertion or during emotional stress, but in a healthy body it will return to normal quite quickly. A number of lifestyle and dietary changes can be made to help reduce the risk of hypertension, for example increasing exercise, reducing salt intake, stopping smoking, and reducing stress and stimulants. A relaxing massage can help to combat the cumulative effects of stress and tension.

If you have been diagnosed with high blood pressure, talk to your doctor before using any complementary remedy to make sure that your condition is being monitored medically. Continue to take your usual prescribed medication alongside remedies unless directed otherwise by your doctor.

Lavender and marjoram massage

Essential oils that have a hypotensive action (meaning they help to lower blood pressure), as well as calming and sedating effects, can be used to alleviate mild hypertension. Here, lavender, marjoram, and ylang ylang essential oils are combined to make a therapeutic massage blend that can be used to help combat mild hypertension.

Ingredients

Makes 30ml (1fl oz)
Almond oil 2 tbsp
Lavender essential oil 6 drops
Marjoram essential oil 6 drops
Ylang ylang essential oil 3 drops

How to **make**

1 Combine all the ingredients together in a bowl. Transfer to a sterilized dark glass bottle and seal with a cap or dropper.

2 Gently massage into the body. Allow the oil to absorb into the skin before you get dressed. Store remaining oil in a cool, dark place. Keeps for up to 3 months.

Sluggish circulation

There are many different symptoms that can indicate poor circulation.

For example, cold extremeties such as the feet and toes and fingers and hands, water retention, and cramps, all suggest that general circulation is sluggish. Apart from the daily discomfort that poor circulation can cause, there are some potentially more serious consequences. Simple dietary and lifestyle changes can help to improve the circulation. For example, if you sit at a desk all day, ensure that you take regular breaks and move around, stop eating convenience foods, and try to give up smoking. The massage below can help to stimulate circulation.

Stimulating rosemary massage

Some essential oils are stimulating and can help to improve circulation. These warming oils dilate the capillaries to increase blood flow. This in turn stimulates the flow of lymph, which helps control the passage of fluids around the body. Poor lymphatic drainage results in a build-up of fluid in the tissues.

Ingredients

Makes 30ml (1fl oz)
Almond oil 2 tbsp
Rosemary essential oil 3 drops
Thyme essential oil 3 drops
Black pepper essential oil 3 drops
Ginger essential oil 3 drops
Clove essential oil 1 drop

How to **make**

1 Combine all the ingredients together in a bowl. Transfer to a sterilized dark glass bottle and seal with a cap or dropper.

2 Gently massage into the body. Allow the oil to absorb into the skin before you get dressed. Store remaining oil in a cool, dark place. Keeps for up to 3 months.

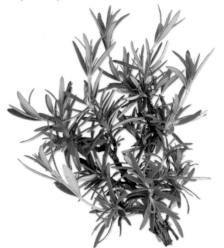

Rosemary *helps improve poor circulation.*

Fluid retention and urinary tract infections

Swelling and puffiness, known as oedema, indicate **fluid retention**, which can have a number of causes. Infections in the urinary system can cause bladder inflammation. Certain essential oils have **diuretic**, anti-inflammatory, and **antiseptic** properties that can help to ease symptoms.

Swelling

Swelling is typically the result of inflammation or a buildup of fluid that can occur internally or that can affect your outer skin and muscles. Using essential oils that have detoxifying properties helps to flush out excess fluids and reduce inflammation. Consult your doctor if you have any unexplained swelling.

Geranium compress

A number of essential oils work as circulatory tonics that can help to reduce swelling and fluid retention and are effective used in massage, in the bath or as a compress, as in the remedy here.

Ingredients

Makes 1 compress
Almond oil 1 tbsp
Geranium essential oil 5 drops
Cypress essential oil 4 drops
Yarrow essential oil 3 drops
Lemon essential oil 3 drops

How to **make**

1 Fill a bowl with cold water. Add the essential oils to the almond oil, then add to the water.

2 Soak a flannel in the bowl, then remove the flannel and squeeze out the excess water.

3 Place the compress on the affected area. Leave the flannel in place while it reaches body temperature, then repeat the process 3 times.

Detox massage

The lymphatic system is responsible for removing the waste products created by the body's organs and tissues. The blend of detoxifying essential oils used in this massage supports the action of the lymphatic system. Grapefruit specifically encourages lymphatic drainage and acts as a diuretic when it is massaged directly into the skin, helping to combat areas of puffiness caused by water retention. Rosemary helps to stimulate lymphatic circulation, helping the body to remove waste products and also relieving water retention. These two potent oils are combined here with black pepper, which works as a mild diuretic. To maximize the effect of this detox massage, use the oils in combination with a body brush to stimulate the circulation.

Ingredients

Grapeseed oil 2 tbsp
Grapefruit essential oil 5 drops
Rosemary essential oil 5 drops
Black pepper essential oil 5 drops

How to **make**

1 Combine all the ingredients together in a bowl. Transfer to a sterilized dark glass bottle and seal with a cap or dropper.

2 Gently massage into the skin in upwards circular movements. Allow the oil to absorb into the skin before you get dressed. Store the remaining oil in a cool, dark place. Keeps for up to 3 months.

Black pepper *helps to flush out waste products.*

Urinary tract infection

Urinary tract infections (UTIs) are very common. They can be painful and uncomfortable, but they usually pass within a few days, though sometimes you may need a course of antibiotics. UTIs are more common in women than in men. Children can also get UTIs, but this is less common.

A UTI develops when part of the urinary tract becomes infected, usually by bacteria, which can enter the urinary tract through the urethra or, more rarely, through the bloodstream. There is usually no obvious reason why the urinary tract becomes infected, although some women find they develop a UTI after having sex. As UTIs are far less common in men than in women these need investigating to find an underlying cause.

Cystitis is inflammation of the bladder, usually caused by an infection. Most cases are thought to occur when bacteria that live harmlessly in the bowel or on the skin enter the bladder through the urethra. It's a common type of UTI, particularly in women, and is usually more of a nuisance than a cause for serious concern. Mild cases will often get better by themselves within a few days. However, some people experience episodes of cystitis frequently and may need regular or long-term treatment. There's also a chance that cystitis could lead to a more serious kidney infection, so it's important to seek medical advice if your symptoms don't improve over a few days, or if you have a fever, severe pain, or blood or pus in the urine. Try the following remedies to help ease symptoms and bring relief.

Bergamot sitz bath

As UTIs are caused by infection, essential oils with antibacterial activity are recommended to help fight the infection and support your recovery. Here, antiviral and antibacterial bergamot is combined with astringent chamomile and soothing lavender. The oils are added to a shallow "sitz" bath, which is waist height only and ideal for treating UTIs.

Ingredients

Makes enough for 1 sitz bath
Bergamot essential oil 4 drops
German chamomile essential oil 3 drops
Lavender essential oil 2 drops

How to **make**

1 Fill the bath to waist height. Adjust the temperature depending on how long you wish to remain in the bath. For a bath of up to five minutes, run hot water at a temperature of 40–45°C (104–113°F). If you want to stay in the bath for up to 15 minutes, keep the water at 33–35°C (91–95°F). Alternatively, fill a bowl with warm water, add the essential oils, then soak a clean flannel in the water. Remove the flannel and squeeze out the excess water, then gently wash the affected area with the flannel. After washing, pat dry the area carefully.

2 If using the oils in a shallow bath, add the essential oils to the bath once run, then soak as required.

Tea tree wash

The antiseptic properties of tea tree essential oil are especially useful for treating UTIs. Try this simple wash to ease discomfort. Always ensure your flannels and towels are clean before using and are washed immediately after every use.

Ingredients

Makes enough for 1 wash
Almond oil 1 tsp
Tea tree essential oil 3 drops
Bergamot essential oil 3 drops

How to **make**

1 Fill a large bowl with warm water. Add the essential oils to the almond oil, then add to the water.

2 Soak a clean flannel in the water, then remove the flannel and wring it out.

3 Gently wash the affected area with the flannel, patting the area dry carefully afterwards.

Antiseptic and soothing essential oils are useful for easing the symptoms of UTIs.

Muscle and joint problems and general aches and pains

Healthy muscles and joints help ensure strength and manoeuvrability. Old age can put a strain on joints and muscles, but **activity** helps maintain **flexibility**. Aches and pains can be due to muscle tension or other causes. Try oils that are **anti-inflammatory**, detoxifying, and **pain-relieving**.

Backache, neck pain, and sciatica

Back pain is a common problem that affects most people at some point in life. It may be triggered by bad posture, by bending awkwardly, or by lifting heavy loads and objects incorrectly. In most cases, back pain improves over a period of weeks or months, although some experience recurrent long-term pain.

Neck pain, or a stiff neck, is a common problem and usually nothing to worry about. You can get a painful or stiff neck if you sleep awkwardly, use a computer for a prolonged period of time, or strain a muscle because of bad posture. The pain and stiffness usually get better after a few days or weeks. Anxiety and stress can also cause tension in the neck muscles that can lead to neck pain. If pain is acute or long-lasting, consult your doctor.

A stiff neck accompanied by other symptoms such as fever, headache, or intolerance to bright lights, should be investigated immediately.

Sciatica is the name for pain that is caused by irritation or compression of the sciatic nerve, which is the longest nerve in the body. It runs from the back of the pelvis, through the buttocks, and all the way down the legs, ending at the feet. When this nerve is compressed or irritated, it can cause pain, numbness, and a tingling sensation that radiates from the lower back down one leg to the foot and toes. While sciatica pain can also be accompanied by general back pain, the pain of sciatica usually affects the buttocks and legs more than the back. Try the following pain-relieving remedies.

Muscle-relaxing massage

Essential oils and massage can be extremely effective in treating backache and neck pain where the pain is due to tension or muscular fatigue. Regular massage with oils and essential oil baths can help to prevent backache by reducing stress, relaxing tight muscles, and improving general wellbeing, which helps to relieve held-in tension. The following massage blend can also be added to a bath for a relaxing soak, combining the essential oils with just a tablespoon of arnica oil, or alternatively with a tablespoon of full-fat milk or vodka.

Ingredients

Makes 30ml (1fl oz)
Arnica macerated oil 2 tbsp
Rosemary essential oil 5 drops
Marjoram essential oil 5 drops
Ginger essential oil 5 drops

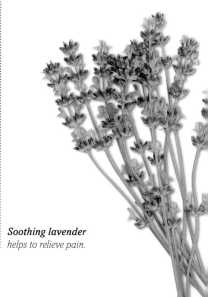

Soothing lavender
helps to relieve pain.

How to **make**

1 Combine the ingredients in a bowl. Transfer to a sterilized dark glass bottle. Sseal with a cap or dropper.

2 Massage into the back and neck. Allow the oil to absorb into the skin before you get dressed. Store the remaining oil in a cool, dark place. Keeps for up to 3 months.

Soothing lavender compress

Lavender is mildly analgesic and antispasmodic so can soothe sciatic pain.

Ingredients

Makes 1 compress
Almond oil 1 tsp
Lavender essential oil 5 drops
Coriander essential oil 2 drops
Black pepper essential oil 5 drops

How to **make**

1 Fill a bowl with warm water. Add the essential oils to the almond oil, then add to the water.

2 Soak a flannel in the bowl, then remove the flannel and squeeze out the excess water.

3 Wrap the flannel in a towel or cling film to insulate it. Place the compress on the affected area. Leave it in place while it cools to body temperature, then repeat the process 3 times.

Headaches and migraines

Headaches are one of the most common health complaints. In many cases they can be easily treated with small lifestyle changes, such as getting more rest and drinking enough fluids so that you stay well hydrated. Tension headaches are often described as a constant ache that affects both sides of the head, and these are commonly linked to stress, poor posture, skipping meals, and dehydration. Migraines are less common than headaches. They're usually felt as a severe, throbbing pain at the front or side of the head. Other symptoms of migraines may include nausea, vomiting, and increased sensitivity to light or sound. A soothing compress or head massage can bring relief.

Calming peppermint and lavender compress

With its gently stimulating and analgesic properties, peppermint is an established treatment in aromatherapy for tension headaches, working in a similar way to drugs such as paracetamol. Its cooling action clears and refreshes the mind. Relaxing lavender helps to bring relief to headaches caused by anxiety and stress.

Ingredients

Makes 1 compress
Almond oil 1 tsp
Peppermint essential oil 3 drops
Lavender essential oil 2 drops

How to **make**

1 Fill a bowl with warm water. Add the essential oils to the almond oil, then add to the water.

2 Soak a flannel in the bowl, then remove the flannel and squeeze out the excess water.

3 Place the compress on the forehead. Leave the flannel in place while it cools to body temperature, then repeat the process 3 times.

Warming marjoram compress

Marjoram essential oil has both a sedative and analgesic effect, so as well as relieving pain, it can also help to reduce the anxiety and tension that lead to headaches and migraine.

Ingredients

Makes 1 compress
Almond oil 1 tsp
Lavender essential oil 3 drops
Marjoram essential oil 2 drops

How to **make**

1 Fill a bowl with warm water. Add the essential oils to the almond oil, then add to the water.

2 Soak a flannel in the bowl, then remove the flannel and squeeze out the excess water.

3 Wrap the flannel in a towel or piece of cling film to insulate it. Place the compress on the temples. Leave the flannel in place while it cools to body temperature, then repeat the process 3 times.

Rosemary and eucalyptus temple massage

Tension headaches caused by mental effort can be treated with rosemary. Eucalyptus is useful for soothing headaches caused by sinus congestion or allergic reactions. Here, the two oils are combined with refreshing peppermint and relaxing lavender.

Ingredients

Makes 30ml (1fl oz)
Almond oil 2 tbsp
Rosemary essential oil 5 drops
Peppermint essential oil 3 drops
Lavender essential oil 2 drops
Eucalyptus essential oil 2 drops

How to **make**

1 Combine all the ingredients together in a bowl. Transfer to a sterilized dark glass bottle and seal with a cap or dropper.

2 Massage gently into the temples in a circular motion. Store the remaining oil in a cool, dark place. Keeps for up to 3 months.

Arthritis

Arthritis is caused by joint inflammation. The two most common types are rheumatoid arthritis and osteoarthritis. Rheumatoid arthritis is a chronic autoimmune disease that causes swelling, pain, and stiffness in joints, commonly affecting the hands, wrists, and feet. Osteoarthritis makes joints painful and stiff. It occurs when there is damage in and around joints. Most joints can be affected with arthritis, but the condition commonly causes problems in the knees, hips, and the small joints of the hands. Massage and bath soaks can ease the stiffness caused by arthritis.

Circulation-boosting massage

Warming, relaxing, and pain-relieving oils such as marjoram, help to relieve the pain of arthritis. Black pepper and ginger stimulate circulation, in turn revitalizing tired, aching joints. Black pepper also has anti-inflammatory properties, making it an ideal oil for soothing arthritis. Ginger also has an anti-infammatory effect and is naturally reviving and stimulating when applied locally. Try using this massage oil blend locally to bring relief to affected areas.

Ingredients

Makes 30ml (1fl oz)
Almond oil 2 tbsp
Marjoram essential oil 6 drops
Black pepper essential oil 5 drops
Ginger essential oil 4 drops

How to **make**

1 Combine all the ingredients together in a bowl. Transfer to a sterilized dark glass bottle and seal with a cap or dropper.

2 Massage into the affected joints. Allow the oil to absorb into the skin before you get dressed. Store the remaining oil in a cool, dark place. Keeps for up to 3 months.

Soothing yarrow soak

Nutmeg and yarrow oils help to reduce inflammation. Adding these oils to a warm bath combines the soothing effects of warm water with the oils' benefits.

Ingredients

Makes 15ml (½fl oz)
Base oil or full-fat milk 1 tbsp
Nutmeg essential oil 3 drops
Yarrow essential oil 3 drops
Lavender essential oil 5 drops

How to **make**

1 Combine all the ingredients together in a bowl.

2 Disperse immediately in the bath and enjoy a relaxing soak.

Muscular aches and pains

Muscular aches and pains are common and can involve several muscles. Muscle pain can also involve ligaments, tendons, and fascia (the soft tissues that connect muscles, bones, and organs). It's usually related to tension, overuse, or injury from exercise or movement. Muscle pain may be a sign of another condition. For example, certain infections and disorders, such as lupus, affect connective tissues and cause muscle pain. Another cause of muscular aches and pains is fibromyalgia, a condition that causes tenderness in the muscles and surrounding tissue, sleep difficulties, fatigue, and headaches. A targeted massage or compress can reduce pain.

"Unknotting" massage

An essential oil massage can help to stimulate the circulation, relieve pain, and reduce inflammation. The blend here with pain-relieving plai and stimulating black pepper can also be added to a bath with 1 tablespoon of either full-fat milk or base oil.

Ingredients

Makes 30ml (1fl oz)
Arnica macerated oil 1 tbsp
Almond oil 1 tbsp
Plai essential oil 5 drops
Lemongrass essential oil 2 drops
Black pepper essential oil 3 drops

How to **make**

1 Combine all the ingredients together in a bowl. Transfer to a sterilized dark glass bottle and seal with a cap or dropper.

2 Massage into the affected area. Allow the oil to absorb into the skin before you get dressed. Store the remaining oil in a cool, dark place. Keeps for up to 3 months.

Hot ginger compress

Alternating hot and cold compresses can be an effective way to deal with aches and pains. This warming ginger blend boosts circulation and soothes sore, aching muscles.

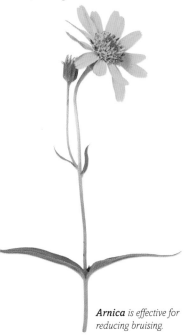

Arnica *is effective for reducing bruising.*

Ingredients

Makes 1 compress
Almond oil 1 tsp
Ginger essential oil 7 drops
Lavandin essential oil 4 drops
Rosemary essential oil 4 drops

How to **make**

1 Fill a bowl with warm water. Add the essential oils to the almond oil, then add to the water.

2 Soak a flannel in the bowl, then remove the flannel and squeeze out the excess water.

3 Wrap the flannel in a towel or cling film to insulate it. Place the compress on the affected area. Leave it in place while it cools to body temperature, then repeat the process 3 times.

Sprains and strains

Sprains are torn ligaments, which join bone to bone, and strains are injuries to tendons, which connect muscle to bone. Sprains are more serious. They can be inflamed, painful, and hot to touch. The initial treatment for both is PRICE: "protection, rest, ice, compression, elevation". Try the following soothing remedies.

Anti-inflammatory lemongrass compress

Try this cold compress on a sprain. This compress uses pain-relieving lemongrass and the anti-inflammatory oils, ginger and black pepper.

Ingredients

Makes 1 compress
Almond oil 1 tsp
Black pepper essential oil 5 drops
Lemongrass essential oil 2 drops
Ginger essential oil 5 drops

How to **make**

1 Fill a bowl with cold water. Add the essential oils to the almond oil, then add to the water.

2 Soak a flannel in the bowl, then remove the flannel and squeeze out the excess water.

3 Place the compress on the affected area. Leave the flannel while it cools to body temperature, then repeat the process 3 times.

Analgesic rosemary massage

A massage with analgesic and anti-inflammatory oils promotes healing. Here, arnica is also used, a traditional remedy to reduce bruising and swelling.

Ingredients

Makes 30ml (1fl oz)
Arnica oil 1 tbsp
Almond oil 1 tbsp
Marjoram essential oil 5 drops
Rosemary essential oil 5 drops
Thyme essential oil 5 drops

How to **make**

1 Combine all the ingredients together in a bowl. Transfer to a sterilized dark glass bottle and seal with a cap or dropper.

2 Massage into the affected area. Allow the oil to absorb into the skin before you get dressed. Store the remaining oil in a cool, dark place. Keeps for up to 3 months.

Skin and hair

Our skin has a protective function, forming a **barrier** against our external environment. Sometimes, though, skin can become irritated, clogged or affected by hormonal changes, or can become damaged by the weather or by being broken. Essential oils can **tone**, balance, and **soothe** a wide range of skin problems, and can also help to **nourish** and hydrate skin.

Acne

Acne is a common skin condition caused by chronic inflammation of the hair follicles and sebaceous glands. It affects many people at some point, but is most common in adolescence. Acne causes spots to develop usually on the face, back, and chest. The spots can range from blackheads and whiteheads to deep, inflamed, pus-filled pustules and cysts, which can be severe and long-lasting, sometimes leading to scarring. It's very important to keep skin clean using a mild cleanser. Be careful not to scrub the skin too hard as it could cause irritation. These skin-soothing remedies can help calm problem skin.

Lavender massage

Skin-regenerating oils help to promote healing and minimize scarring. Lavender, is antiseptic and calming on the skin. Here it is combined with palmarosa, which is gently astringent and anti-inflammatory, helping to soothe inflamed skin.

Ingredients

Makes 15ml (½fl oz)
Wheatgerm oil 1 tsp
Rosehip seed oil 1 tsp
Calendula macerated oil 1 tsp
Palmarosa essential oil 3 drops
Lavender essential oil 1 drop

How to **make**

1 Combine all the ingredients together in a bowl. Transfer to a sterilized dark glass bottle and seal with a cap or dropper.

2 Massage into the skin on the body or face. Allow the oil to absorb into the skin before you get dressed. Store the remaining oil in a cool, dark place. Keeps for up to 3 months.

Lemon and bergamot facial sauna

Essential oils can help to bring acne and pimples under control by helping to clear infection and reduce inflammation. The oils can also help mentally, reducing the stress and anxiety that can often accompany skin conditions. For a deep-pore cleanse, try this essential oil facial steam. The skin-clarifying and toning effects of lemon are combined with the antiseptic and skin-balancing properties of petitgrain, and soothing and antibacterial bergamot.

Ingredients

Makes 1 facial sauna
Bergamot essential oil 3 drops
Lemon essential oil 2 drops
Petitgrain essential oil 1 drop

How to **make**

1 Add the essential oils to a bowl of hot water. Cover your head with a towel, make a tent over the bowl of hot water, and then lean forwards over the bowl.

2 Allow the steam to act on the face for 5 minutes, taking a break from the steam if necessary. Wash your skin with cool water and pat dry with a clean towel.

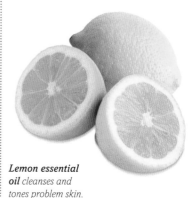

Lemon essential oil *cleanses and tones problem skin.*

Palmarosa massage

The essential oils geranium and palmarosa have skin-balancing properties that naturally help to reduce the amount of sebum produced by the oil glands. Combining these essential oils with skin-conditioning base oils helps to create a nourishing and toning massage oil that can help to calm outbreaks.

Ingredients

Makes 15ml (½fl oz)
Jojoba oil 1 tsp
Grapeseed oil 2 tsp
Palmarosa essential oil 3 drops
Geranium essential oil 2 drops

How to **make**

1 Combine all the ingredients together in a bowl. Transfer to a sterilized dark glass bottle and seal with a cap or dropper.

2 Massage into the skin on the body or face. Allow the oil to absorb into the skin before you get dressed. Store the remaining oil in a cool, dark place. Keeps for up to 3 months.

Tea tree hot compress

Tea tree essential oil is renowned for its antiseptic properties, making it an excellent choice for treating problem skin conditions. Added to a hot compress, it can help to soothe and cleanse skin. If you wish, you can also apply it neat on spots and pimples as an antiseptic ointment.

Ingredients

Makes 20 to 30 treatments
Grapeseed oil 1 tbsp
Tea tree essential oil 3 drops
Cajuput essential oil 2 drops
Lavender essential oil 1 drop

How to **make**

1 Fill a bowl with warm water. Add a few drops of the essential oil blend. Transfer the remaining blend to a sterilized glass jar and store in a cool, dark place. The blend keeps for up to 3 months.

2 Soak a flannel in the bowl, then remove the flannel and squeeze out the excess water.

3 Wrap the flannel in a towel or piece of cling film to insulate it. Place the compress on the area requiring treatment. Leave the flannel while it cools to body temperature, then repeat the process 3 times.

Athlete's foot

Athlete's foot is caused by fungi growing on the skin. The fungi thrive in warm, dark, moist places such as the feet, usually between the toes. Affected skin may be itchy, red, scaly, dry, cracked, or blistered. It's not usually serious, but should be treated to stop it spreading to other parts of the body or to other people. Keep feet clean, carefully dry the feet, especially between the toes, and go barefoot when possible. Try the massage below to help combat this fungal infection.

Geranium foot massage

Antifungal essential oils, such as tea tree and geranium, are ideal for athlete's foot. Here, these oils are blended with lavender essential oil, which helps to heal skin conditions and rejuvenate skin.

Ingredients

Makes 30ml (1fl oz)
Neem oil 2 tbsp
Geranium essential oil 4 drops
Tea tree essential oil 4 drops
Lavender essential oil 3 drops

How to **make**

1 Combine all the ingredients together in a bowl. Transfer to a sterilized dark glass bottle and seal with a cap or dropper.

2 Massage into clean, dry skin on the feet. Allow the oil to absorb into the skin before you get dressed. Store the remaining oil in a cool, dark place. Keeps for up to 3 months.

Bruising

Bruises are bluish or purple-coloured patches. They appear on unbroken skin when tiny blood vessels under the skin, known as capillaries, break. The blood leaks into the tissues, causing discolouration, which fades through shades of yellow or green. Try these healing remedies.

Cooling lavender compress

Applying an ice-cold compress with healing oils as quickly as possible can help to reduce bruising.

Ingredients

Makes 1 compress
Almond oil 1 tsp
Yarrow essential oil 3 drops
Lavender essential oil 5 drops

How to **make**

1 Fill a bowl with ice and cold water. Add the essential oil blend to the almond oil, then add to the water.

2 Soak a flannel in the bowl, then remove the flannel and squeeze out the excess water.

3 Place the compress on the area requiring treatment. Leave the flannel in place while it reaches body temperature. Repeat 3 times.

Arnica massage

Arnica macerated oil, ideal for bruising, is blended here with regenerative and rejuvenating helichrysum and lavender oils for a massage blend that can help to reduce the appearance of bruises.

Ingredients

Makes 30ml (1fl oz)
Arnica oil 2 tbsp
Helichrysum essential oil 3 drops
Lavender essential oil 3 drops

How to **make**

1 Combine all the ingredients together in a bowl. Transfer to a sterilized dark glass bottle and seal with a cap or dropper.

2 Gently massage the affected area. Allow the oil to absorb into the skin before getting dressed. Store the remaining oil in a cool, dark place. Keeps for up to 3 months.

Body odour

Body odour is the unpleasant smell that can occur when the body sweats. The sweat doesn't

smell, but bacteria on the skin break down the sweat into acids that produce the odour. Deodorizing oils help to regulate perspiration and reduce and control unwelcome body odour.

Lemon deodorant

Deodorants work to cover the smell of body odour. The essential oils grapefruit and lemon combine fantastic deodorizing properties with an appealing aroma to keep you smelling fresh throughout the day.

Ingredients

Makes 100ml (3½fl oz)
Witch hazel 90ml (3fl oz)
Glycerine 1 tsp
Aloe juice 1 tsp
Palmarosa essential oil 5 drops
Lemon essential oil 5 drops
Coriander essential oil 3 drops
Grapefruit essential oil 3 drops

How to **make**

1 Mix all the ingredients together in a bowl. Pour into a sterilized bottle with an atomizer.

2 Shake before use. Apply to clean underarms and use whenever it is required.

Safe usage *Do not use on freshly shaved skin.*

Pine-fresh shower gel

The best way to avoid developing unwelcome body odour is to keep the areas of your body that are prone to sweating, such as the armpits, feet, and genital area, clean and free of bacteria. Changing your clothes regularly and

washing daily will also help to avoid a buildup of sweat and bacteria.

Ingredients

Makes 30ml (1fl oz)
Unscented shower gel 2 tbsp
Lemongrass essential oil 7 drops
Pine essential oil 7 drops
Vetiver essential oil 1 drop

How to **make**

1 Make a fresh and revitalizing shower gel by adding the essential oils to an unfragranced shower gel.

2 Use the gel once or twice a day to keep skin clean and odour-free.

Eczema and psoriasis

Eczema is when skin becomes itchy, red, dry, and cracked. It is often long-term (chronic), although it can improve, especially in young children. Atopic eczema ("atopic" means a tendency to develop a sensitivity to allergens), also known as atopic dermatitis, is the most common type

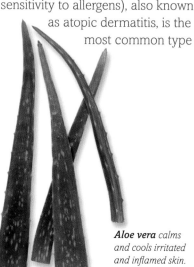

Aloe vera *calms and cools irritated and inflamed skin.*

of eczema. It mainly affects children, but can affect adults, too. Its exact cause is unknown, but it often occurs in people who are prone to allergic reactions, or who have a family history of allergies, and it can be linked to stress. Psoriasis is an inflammatory skin disease that is linked to stress and diet. Sufferers develop red, crusty patches of skin, usually on the elbows, knees, scalp, and back.

Soothing essential oils can be used to treat eczema and psoriasis to help control itching and reduce inflammation.

Calming chamomile compress

Chamomile has been found to be very effective for treating eczema due to its anti-inflammatory and soothing effects that help to relieve and calm itchy and inflamed skin. Sandalwood and lavender are both soothing essential oils that are especially effective on dry, itchy skin. Apply this compress to affected areas to help balance and soothe the skin.

Ingredients

Makes 1 compress
Sunflower or almond oil 1 tsp
German chamomile essential oil 1 drop
Lavender essential oil 3 drops
Sandalwood essential oil 3 drops

How to **make**

1 Fill a bowl with cold water. Add the essential oils to the base oil, then add to the water.

2 Soak a flannel in the bowl, then remove the flannel and squeeze out the excess water.

3 Place the compress on the area requiring treatment. Leave the flannel in place while it reaches body temperature. Repeat 3 times.

Lavender bath float

Create a relaxing bath float with this mix of skin-soothing oats and bran, dried flowers, and uplifting oils. Helichrysum is calming on itchy breakouts, and cistus is mildy astringent, helping to tone skin.

Ingredients

Makes 45g (1½oz)
Organic jumbo oats 1 tbsp
Bran 1 tbsp
Dried lavender flowers 1 tbsp
Helichrysum 4 drops
Lavender essential oil 4 drops
Cistus essential oil 1 drop

How to **make**

1 Make a herb bag using a muslin cloth. Lay the cloth out and place 1 tablespoon each of organic jumbo oats, bran, and dried lavender flowers on the cloth. Add the essential oils.

2 Gather the cloth around the bath mix and tie a ribbon around the corners to keep all the ingredients together.

3 Place the float in a warm bath and dab on the skin to soothe affected areas.

Stress-busting diffusion

Aromatherapy is especially effective in reducing stress and anxiety, making it helpful for dealing with stress-related cases of psoriasis and eczema. The calming oils in this diffusion will help to soothe the anxiety that can be caused by and exacerbate skin conditions.

Ingredients

Makes 1 diffusion
Cedarwood essential oil 4 drops
Frankincense essential oil 3 drops
Geranium essential oil 2 drops

How to **make**

1 Add the essential oil blend to a diffuser, vaporizer or oil burner.

2 Gently fragrance your chosen environment.

Eczema ointment

Chamomile and rose cool and balance skin. Combined with an unscented base they can be applied to affected areas to take the heat out of itchy skin.

Ingredients

Makes 15ml (½fl oz)
Unfragranced lotion 1 tbsp
Roman chamomile essential oil 3 drops
Rose absolute essential oil 2 drops

How to **make**

1 Mix the essential oils into the lotion or ointment.

2 Dab on to affected areas of skin.

Stretch marks

Stretch marks are caused by excessive and rapid weight gain, for example during pregnancy, which over-stretches skin and causes the fibres in the deeper layers to tear.
This leaves wavy reddish stripes that gradually turn white. The

marks usually appear on the thighs, breasts, abdomen, and buttocks. Massage tones skin, which may limit the effects and severity of stretch marks. However, once they appear they are permanent, although they do fade over time.

Skin-toning massage

A massage with nourishing oils improves skin tone, encourages the renewal of skin cells, and makes skin look and feel smoother. Here, moisturizing base oils are blended with toning frankincense and skin-cell regenerating mandarin and neroli essential oils.

Ingredients

Makes 30ml (1fl oz)
Almond oil 1tbsp
Wheatgerm oil 1tsp
Apricot kernel oil 1tsp
Avocado oil 1tsp
Frankincense essential oil 7 drops
Mandarin essential oil 5 drops
Neroli essential oil 3 drops

How to **make**

1 Combine all the ingredients together in a bowl. Transfer to a sterilized dark glass bottle and seal with a cap or dropper.

2 Gently massage the affected area. Allow the oil to absorb into the skin before you get dressed. Store the remaining oil in a cool, dark place. Keeps for up to 3 months.

Sunburn

Sunburn occurs when skin is damaged by the sun's ultraviolet rays. Skin

becomes red, sore, warm, tender, and, occasionally, itchy, and starts to flake and peel after a few days. It is extremely important to try to avoid getting sunburnt in the first place as damaging the skin in this way increases the chances of developing serious health problems later on, for example skin cancer. If skin does become burnt, try to keep the affected area cool and moist. Essential oil remedies that are calming and cooling are ideal.

Cooling lavender compress

Skin-healing oils, such as lavender and chamomile essential oils, and cooling peppermint essential oil are combined here to make a cooling compress that can be applied to help bring relief to tender, sunburnt skin.

Ingredients

Makes 1 compress
Aloe vera juice 1 tbsp
Lavender essential oil 4 drops
Peppermint essential oil 1 drop
German chamomile essential oil 2 drops

How to **make**

1 Fill a bowl with cold water. Add the aloe vera juice and essential oil blend.

2 Soak a flannel in the bowl, then remove the flannel and squeeze out the excess water.

3 Place the compress on the affected area of skin. Leave the flannel on the skin while it reaches body temperature. Repeat 3 times.

Cradle cap

Cradle cap, also known as seborrhoeic dermatitis, is a condition that causes greasy, yellow scaly patches on babies' scalps. It's a harmless condition that doesn't usually itch or cause any discomfort. Most cases clear up on their own over a period of weeks or months. The cause of cradle cap is unknown, but may be linked to an excess of sebum. Essential oils blended with base oils, or with an unfragranced baby shampoo, can help it to clear.

Gentle scalp massage

Massaging almond or olive oil into the scalp at night loosens crusts. Patchouli is astringent and tones skin; palmarosa is skin-balancing; and lavender heals and soothes skin if crusts peel off. This blend is suitable for infants over 12 months; for babies 3-12 months, use just one drop of lavender; under 3 months just the base oil.

Ingredients

Makes 30ml (1fl oz)
Olive oil 2 tbsp
Lavender essential oil 1 drop
Palmarosa essential oil 1 drop
Patchouli essential oil 1 drop

How to **make**

1 Combine all the ingredients together in a bowl. Transfer to a sterilized dark glass bottle and seal with a cap or dropper.

2 Gently massage into your baby's scalp. Leave the oil overnight, then use a soft-bristled baby brush to gently remove loose flakes in the morning before washing with a baby shampoo. Don't be tempted to pick at or remove flakes that aren't already lose as this could damage skin and lead to infection.

3 Store the oil in a cool, dark place. Keeps for up to 3 months.

Lavender shampoo

Gently washing your baby's hair and scalp with a mild shampoo can help prevent a build-up of scales. In addition to its skin-healing properties, lavender is a gentle oil to use on your baby's scalp.

Ingredients

Makes 2 applications
Unscented baby shampoo 1 tbsp
Lavender essential oil 2 drops

How to **make**

1 Mix 2 drops of lavender essential oil in an unfragranced shampoo.

2 Gently wash your baby's hair, taking care not to remove flakes that aren't already loose. Rinse with just warm water.

Dandruff

The body continually sheds dead skin cells as new cells are formed.

In most cases, this is a gradual process that goes unnoticed. However, if the process speeds up, it can produce a buildup of dead skin cells that appear prominent and feel unsightly. Dandruff is a common skin condition that causes dry white or grey flakes of dead skin to appear on the

scalp or attached to hair. The scalp may feel dry and itchy. It's not always clear why this happens, but possible causes include seborrhoeic dermatitis, which is a common skin condition that causes oily skin. Certain factors can make dandruff worse, for example, an overuse of hair products, emotional stress, and washing hair too much or too little. The following treatments can help to condition the scalp.

Invigorating scalp massage

The stimulating action of a scalp massage can be used with essential oils to create an effective dandruff treatment. Thyme essential oil has an anti-fungal action that is useful for treating conditions such as dandruff, while tea tree helps to balance oils and keep the scalp healthy.

Ingredients

Makes 2 applications
Coconut oil solid 1 tbsp
Tea tree essential oil 3 drops
Lavender essential oil 2 drops
Thyme essential oil 2 drops

How to **make**

1 Melt the coconut oil solid in a bain marie (see p188), then add the essential oils and pour the blend into a sterilized glass jar. Massage half the oil blend into the scalp. Do this before bed, then cover the pillow with a towel to avoid the oil blend staining the pillowcase.

2 Leave the oil on overnight and then rinse it out in the morning, applying shampoo before wetting and rinsing the hair.

Peppermint hair rinse

Combining essential oils with dried herbs creates a natural hair tonic that can add shine and help to tone and balance oils on the scalp and control flaky dandruff. Adding soothing peppermint to stimulating rosemary can help to condition the scalp and combat dandruff.

Ingredients

Makes 45ml (1½fl oz)
Dried peppermint 1 tbsp
Dried rosemary herb 1 tbsp
Cider vinegar 1 tbsp
Peppermint essential oil 2 drops
Rosemary essential oil 1 drop

How to **make**

1 To make the infusion, place the dried herbs in a teapot and add 200ml (7fl oz) boiling water. Leave to infuse for around 10 minutes then strain the water.

2 Add the essential oils to the cider vinegar, then to the herbal infusion.

3 Use the infusion as a final hair rinse after shampooing. Finish with a final rinse of warm water only.

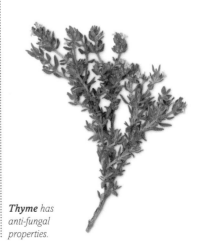

Thyme has anti-fungal properties.

Allergic reactions

Our immune system is designed to **protect** the body against harmful foreign substances. Sometimes, however, the body develops a **sensitivity** to a substance that doesn't pose a threat and reacts as though it is harmful, releasing the substance histamine, which triggers an allergic reaction. Essential oils can help to **calm** allergic responses and **soothe** symptoms.

Allergies and hay fever

An allergy is the body's reaction to a particular food or substance, known as an allergen. Allergic reactions are most common in children. The severity of a reaction can vary. Most are mild, but occasionally a severe reaction, called anaphylaxis, or anaphylactic shock, can occur, which is a medical emergency and requires urgent treatment. Allergic reactions can usually be kept under control with careful management. Common allergens include dust mites, medication, food such as nuts, shellfish, fruit, and cows' milk, and animal fur.

Hay fever is a common allergic reaction to pollen in the warmer months. Many types of pollen are released by plants at different times of the year, causing symptoms such as sneezing, a runny nose, and itchy eyes. Remedies with calming oils can help control symptoms.

Clearing eucalyptus inhalation

Essential oils can help open the airways. Here, the sharp aroma of eucalyptus blends with ravensara for an effective decongestant. The addition of calming lavender helps to quell the stress and anxiety caused by allergic reactions.

Ingredients

Makes 1 inhalation
Eucalyptus radiata essential oil 5 drops
Lavender essential oil 3 drops
Ravensara essential oil 2 drops

How to **make**

1 Add the essential oils to a bowl of hot water. Cover your head with a towel, make a tent over the bowl of hot water, and then lean forwards over the bowl. For children or asthma sufferers, don't cover the head with a towel.

2 Inhale the steam for 5 minutes, taking a break if needed.

Chamomile nose balm

Essential oils provide a simple yet effective way to reduce hay fever and allergy symptoms. Using calming oils, such as chamomile, in a balm can trap pollen and soothe irritated skin.

Ingredients

Makes 20 to 30 applications
Beeswax 1 tbsp
Sunflower oil 1 tbsp
German chamomile essential oil 1 drop
Lavender essential oil 1 drop
Peppermint essential oil 1 drop

How to **make**

1 Gently melt the wax and sunflower oil in a bain marie (see p.188).

2 Add the essential oils and mix together. Pour into a sterilized jar and leave to cool, then seal with a lid.

3 Apply the balm around the nose as required to soothe irritated skin.

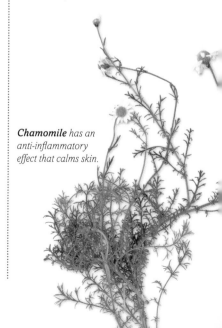

Chamomile has an anti-inflammatory effect that calms skin.

Mind and wellbeing

Stress is a common modern-day malady and it can have profound effects on mental health. Addressing over-hectic lifestyles can help to **combat stress**, and essential oils can be a great support here as their numerous therapeutic benefits work **holistically** to **soothe** and calm emotions, ease anxiety and tension, and **balance moods**, creating an enhanced sense of wellbeing.

Anxiety

We all experience anxiety at some point in life. The feeling of unease or worry that can be mild or severe is a normal response to the stresses of life. For example, you may feel worried about an exam, or anxious about a medical test or an interview. Feeling anxious at stressful times is normal, but if it becomes hard to control worries, and feelings of anxiety become constant, talk to your doctor. Using oils in a diffuser creates a reassuring and calm environment.

Lemon balm diffusion

There are a number of relaxing oils for reducing anxiety that can be used in a massage, in the bath, or diffused into a room to create a peaceful environment.

Ingredients

Makes 1 diffusion
Lemon balm essential oil 5 drops
Lemon essential oil 3 drops
Cypress essential oil 3 drops
Bergamot essential oil 2 drops

How to **make**

1 Add the essential oil blend to a diffuser, vaporizer or oil burner.

2 Gently fragrance your chosen environment.

Depression

Difficult events and experiences can leave us feeling in low spirits. If this low feeling persists we can develop depression.

Some common causes of depression include relationship problems, bereavement, sleep problems (which may arise from stress and other concerns), stress at work, bullying, and chronic illness and pain. Sometimes it's possible to feel down without there being an obvious reason. Depression can also come on at specific points in life or at specific times, for example after the birth of a child or during the winter months.

A low mood that lasts for two weeks or more can be a sign of depression. Other symptoms of depression include: not getting any enjoyment out of life, feeling hopeless, feeling tired or lacking energy, not being able to concentrate on everyday tasks such as reading the paper or watching television, comfort eating or losing one's appetite, sleeping more than usual or being unable to sleep, having suicidal thoughts or thoughts about harming yourself. It's always important to talk to your doctor about how you are feeling if you are experiencing any of the above symptoms and a low mood persists for an extended period of time.

Therapeutic essential oils can be very beneficial for helping to lift feelings of depression and bring a feeling of calm that can release anxiety and tension.

Calming diffusion

Essential oils can be wonderful remedies for providing emotional support. In this diffusion, calming frankincense helps to lift the spirits and is especially helpful when you are feeling tired or overwhelmed, while mandarin soothes frayed nerves, promoting relaxation, and uplifting neroli helps to balance emotions and is effective for relieving stress.

Ingredients

Makes 1 diffusion
Frankincense essential oil 5 drops
Neroli essential oil 3 drops
Mandarin essential oil 2 drops

How to **make**

1 Add the essential oil blend to a diffuser, vaporizer or oil burner.

2 Gently fragrance your chosen environment.

Grief and shock

Times of emotional crisis and upset often involve some kind of loss or bereavement. This may be the loss of a loved one, or the end of a marriage or important relationship. Most people grieve when they lose something or someone important to them. Grieving can feel unbearable at times, but it's a necessary process to work through. There are many different reactions to loss, and no one right reaction, but grief usually does consist of a few key emotions: these include anxiety and helplessness, and anger and sadness. Eventually, you adjust to a loss and though your feelings can remain as intense, they tend to become less frequent. Essential oils can be especially helpful at times of loss or trauma, helping to lift spirits and ground emotions.

Neroli "rescue" remedy

Neroli essential oil is considered to be the "rescue remedy" of essential oils and is particularly helpful during times of grief and shock. Here, its effects are supported by uplifting bergamot and calming petitgrain essential oils. Disperse this blend of oils in your environment to help calm emotions and ease feelings of anxiety.

Ingredients

Makes 1 diffusion
Neroli essential oil 5 drops
Petitgrain essential oil 3 drops
Bergamot essential oil 2 drops

How to **make**

1 Add the essential oil blend to a diffuser, vaporizer or oil burner.

2 Gently fragrance your chosen environment.

Soothing rose and geranium massage

Essential oils with uplifting and euphoric properties are very useful for helping to deal with grief. Geranium is uplifting and calming at the same time, which makes it useful for warding off the feelings of depression that often accompany grief. Frankincense essential oil also helps to lift the spirits, and the calming aroma of rose promotes relaxation and helps to reduce feelings of anxiety and releases tension, helping to create a sense of wellbeing that can punctuate the grief.

Ingredients

Makes 2 tbsp of massage oil
Almond oil 2 tbsp
Frankincense essential oil 4 drops
Rose absolute or essential oil 3 drops
Geranium essential oil 1 drop

How to **make**

1 Combine all the ingredients together in a bowl. Transfer to a sterilized dark glass bottle and seal with a cap or dropper.

2 Massage into the skin (avoiding the face). Allow the oil to absorb into the skin before you get dressed. Store the remaining oil in a cool, dark place. Keeps for up to 3 months.

Uplifting jasmine bath

This combination of oils provides a revitalizing bath soak that can create a feeling of wellbeing. Jasmine essential oil or absolute helps to increase optimism, combating the feelings of listlessness, while sandalwood promotes restful sleep and helps to restore vitality.

Ingredients

Makes 1 tbsp
Almond oil or full-fat milk 1 tbsp
Sandalwood essential oil 4 drops
Jasmine absolute or essential oil 4 drops
Grapefruit essential oil 2 drops

How to **make**

1 Combine all the ingredients together in a bowl.

2 Disperse the blend immediately in the bath and enjoy a reviving and soothing soak.

Stress and insomnia

Stress is one of the major health problems in the Western world and is responsible for many

of our illnesses. It has numerous causes and can affect us in a number of different ways, both mentally and physically. The body's natural response to stress is controlled by the autonomic nervous system and involves the release of the hormones adrenaline and cortisol, which also control the "fight or flight" mechanism – the body's inbuilt reaction to dangerous or threatening situations. While a certain amount of stress is good for us, helping to keep us motivated and interested in tasks, if stress starts to impact on our moods, digestion, and sleep, it becomes more of an issue. Try these relaxing and soothing remedies to help yourself wind down and let go of tension.

De-stressing clary sage massage

Using therapeutic essential oils in a massage blend is an excellent way to help the body to manage chronic stress, promote relaxation, and improve the quality of sleep if stress is causing insomnia. You can also enjoy this oil blend in a soothing bedtime bath by adding the essential oils to 1 tablespoon of either base oil or full-fat milk, and dispersing immediately in the bath, then enjoy a relaxing pre-bedtime soak.

Ingredients

Makes 2 tbsp
Almond oil 2 tbsp
Clary sage essential oil 5 drops
Frankincense essential oil 5 drops
Geranium essential oil 5 drops

How to **make**

1 Combine all the ingredients together in a bowl. Transfer to a sterilized dark glass bottle and seal with a cap or dropper.

2 Massage into the skin (avoiding the face). Allow the oil to absorb into the skin before you get dressed. Store the remaining oil in a cool, dark place. Keeps for up to 3 months.

Litsea and bergamot calming diffusion

Litsea essential oil is a useful stress buster. Its naturally soothing properties calm the rapid heartbeat that can accompany stress and panic, helping you to think more rationally. Bergamot is grounding and helps to balance the mind. The addition of uplifting orange adds to the calming effect of this blend.

Ingredients

Makes 1 diffusion
Litsea essential oil 6 drops
Orange essential oil 4 drops
Bergamot essential oil 4 drops

How to **make**

1 Add the essential oil blend to a diffuser, vaporizer or oil burner.

2 Gently fragrance your chosen environment.

Ylang ylang bedtime spray

If stress and anxiety keep you awake at night, or you find it difficult to switch off at bedtime and find that you wake in the morning feeling groggy, try this wonderfully relaxing pillow spray. Calming chamomile and rose essential oils are joined by the uplifting, sweetly scented ylang ylang, which helps to calm breathing, and grounding vetiver, which has a profoundly calming effect when you feel overwhelmed by stress.

Ingredients

Makes 30ml (1fl oz)
Ylang ylang essential oil 6 drops
Rose essential oil 6 drops
Vetiver essential oil 2 drops
Roman chamomile essential oil 1 drop

How to **make**

1 Mix the essential oils with 2 tablespoons cold water and pour into a sterilized bottle with an atomizer.

2 Spritz your room before bedtime. Shake before use, and avoid spraying directly onto fabric.

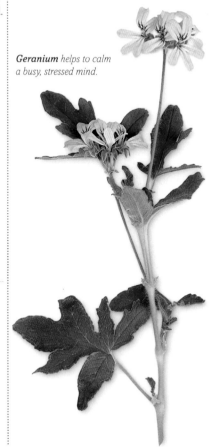

Geranium helps to calm a busy, stressed mind.

Women's health

Women's hormones go through a number of changes throughout life, causing physical and **emotional** symptoms, many of which can be helped by essential oils. Premenstrual fluid retention can be alleviated using oils and massage, and premenstrual tension can be **soothed** with **calming oils.** Uplifting oils can alleviate depression after birth and during the menopause.

Premenstrual symptoms

Many women experience a mix of emotional and physical symptoms in the run up to menstruation.

For some women, these symptoms are mild and occur for just a couple of days before menstruation begins. For others, symptoms can be wider ranging, more pronounced, and can start as early as two weeks before the onset of menstruation.

Physical premenstrual symptoms include fluid retention and bloating, fatigue, breast tenderness, lower back ache, and abdominal discomfort. Emotional symptoms include general anxiety, irritability, stress, and a low mood, or unpredictable mood swings. Therapeutic essential oils are a great help for premenstrual complaints as their holistic nature helps to treat the whole range of symptoms, relieving physical complaints and providing emotional support by calming and balancing emotions.

Juniper compress for fluid retention

Essential oils with a mild diuretic action, such as juniper, geranium, and fennel, are effective for flushing out toxins and reducing the uncomfortable fluid retention and puffiness commonly experienced before menstruation. As well as their physical benefits, the oils relieve emotional premenstrual symptoms, too. Juniper helps to revive flagging spirits and calms nervous tension, and geranium balances the emotions, which can ward off mood swings. A hot or cold compress using this essential oil blend makes a soothing and effective premenstrual remedy. Avoid this blend in pregnancy.

Ingredients

Makes 1 compress
Almond oil 1 tsp
Calendula macerated oil 2 tsp
Wheatgerm oil 1 tsp
Juniper essential oil 5 drops
Fennel essential oil 5 drops
Geranium essential oil 5 drops

How to **make**

1 Fill a bowl with hot or cold water, whichever is your preference. Add the oil blend.

2 Soak a flannel in the bowl, then remove the flannel and squeeze out the excess water.

3 If the flannel is hot, place a towel or piece of cling film over it to insulate it, if you wish. Place the compress on the area requiring treatment. Leave the flannel in place while it reaches body temperature. Repeat 3 times.

Pre-menstrual rose and geranium bath

Pre-menstrual tension (PMT) can be stressful and tiring as hormonal changes lead to sudden mood swings, or bring on a general low mood, and feelings of tension and anxiety can feel overwhelming. Try this soothing and grounding essential oil bath soak for a pre-menstrual stress-reducing tonic that will leave you feeling more grounded, calm, and uplifted.

Ingredients

Makes 1 tbsp
Base oil or full-fat milk 1 tbsp
Rose essential oil 5 drops
Clary sage essential oil 2 drops
Geranium essential oil 2 drops

How to **make**

1 Combine all the ingredients together in a bowl.

2 Disperse the oil blend immediately in a hot bath, and then enjoy a reviving and uplifting soak that can leave you feeling revived.

Pregnancy

Many essential oils aren't advised in pregnancy (see Safe usage in the A–Z for each oil), but some are safe and help with relaxation and some pregnancy symptoms. For example, juniper, mandarin, rose, rosemary, marjoram, and neroli are popular pregnancy oils. See page 37 for a list of oils that are safe in pregnancy.

Skin-nourishing pregnancy massage

Enjoy a backache-relieving massage or a calming facial massage. Stick to 1 per cent dilutions as your sense of smell is heightened in pregnancy. The massage blend below nourishes skin and improves elasticity. Used daily from the fifth month of pregnancy, it can help to prevent stretch marks. It is best not to use essential oils until you are past the first trimester (unless you have had advice from a qualified aromatherapy practitioner).

Ingredients

Makes 30ml (1fl oz)
Almond oil 1 tbsp
Wheatgerm oil 1 tbsp
Mandarin essential oil 2 drops
Lavender essential oil 2 drops
Neroli essential oil 2 drops

How to **make**

1 Combine the ingredients in a bowl. Transfer to a sterilized dark glass bottle. Seal with a cap or dropper.

2 Gently massage the skin. Allow the oil to absorb into the skin before you get dressed. Store the remaining oil in a cool, dark place. Keeps for up to 3 months.

Postnatal and menopause

Hormonal swings after birth can affect mood, leading to the baby blues, and sometimes longer-lasting postnatal depression. Similarly, hormonal changes in the menopause can affect mood, causing irritability and depression. Menopause also has a range of physical symptoms, one of the best-known being hot flushes, characterized by a sudden feeling of heat sweeping over the body. Calming and relaxing essential oils can help to ease symptoms and lift the spirits.

Soothing blend for hot flushes and irritability

This cooling blend of oils is ideal for hot flushes and general irritability. Bergamot is particularly helpful when the body is overheated. Roman chamomile calms and soothes, while rose and geranium enhance wellbeing.

Ingredients

Makes 90ml (3fl oz)
Bergamot essential oil 5 drops
Rose absolute oil 5 drops
Geranium essential oil 2 drops
Roman chamomile essential oil 2 drops

How to **make**

1 Add the oils to 90ml (3fl oz) water. Transfer to an atomizer bottle.

2 Spritz the face to cool hot flushes, or spray a room to create a calming environment. Alternatively, add the blend to a diffuser and gently fragrance your chosen environment.

Hormone-balancing fennel massage

Cooling fennel is blended with soothing rose and geranium oils here to create a gentle balancing and grounding blend. Avoid this blend in pregnancy.

Ingredients

Makes 2 tbsp
Almond oil 2 tbsp
Fennel essential oil 3 drops
Rose absolute oil 5 drops
Geranium essential oil 5 drops

How to **make**

1 Combine all the ingredients together in a bowl. Transfer to a sterilized glass dark bottle and seal with a cap or dropper.

2 Gently massage the body (avoid the face). Allow the oil to absorb into the skin before getting dressed. Store the remaining oil in a cool, dark place. Keeps for up to 3 months.

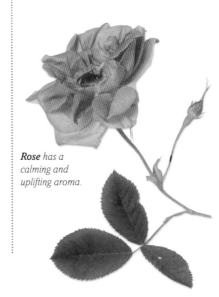

Rose has a calming and uplifting aroma.

Men's health

As with women, men can encounter specific health issues. Prostate health is important for men, and the effects of stress can feature prominently. Essential oils have clear benefits for these areas. Remedies that work **holistically** on **body** and **mind** help to counter the negative effects of stress, and antiseptic and diuretic oils target prostate problems **alongside medical treatments**.

Heart health and stress

Cardiovascular disease is one of the leading causes of death for men in the United States and is a growing health concern worldwide. General heart health can be improved by exercising regularly, eating a healthy, balanced diet, giving up smoking, and finding ways to reduce and manage everyday stress. See pages 222–23 for other remedies for circulation. Essential oils have numerous properties that can help with problems that are associated with the cardiovascular system, such as high blood pressure and sluggish circulation.

Bergamot and neroli bath oil blend

This bath oil remedy can also be used as a massage blend, added to a shower gel, or the essential oils can be added to a diffuser. Here, relaxing essential oils are used in a warm bath to help release tension in the body and combat the effects of stress and anxiety.

Ingredients

Makes 15ml (½fl oz)
Almond oil 1 tbsp
Bergamot essential oil 5 drops
Neroli essential oil 2 drops
Sandalwood essential oil 5 drops

How to **make**

1 Combine all the ingredients together in a bowl.

2 Disperse the oil blend immediately in the bath and enjoy a relaxing soak.

Prostate problems

Problems with the prostate are increasingly common in older men. The prostate gland can become enlarged, which can sometimes be due to bacterial infection. Anti-inflammatory and antiseptic essential oils can help to calm swelling and kill off bacteria. It's also important that men get the prostate checked regularly so that changes in size are spotted and any necessary treatment given.

Prostate massage

Antiseptic and anti-inflammatory frankincense blends well with myrrh and anti-bacterial rosemary. Massage around the genital area regularly to stimulate circulation and improve prostate health.

Ingredients

Makes 15ml (½fl oz)
Almond essential oil 1 tbsp
Rosemary essential oil 1 drop
Frankincense essential oil 1 drop
Myrrh essential oil 1 drop

How to **make**

1 Combine all the ingredients together in a bowl. Transfer to a sterilized dark glass bottle and seal with a cap or dropper.

2 Gently massage into the area around and below the genitals. Allow the oil to absorb into the skin before getting dressed. Store the remaining oil in a cool, dark place. Keeps for up to 3 months.

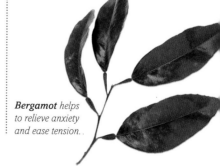

Bergamot helps to relieve anxiety and ease tension.

First aid

Essential oils are a valuable addition to a home first-aid kit. Alongside the bandages and plasters, oils act as antiseptics for cuts and wounds and can **soothe** and **calm** irritated skin, bites and stings, and minor burns and scalds. Oils such as tea tree can be applied neat to protect wounds from infection, while **cooling** and **warming oils** can counter the effects of weather.

Blisters

Blisters on the skin often occur after an injury, burning, scalding, repetitive rubbing or an insect sting. They can be painful and also very annoying. A blister develops when there is an accumulation of fluid underneath the skin. When the blister bursts, the revealed tissue beneath may be sore and become infected.

Tea tree and lavender ointment

Regular application of lavender essential oil directly onto the affected area can help reduce swelling and prevent infection and ease pain.

Ingredients

Makes 1 application
Tea tree essential oil 1 drop
Lavender essential oil 1 drop

How to **make**

1 Apply the essential oils directly to the blister with a cotton bud.

2 Cover the blister carefully with a plaster to reduce the chance of an infection.

Heat exhaustion and fever

Heat exhaustion is when too much heat or sunlight causes lethargy, dizziness, nausea, vomiting, and a headache. A person with heat exhaustion should be moved to a cool place and given water.

Fever is the body's defence against infections. Seek medical help if a temperature rises quickly.

Cooling compress

Cool the body with this compress.

Ingredients

Makes 1 compress
Witch hazel 1 tbsp
Peppermint essential oil 2 drops
Lavender essential oil 3 drops

How to **make**

1 Fill a bowl with cold water. Add the essential oils to the witch hazel and then to the water.

2 Soak a flannel in the bowl, remove and wring out.

3 Place the compress on the skin. Leave in place while it reaches body temperature. Repeat 3 times.

Insect bites and stings

The severity of bites and stings depends on the type of insect and a person's sensitivity. A serious allergic reaction will require immediate medical help.

Lavender compress

This soothing compress reduces itching.

Ingredients

Makes 1 compress
Witch hazel 1 tbsp
Lavender essential oil 3 drops
Roman chamomile essential oil 1 drop

How to **make**

1 Fill a bowl with cold water. Add the essential oils to the witch hazel and then to the water.

2 Soak a flannel in the bowl, remove and wring out.

3 Place the flannel on the skin. Leave it in place while it reaches body temperature. Repeat 3 times.

Treatment reference charts

Essential oils are versatile and the choice can be overwhelming, which can make it hard to decide which oils have the right properties for your specific needs. The quick reference charts below are designed to help you rapidly pinpoint the essential oils particularly suited to your requirements. The chart on pages 244–6 lists essential oils for common complaints, while the charts on page 247 recommend essential oils for mind and wellbeing and essential oils for cosmetic use.

Common **complaints**

Everyday common complaints include chronic conditions that require long-term management, such as arthritis, depression, and stress; occasional problems, such as headaches or diarrhoea; one-off first-aid situations; skin complaints, such as eczema, athlete's foot, and dandruff; and menstrual and menopausal complaints. This chart helps you to identify at a glance which essential oils are especially recommended to help with specific concerns. Always consult your doctor about symptoms and use essential oils as complementary treatments alongside medications when necessary. For information on each essential oil, check the A–Z listings on pages 40–145.

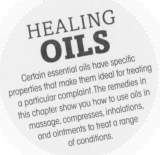

HEALING OILS

Certain essential oils have specific properties that make them ideal for treating a particular complaint. The remedies in this chapter show you how to use oils in massage, compresses, inhalations, and ointments to treat a range of conditions.

Common complaint	Recommended essential oils
Allergies	Yarrow, Helichrysum, Lavender, Chamomile
Appetite loss	Buchu, Galangal, Dill, Tarragon, Cinnamon, Lemon, Lemongrass, Fennel, Wintergreen, Litsea, Peppermint, Nutmeg, Ginger
Arthritis	Yarrow, Lemon verbena, Mugwort, Birch leaf, Frankincense, Cedarwood, Cypress, Wintergreen, Helichrysum, Star anise, Juniper, Lavender, Nutmeg, Marjoram, Parsley, Black pepper, Benzoin, Plai, Ginger
Asthma	Frankincense, Caraway, Lemon, Eucalyptus, Lavender, Roman chamomile, Niaouli, Lemon balm, Peppermint, Myrtle, Sandalwood, Clove
Athlete's foot	Galangal, Cedarwood, Lemongrass, Palmarosa, Eucalyptus, Wintergreen, Star anise, Lavender, Manuka, Tea tree, Cajuput, Oregano, Geranium, Patchouli, Summer savory, Tagetes, Thyme
Backache and neck pain	Tarragon, Coriander, Camphor, Grapefruit, Bay laurel, Lavender, Niaouli, Marjoram, Geranium, Allspice, Black pepper, Rosemary, Ginger
Bites and stings	Lime, Lavender, Manuka, Roman chamomile, Lemon balm, Peppermint, Allspice, Patchouli, Summer savory
Blisters	Lavender, Tea tree
Body odour	Galangal, Tarragon, Petitgrain, Lemon, Grapefruit, Coriander, Cypress, Lemongrass, Palmarosa, Cardamom, Star anise, Manuka, Litsea, Pine, Sage, Vetiver

Common complaint	Recommended essential oils
Bruising	Yarrow, Lavender
Constipation	Orange, Fennel, Marjoram, Peppermint, Pine, Black Pepper, Rosemary
Coughs and colds	Frankincense, Cedarwood, Lemon, Cypress, Eucalyptus, Fennel, Helichrysum, Lavender, Tea tree, Peppermint, Marjoram, Pine, Ravintsara, Rosemary, Clary sage, Thyme
Cradle cap	Palmarosa, Lavender, Patchouli
Dandruff	Birch, Cedarwood, Lime, Lemon, Wintergreen, Juniper, Bay laurel, Lavender, Tea tree, Peppermint, Geranium, Rosemary, Sage, Thyme
Depression	Frankincense, Ylang ylang, Cedarwood, Cinnamon, Neroli, Bergamot, Mandarin, Orange, Lemongrass, Helichrysum, Jasmine, Litsea, Basil, Geranium, Tuberose, Ravintsara, Clary sage, Benzoin
Diarrhoea	Neroli, Mandarin, Cypress, Eucalyptus, Fennel, Chamomile, Peppermint, Black pepper, Ginger
Eczema and psoriasis	Yarrow, Frankincense, Cedarwood, Cistus, Cumin, Helichrysum, Juniper, Lavender, German chamomile, Lemon balm, Geranium, Sandalwood, Benzoin, Fenugreek
Fluid retention	Yarrow, Buchu, Dill, Cedarwood, Cistus, Lime, Lemon, Grapefruit, Mandarin, Orange, Cypress, Carrot seed, Juniper, Geranium, Parsley seed, Rosemary
Grief	Frankincense, Cistus, Neroli, Petitgrain, Bergamot, Geranium, Rose
Headaches and migraines	Rosewood, Grapefruit, Coriander, Lemongrass, Eucalyptus, Bay laurel, Lavender, Lemon balm, Peppermint, Marjoram, Rosemary, Ginger
Heat exhaustion and fever	Lime, Bergamot, Lavender, Lemon balm, Peppermint, Vetiver
High blood pressure	Ylang ylang, Cumin, Lavender, Marjoram, Clary sage, Valerian
Hot flushes	Bergamot, Roman chamomile, Geranium, Rose, Clary sage

Essential oils make useful additions to your home remedy cabinet.

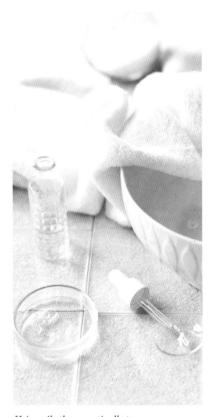

Using oils therapeutically in steam inhalations can be an excellent way to relieve congestion.

Common complaint	Recommended essential oils
Insomnia	Yarrow, Dill, Neroli, Petitgrain, Bergamot, Lemon, Orange, Star anise, Bay laurel, Lavender, Roman chamomile, Nutmeg, Myrtle, Marjoram, Allspice, Tuberose, Sandalwood, Valerian, Vetiver
Mouth and gum care	Cistus, Myrrh, Cardamom, Fennel, Tea tree, Peppermint, Nutmeg, Clove
Muscular aches and pains	Eucalyptus, Lavender, Peppermint, Nutmeg, Rosemary, Clove, Thyme, Ginger
Nausea and sickness	Buchu, Lemon verbena, Galangal, Dill, Mandarin, Cardamom, Litsea, Roman chamomile, Lemon balm, Peppermint, Nutmeg, Parsley seed, Allspice, Black pepper, Rose, Clary sage, Fenugreek, Ginger
Pre-menstrual tension	Fennel, Juniper, Marjoram, Geranium, Rose, Clary sage
Prostate health	Frankincense, Myrrh, Rosemary
Reflux and indigestion	Dill, Mandarin, Coriander, Cardamom, Fennel, Chamomile, Peppermint, Basil, Parsley, Ginger
Sprains and strains	Lemongrass, Marjoram, Black pepper, Rosemary, Thyme, Ginger
Stress and anxiety	Frankincense, Ylang ylang, Cedarwood, Neroli, Petitgrain, Bergamot, Lemon, Mandarin, Orange, Jasmine, Lavender, Litsea, Chamomile, Lemon balm, Basil, Marjoram, Geranium, Patchouli, Rose, Rosemary, Clary sage, Sandalwood, Vetiver
Sunburn	Bergamot, German chamomile, Lavender, Tea tree
Urinary tract infections	Lavender, German chamomile, Peppermint
Varicose veins/ haemorrhoids	Lemon, Cypress, Helichrysum, Juniper, Geranium

Each essential oil has a range of therapeutic properties.

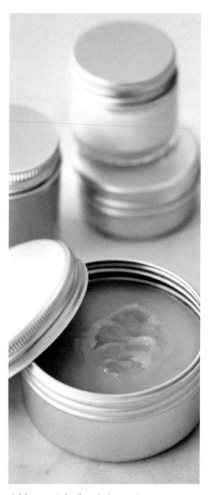

Add essential oils *to balms and creams to create healing remedies and nourishing cosmetic products.*

Mind and **wellbeing**

An important and key element of aromatherapy is its ability to treat holistically, looking beyond isolated symptoms and treating both body and mind. For example, when oils are used to promote relaxation or to energize, they can also help the body to deal with other specific complaints. The chart, right, suggests key oils for mental and physical wellbeing.

Mind and wellbeing	Recommended essential oils
Calming and soothing	Ylang ylang, Cypress, Palmarosa, Helichrysum, Lavender, Chamomile, Patchouli, Rose, Clary sage, Sandalwood
Concentration and focus	Cardamom, Peppermint, Basil, Thyme
Energizing	Lemongrass, Juniper, Pine, Rosemary, Clove, Thyme
Relaxation	Ylang ylang, Neroli, Orange, Lavender, Rose, Sandalwood, Vetiver
Stimulating and invigorating	Citronella, Basil, Black pepper, Rosemary, Ginger
Uplifting	Lime, Neroli, Petitgrain, Bergamot, Lemon, Grapefruit, Orange, Lemongrass, Palmarosa, Litsea, Lemon balm, Peppermint, Geranium, Rose
Warming	Cinnamon, Nutmeg, Marjoram, Black pepper, Clove

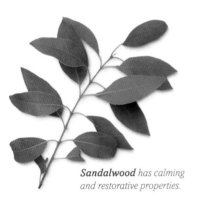

Sandalwood has calming and restorative properties.

Cosmetic **treatments**

Essential oils can play a key role in cosmetics, where their properties prove extremely useful for balancing and enhancing skin. The chart, right, helps you to choose oils and tailor blends to suit your particular skin type. When using oils cosmetically, ensure you first dilute them in a base oil or combine them with a cream or lotion base. The recipes in chapter five show you how to create cosmetic products using essential oils.

Skin conditions	Recommended essential oils
Dry and mature skin	Frankincense, Ylang ylang, Neroli, Palmarosa, Jasmine, Lavender, Chamomile, Patchouli, Rose, Sandalwood
Dry/oily hair	Cedarwood, Grapefruit, Tea tree, Rosemary
Oily and acne-prone skin	Ylang ylang, Petitgrain, Bergamot, Lime, Neroli, Lemon, Mandarin, Cypress, Palmarosa, Juniper, Bay laurel, Lavender, Tea tree, Niaouli, Geranium, Rose, Rosemary, Clary sage, Sandalwood
Scars/stretch marks	Frankincense, Neroli, Mandarin, Palmarosa, Jasmine, Lavender, Patchouli, Sandalwood, Vetiver, Plai
Sensitive skin	Neroli, Helichrysum, Lavender, Chamomile, Sandalwood

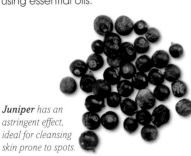

Juniper has an astringent effect, ideal for cleansing skin prone to spots.

Glossary

Absolute Concentrated aromatic oils extracted from a single plant source by solvent extraction. None of the solvent remains after the process. Absolutes can be used like essential oils.

Adaptogen A substance that can relax or stimulate to help balance body systems, especially in times of stress.

Adrenaline *See epinephrine*

Analgesic A substance that reduces or eliminates pain.

Antibacterial A substance that inhibits bacterial growth.

Antidepressant A medication or compound that alleviates depression.

Antifungal Inhibits the growth of mould and fungi.

Antihistamine A substance or medication that counters allergic reactions. Commonly used in the treatment of hay fever, hives, itching, and insect bites and stings.

Anti-inflammatory A substance that prevents or reduces inflammation.

Antimicrobial A substance that reduces or resists microbes, commonly used to refer to substances that are active against a wide range of bacteria, viruses, and fungi.

Antioxidant Substances that inhibit the oxidation of other molecules. Oxidation is a chemical reaction that can produce free radicals, which damage body tissues. It is also a process that can cause oils and fats to become rancid.

Antispasmodic Provides relief from muscle spasms and cramps.

Antiviral Capable of killing some viruses.

Aphrodisiac Something that arouses or increases sexual desire.

Aromatherapy The therapeutic use of essential oils. Aromatherapy can involve inhalation or application of essential oil blends to the skin.

Aromatic Refers to the unique aroma emitted by a plant or substance.

Astringent A substance that produces a localized tightening effect on body tissues. Used in preparations to tone the skin and close pores, or to reduce secretions and bleeding from abrasions. Astringents also help to close wounds and ulcers.

Base oil An oil used to dilute essential oils before a massage.

Carrier oil *See Base oil*

Compound A substance formed when two or more chemical elements bond together.

Compress A wet cotton pad or flannel pressed onto the body to relieve pain, inflammation, or to stop bleeding. Can be used hot or cold.

Concentrated Essential oils are concentrated because they are the essence of a large volume of plants distilled into a small amount of oil. For example, it takes around 136kg (300lb) rose petals to produce 30ml (1oz) rose essential oil.

Concrete The first products of solvent extraction; a concrete is a semi-solid mix of plant waxes and essential oils that are used to make solid perfumes.

Decongestant A substance or process that reduces congestion in the nasal passages or lungs.

Detoxifying Aids the body in eliminating waste and impurities.

Diffusion/diffuser In aromatherapy, the process by which concentrated essential oil molecules are dispersed/diluted into the air. This can be via a device, such as an electronic diffuser, or a process, such as using a room spray, which releases fragrance molecules into the air.

Dilution The process of making something less concentrated.

Diuretic Increases urine production and output.

Dopamine A neurotransmitter that helps control the brain's reward and pleasure centres.

Elixir In aromatherapy, a blend of essential oils in a base oil. Usually refers to a mixture used on the face for the purposes of improving skin tone.

Emollient Any substance that prevents water loss from the skin. Most natural oils perform this function.

Emulsifier A substance that holds oil and water together, necessary for the production of lotions and creams.

Epinephrine A hormone, commonly called adrenaline, released by the body when a person feels a strong emotion, such as excitement, fear, or anger. It causes the heart to beat faster and prepares the body for a "fight or flight" response.

Esters Chemical compounds derived from an acid. One of a number of constituents of essential oils. Most esters have fruity aromas.

Exfoliate To remove surface layers of the skin, especially dead skin cells, by using an abrasive agent.

Expectorant Encourages mucus to be expelled from the lungs.

Expression The "cold press" method by which essential oils are extracted from citrus peels.

Extraction In aromatherapy, any one of a number of methods by which essential oils are obtained from plant materials. *See also Expression, Steam-distillation,* and *Solvent extraction.*

Holistic Treatment of the whole person, taking into account mental and social factors, rather than just the symptoms of a disease.

Hypotensive Having low blood pressure.

Infusion When the active constituents of a plant are extracted into a solvent such as water, alcohol, or oil. The process can be aided by heat and/or time. *See also Macerate.*

Irritant A substance that can irritate the skin or mucous membranes.

Macerate A type of infusion made by steeping chopped-up parts of a plant in a base oil to extract the plant's therapeutic properties.

Neurotransmitter Chemicals released by the brain that act like messengers, carrying information and instructions to other parts of the body.

Ointment An oily substance that is rubbed on the skin for medicinal or cosmetic purposes.

Olfactory Refers to the sense of smell. The olfactory system collects aromatic compounds from the environment and translates these into neural signals that help our brains identify individual aromas.

Organic A method of farming and growing using practices that strive to work with nature and seasonal cycles, promote ecological balance, and conserve biodiversity. Organic farmers and growers, for instance, do not use synthetic pesticides and fertilizers.

Photo-allergy A skin reaction, often slow to develop (1–3 days), caused when the sun's UV rays change a substance such as an essential oil into one that the immune system considers

foreign. The reaction can spread beyond the sun-exposed area.

Photo-sensitive Referring to any substance that can increase skin damage on exposure to UV rays. *See also Photo-allergy* and *Photo-toxicity.*

Photo-toxicity A skin reaction, often immediate, caused by the interaction of a substance with UV rays, which produces free radicals that damage skin. This is the most common type of photo-sensitive reaction; rashes tend to be limited to the sun-exposed area.

Regenerative Supports healing and the regeneration of cells and tissues.

Sedative A substance that has a tranquillizing effect, reducing irritability and over-excitement.

Sensitizer Something that causes an allergic reaction. Often an initial application will not produce an effect, but used over time it may induce a severe inflammatory response.

Solvent extraction A method of extracting essential oils from delicate plant materials that cannot withstand heat. With this method, the oil is infused in a solvent. The solvent is then removed leaving behind a waxy substance, a "concrete", from which a thick essential oil known as an absolute is extracted. *See also Concrete* and *Absolute.*

Steam-distillation A process by which steam is used to extract an essential oil from plant material. Steam flows into a container that holds the raw plant material. The heat encourages the release of the oil into the steam, which passes into another container where the steam is condensed back into water. The essential oil is then separated out from the water.

Steam inhalation The process of inhaling steam deep into the lungs. Adding essential oils to hot water creates an aromatic steam which,

once in the lungs, has a range of medicinal effects.

Sustainability Refers to the way we produce and use goods, specifically to systems that are regenerative and that work to conserve the natural balance of ecosystems.

Synergy When several elements work together to produce an effect that is greater than the sum of each part. Synergy usually refers to compounds in a single essential oil, but the way an oil blends with other oils to produce a therapeutic or aromatic effect is also sometimes referred to as synergy.

Terpenes One of the naturally occurring constituents of essential oils. A large and diverse class of organic compounds, often strong-smelling, produced by a variety of plants, particularly conifers.

Therapeutic Having a healing effect on the body and/or mind.

Toxic Something that can cause damage to living organisms.

Vaporizer A device used to disperse an essential oil mist into the air. *See also Diffusion.*

Volatile In aromatherapy, refers to volatile aromatic compounds: the molecules that make up individual essential oils. They are very light and mobile and quickly disperse into the air, even at room temperature.

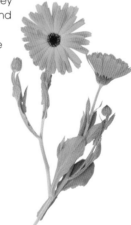

Index

Bold type indicates ingredients with their own directory entry

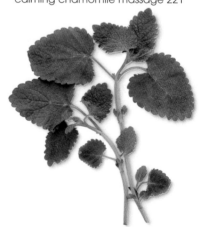

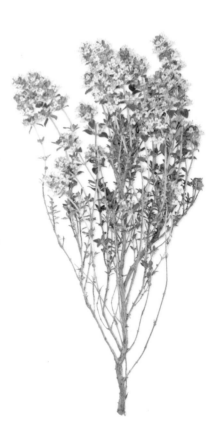

Resources

Neal's Yard Remedies

www.nealsyardremedies.com
Supplier of essential oils and essential oil products. Also provides treatment rooms for consultations with qualified aromatherapists.

For courses in aromatherapy, call 020 3119 5904, or email: courses@nealsyardremedies.com

G. Baldwin & Co

www.baldwins.co.uk
Supplier of essential oils and complementary products.

Aromatherapy Trade Council (ATC)

www.a-t-c.org
Provides information and news on essential oils.

International Federation of Professional Aromatherapists (IFPA)

www.ifparoma.org
Has a register of qualified aromatherapy practitioners.

Essential Oil Safety
Tisserand and Young

Comprehensive reference book for aromatherapy practitioners.

Acknowledgments

The authors at Neal's Yard Remedies would like to thank:
our great editor, Claire Cross, from DK. Our wonderful essential oil suppliers and experts who work so hard to get fairly traded, organic, and amazing quality oils, and share their expertise freely, especially Patrick Collin, Walter De Boeck, Denzil Phillips and Ulli Wentzler. Also the inspiring and dedicated tutors on our aromatherapy courses, especially Victoria Plum and Elaine Tomkins.

Dorling Kindersley would like to thank the great team at Neal's Yard Remedies for their expertise and guidance throughout.

The publisher would like to thank the following for their kind permission to use their photographs:
(Key: a-above; b-below/bottom; c-centre; f-far; l-left; r-right; t-top)

Beniculturali (bc). 13 SuperStock: Eye Ubiquitous (bc). 16 Dorling Kindersley: Barnabas Kindersley (ca). 18 Science Photo Library: Eye of science (c). 40-41 123RF.com: Elena Lifantseva. Paperbark Co., Fragonia p43, 45 Alamy Stock Photo: Blickwinkel (l). 47 Alamy Stock Photo: Valery Voennyy (r). 49 123RF.com: Ekasak Chuenchob (crb). 54-55 Alamy Stock Photo: imageBROKER. 57 123RF.com: Arcticphotoworks (r). 59 123RF.com: Igor Dolgov. 66-67 123RF.com: Varaporn Chaisin. 69 123RF.com: Vitaly Suprun / suprunvitaly (r). 71 Dorling Kindersley: Mockford and Bonetti / Villa Giulia and Beniculturali (r). 72 SuperStock: Eye Ubiquitous. 79 123RF.com: Arthit Buarapa (crb). 82-83 123RF.com: Joemat (c). 87 Alamy Stock Photo: Emilio Ereza (l). 90-91 Alamy Stock Photo: Tim Gainey. 97 Alamy Stock Photo: Yooniq Images (crb). 103 Alamy Stock Photo: Stephanie Jackson - Aust wildflower collection (tr). Alan Buckingham, Peppermint p107, Parsley p114, 119 Alamy Stock Photo: imageBROKER (l). Alan Buckingham, Tuberose p120 122 Alamy Stock Photo: WILDLIFE GmbH (tr). 124-125 Alamy Stock Photo: Steffen Hauser / botanikfoto. 135 Dorling Kindersley: John Glover / Unwins (tr). 143 123RF.com: Anna Bogush. 144 123RF.com: Pittawut Junmee (crb). 154 Getty Images: Image Source (cla). 155 123RF.com: Mohammed Anwarul Kabir Choudhury (cla). 166 Dorling Kindersley: Alan Buckingham (br). Getty Images: Image Source (tr). 218 Getty Images: felipedupouy.com / Photodisc (bc)

All other images © Dorling Kindersley
For further information see: www.dkimages.com

Recipe and ingredient photography William Reavell
Recipe styling Jane Lawrie
Photoshoot prop styling and art direction
Isabel de Cordova
Design/illustration help Steve Marsden
Proofreading Anna Davidson
Indexing Hilary Bird

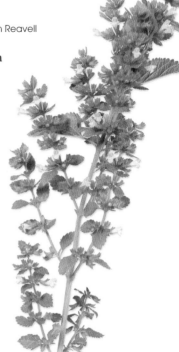

Disclaimer

Essential oils contain natural therapeutic properties and should be treated with respect. This book is not intended as a medical reference book, but as a source of information. Do not use essential oils for conditions if you are undergoing any other course of medical treatment without seeking professional advice. The reader is advised not to attempt self-treatment for serious or long-term problems, during pregnancy, or for children without consulting a qualified aromatherapist. Neither the authors nor the publisher can be held responsible for any adverse reactions to the recipes or remedies, recommendations, and instructions contained herein, and the use of any essential oil is entirely at the reader's own risk.